Forensic Medicine
for Lawyers

Forensic Medicine for Lawyers

by
J. K. MASON, CBE, MD, FRCPath, DMJ

Regius Professor of Forensic Medicine
University of Edinburgh

with Chapters by

A. K. M. MACRAE, MB, FRCPE, FRCPsych
Regius Professor of Forensic Psychiatry
University of Edinburgh

H. V. STREET, DSc, PhD, FRIC, FRCPath
Senior Lecturer in Forensic Chemistry
University of Edinburgh

A. T. PROUDFOOT, BSc, MB, MRCPE
Consultant in charge of the Regional
Poisoning Treatment Centre
The Royal Infirmary, Edinburgh

and a section by

T. J. ANDERSON, MB, PhD, MRCPath
Senior Lecturer in Pathology
University of Edinburgh

BRISTOL: JOHN WRIGHT & SONS LTD
1978

CIP Data

Mason, John Kenyon
   Forensic medicine for lawyers.
   1. Medical jurisprudence – Great Britain
   I. Title
   614'.19'02434   RA1051

   ISBN 0 7236 0455 X

Photoset, printed and bound in Great Britain by
REDWOOD BURN LIMITED
Trowbridge & Esher

This book is dedicated to
the Edinburgh University LL.B Class of 1973–74
who made everything seem worthwhile
and to
the Class of 1974–75
who kept it that way

Preface

IN my inaugural address to the University*, I defined forensic medicine as 'medicine applied to the protection and assistance of individuals in relation to the community'. This concept was based on the 'forum' as being a public place in which those responsible to the public in many spheres argued and defended their views rather than being limited to the criminal court.

It seemed to me that forensic medicine should be taught to medical students in this wide spirit whereas, paradoxically, it was the law students who, in having to decipher and understand the reports of their expert medical witnesses, needed the greater exposure to the details of pathology despite the fact that they had no medical background. I could find no textbook extant which would satisfy their particular needs; what follows is an attempt to fill the gap. One of the main difficulties has been to find the right pitch of knowledge and the book has, in the process of writing, settled into an outline of the LL.B Course in Forensic Medicine presently given at Edinburgh University. It is, however, hoped that it will still be found useful by practising advocates, solicitors, Procurators Fiscal and Coroners.

I recently read a review which stated that 'the day of the single-author textbook has gone', and it is certain that multiple authorship ensures that each facet of the work is covered by an expert practising in that sphere; the single author attempting a wide range must lose a sense of immediacy.

In an effort to compensate for this, I have shown drafts of the majority of chapters to persons particularly well-qualified to criticize and advise. Helpful criticism does not, however, necessarily mean approval and, lest naming one's reviewers might be taken as implying their shared responsibility for, and satisfaction with, the end result, I intend to express my thanks anonymously to the many members of the forensic fraternity, the academic staff of the Faculties of Medicine and of Law in Edinburgh University, the NHS officials, the Government and Local Authority officers and others who have responded so kindly to my calls for help; my gratitude loses no sincerity in its generality.

Three especial personal acknowledgements are, however, called for. Professor Keith Simpson and Mr Alistair R. Brownlie have been good enough to read the whole manuscript from the point of view of the forensic pathologist and of the lawyer respectively. They have given invaluable advice although, again, it should be stressed that their participation does not necessarily imply agreement with the views expressed. Mr Charles N. Stoddart has reviewed the text with particular reference to the legal technicalities. In doing so, he has not only improved the book's acceptability to lawyers but has also offered many helpful

---

* *Ambitions for a Motley Coat* (1973), Inaugural Address No. 56, University of Edinburgh.

vii

criticisms; he has my sincere thanks for undertaking a most time-consuming task.

I owe my secretarial assistant, Mrs Gladys Hamilton, a debt of gratitude for unstinting cooperation and much encouragement. A number of temporary assistants have had a hand in the typing but the great bulk of this has been undertaken by Miss Iris Falconer with great skill and good heart. Many of the illustrations are reproduced with the cooperation of Mr John Orr, Chief Constable, the Lothian and Borders Constabulary, and by permission of the Crown Office; much of the photographic work involved has fallen on Detective Chief Inspector Norman Deland. Miss Daphne Lytton was responsible for the preparation of *Figs.* 2, 3, 4, 6, 7, 13–15 and 17 and Mr Ian Lennox for *Fig.* 12. I am very grateful to Mr Jim Paul, Deputy Director, Department of Medical Illustration, University of Edinburgh, who has been responsible for the great majority of the photographic reproduction.

Finally, I have to thank my wife for letting it happen. At a time of our lives which was, for several reasons, difficult, she spent many lonely hours of televiewing without complaint; I hope this book is worthy of her memory.

Edinburgh, 1977   J.K.M.

Contents

CONTENTS

A Note on Bibliography

THIS textbook is virtually unreferenced as a matter of policy; the alternative would be a massive medical bibliography which would be of little value to the lawyer. In general, I have attempted to confine the medical references to subjects which are in some dispute and, so far as possible, to refer only to review articles which have appeared in journals which are readily available.

I have made much use of published textbooks as sources and the lawyer wishing to improve his knowledge of specialist pathology should consult the many books which are written primarily for doctors. Those which have been most frequently used as authorities include:

Gradwohl's Legal Medicine, 3rd ed. (1976), ed. F. E. Camps, A. E. Robinson and B. G. B. Lucas (Bristol, Wright). This multi-author book corresponds most closely to my concept of the range of forensic medicine.
Essentials of Forensic Medicine, 3rd ed. (1973), by C. J. Polson and D. J. Gee (Oxford, Pergamon). An up-to-date, massive and authoritative work which is particularly well referenced. It includes no toxicology.
Forensic Medicine, 7th ed. (1974), by K. Simpson (London, Edward Arnold). A classic work which compresses an amazing amount of information into a slim volume.
Taylor's Principles and Practice of Medical Jurisprudence, 12th ed. (1965), ed. K. Simpson (London, Churchill). The authoritative English work.
Glaister's Medical Jurisprudence and Toxicology, 13th ed. (1973), ed. E. Rentoul and H. Smith (Edinburgh, Churchill Livingstone). This is the only extant work which presents the subject with due regard to Scots practice. Unfortunately, it virtually ignores the commonest of medico-legal problems – sudden death from natural causes.
Legal Aspects of Medical Practice, 2nd ed. (1976), by B. Knight (Edinburgh, Churchill Livingstone). A highly informative little book but one which is essentially written for general medical practitioners.

I have also drawn heavily on the following monographs in relation to medical jurisprudence:

The Human Body and the Law (1970), by D. W. Meyers (Edinburgh, Edinburgh University Press). A PʰᴅD thesis concerned with the law as it applies to selected problems in medical ethics.
Law of Doctor and Patient (1973), by S. R. Speller (London, H. K. Lewis). An authoritative work on the subject.
The Doctor and the Law (1970), by J. L. Taylor (London, Pitman Medical). A short and easy-to-read account of the doctor's medico-legal responsibilities.

My preference among books on forensic odontology is for:

Dental Identification and Forensic Odontology (1976), by W. Harvey, (London, Kimpton), which appeared during the writing of this volume.

It goes without saying that this list is not exhaustive and it is known that several major new works are in the process of publication.

Introduction

Some Terms used in Medical Evidence

THE basic intention of this textbook is to give the lawyer a better understanding of the evidence provided in Court by medical men. Much of
this must depend on some knowledge of anatomy and physiology. It is
impossible to describe either the natural conditions or the responses
of the body to hurts which occur in forensic practice in entirely
nonmedical terms, and lawyers may well need an explanation of the
phraseology which the medical witness uses. A medical report which
will be satisfactory to all interested parties cannot be written without
using some academic jargon. No apology is made, therefore, for an
introduction which may seem unduly elementary to some readers but
which may be useful – if only as a source of *aides-mémoire* – to others.

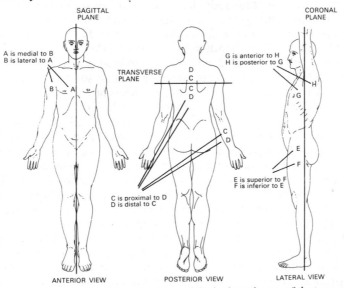

Fig. 1. Line drawings illustrating the planes of the body and some of the terms used for
anatomical reference.

1

For anatomical descriptive purposes the human body should be regarded as standing erect with the palms of the hands facing forward (*Fig.* 1). Everything which can be seen in the mirror is then *anterior* while that which cannot be seen is *posterior.* These views are related to the *coronal* plane – that is, the plane which divides the body vertically through the shoulders. The vertical plane at right angles to this is the *sagittal* plane and that sagittal plane which bisects the body into symmetrical left and right halves is the *midline.* If point A is on the same side of the body as is point B and is nearer the midline, then A is *medial* to and B is *lateral* to A. Thus, while the main torso has anterior, posterior and lateral aspects, the limbs have anterior, posterior, medial and lateral surfaces. The great toe is medial in man as in four-footed animals but the human and primate thumb is on the lateral side of the hand.

Dividing the body horizontally results in the *transverse* section. From a section taken through the middle of the chest, one can move upwards towards the cephalic extremity and downwards to the caudal extremity. If one assumes the limbs extended to form an 'X', then, if point C is nearer to the midchest transverse plane than is point D , it is *proximal* to D whereas D is *distal* to C. These terms can, however, be used functionally rather than anatomically; thus, while anatomically much of the small intestine lies distal to the transverse colon, the former is functionally a proximal portion of gut.

Strictly speaking, the body has also a *superior* surface which is seen from above and an *inferior* surface which is the soles of the feet. The terms 'superior' and 'inferior' are, however, far more important in regard to the surfaces of individual organs; all the above descriptions of the whole body are applicable to its component parts. Points on the body can also be described as superior or inferior to one another depending on whether they are nearer the head or the foot. The terms 'anterior' and 'posterior' can likewise be used relatively.

At its simplest, the body is divided into the limbs and the torso. The latter consists of three cavities – *cranial, thoracic* and *abdominal.* The protection of these cavities differs markedly. The cranial cavity, which contains the brain, is surrounded by the rigid skull which, while giving a high degree of protection, is itself subject to shattering forces which can be propagated through its substance; once fully-developed, it also inhibits expansion of the contents. The thoracic cavity houses the heart and the lungs. The governing functional principle is that of elasticity. The contents have considerable freedom of movement and the chest wall consists of a mobile combination of ribs and muscle which is only partially protective. Except where the massive lumbar spine protects it posteriorly, the abdominal cavity lacks a bony structure and its contents are therefore susceptible to injury both by penetrating and by blunt force. The major contents, which lie within a covering envelope – the *peritoneum* – include the stomach and greater part of the bowel, the liver and the spleen; these are loosely connected by ligaments and have considerable mobility. Those lying behind the peritoneum – including the pancreas and the kidneys – are more rigidly fixed but, in general, are better protected. The lower part of the abdominal cavity is bounded by the two pelvic bones and is known as the *pelvic* cavity which contains the urinary bladder and, in the female, the uterus and ovaries.

The ability of the various organs to move has much importance in relation to accidental injury. A mobile object can, to some extent, slide away from direct violence; the more fixed an organ is, the more susceptible it is to bruising and crushing. On the other hand, even the most mobile organ must be attached at some point to a relatively rigid structure; organs which can move are thus particularly susceptible to shearing forces and to indirect injury. The size of the organ will influence the likelihood of its being directly involved – the liver is a good example – while the extent of air/fluid/solid interfaces will partly determine the damage likely to result from internal vibration and other stresses. The *elasticity* of the organ is another major determinant in this type of trauma, while the condition of an individual organ at the time of stress may affect its response – a diseased spleen for example is more likely to rupture than is a normal organ.

The solid portions of the body are composed of myriads of *cells* held together by *ground substance*. The cells are organized so as to form either *epithelium* or *connective tissues*. Cancerous overgrowth of the former is known as *carcinoma* and, of the latter, as *sarcoma*. Epithelium either lines or cloaks the organs of the body. It is often specialized – for example, to secrete, as in the gut, or to waft particles (e.g., of dust) – in which case the epithelium is said to be *ciliated*. The skin is a most complex epithelium with many functions, perhaps the primary one of which is to retain the body fluids; thus, destruction of the skin by burning leads to a massive loss of fluid – the potentially lethal condition of *dehydration*. The *connective tissue* connects not only the various epithelia but also the major parts of the body – it includes fat, muscle, fibrous tissue including tendons and bones, the whole being permeated by a network of blood vessels. The connective tissues are of great importance in the healing of wounds. When the continuity of part of the body – for example the skin – is interrupted, a variable quantity of bleeding takes place; this is partly stemmed by contraction of the cut ends of the vessels and by the pressure exerted by the extravasated blood. Wandering tissue repair cells then enter the bruise and the dead area is penetrated by new blood vessels which, in turn, provoke the appearance of young fibrous connective tissue cells.

These then age and become tough and bloodless – the result being a *scar*. The recognition of these stages is the basis of 'ageing' of wounds.

The blood itself is a specialized form of connective tissue which consists of cells and fluid, the latter being the *plasma* which carries soluble foodstuffs and electrolytes, waste products and messenger substances, or *hormones,* which provide the body's system of communication between organs. The blood cells are either *red* (erythrocytes) or *white* (leucocytes); the function of the former is the carriage of oxygen while the latter are, in general, concerned with the defence of the body against infection. Sarcomatous overgrowth of the white cells results in *leukaemia. Platelets,* concerned with blood coagulation, also circulate in the plasma.

All cells other than the erythrocytes consist of two main parts – the *nucleus* and the *cytoplasm.* The nucleus controls cell reproduction and contains 23 pairs of *chromosomes,* one of each pair being derived from a parent. Normal cell division and tissue growth results from *mitosis* in which each chromosome reproduces itself; the two new cells therefore contain the same chromosomes as did their progenitor. The exception lies in the sex cells, male spermatozoa or female ova, which divide by a process of *meiosis* and contain only 23 single chromosomes; the fusion of two sex cells thus results in a *zygote* with the normal nuclear configuration. The chromosomes are composed of a number of *genes* which are transmitted hereditarily and which determine the constitution of the body.

One pair of chromosomes dictates the sex of the subject. These sex chromosomes are designated X and Y. The presence of a Y chromosome in the pair indicates maleness.

In addition to describing the body on anatomical grounds, it is often useful to consider it systematically – that is, relating those parts which are functionally integrated irrespective of their position. These 'systems' are referred to frequently in medical reports and most are dealt with in greater detail in the opening chapter. In summary, the medical witness may refer to:

a. The *nervous* system, comprising the brain and spinal cord (central nervous system) and the peripheral nerves.

b. The *musculoskeletal* system, or the bones, tendons and muscles.

c. The *cardiovascular* system, consisting of the heart and blood vessels.

d. The *respiratory* system, running from the nose to the lungs and including the diaphragm and chest muscles.

e. The *gastro-intestinal* system, which includes not only the gut from mouth to anus but also those organs whose function is to control the processing of food – i.e. the salivary glands, the liver and the pancreas.

f. The *genito-urinary* system. Although quite distinct functionally, the genital and urinary systems are commonly combined on anatomical grounds. The genital system includes the ovaries, uterus, vagina and vulva in the female and the testes, ducts and penis in the male. The main components of the urinary system are the kidneys, the ureters, the bladder and the uretha – and the prostate gland in the male.

g. The *lympho-reticular* system, which is responsible for many functions particularly related to defence against infection. The main solid organs are the spleen, the thymus gland and the numerous lymph nodes including specialized nodes such as the tonsils.

h. The *endocrine system,* comprising those glands which control body function by secretion of hormones into the blood stream. The most important from the forensic aspect are the pituitary, the adrenal and the thyroid glands.

All these systems are interlinked – all, for example, are dependent upon their component of the cardiovascular system and its contained blood, while the musculoskeletal system, in particular, cannot function in the absence of a nervous system. They form useful descriptive compartments in so far as the functional result of disease or injury within a system is immediately understandable.

Many medical terms are made up of the Latin name for the organ or tissue associated with a descriptive prefix or suffix. A selected list of these is given at Appendix A.

Chapter 1

Some Aspects of Applied Anatomy and Physiology

THE CARDIOVASCULAR SYSTEM

LIFE depends upon the supply of oxygen to the tissues. This is the function of two biological systems – the respiratory system which collects or harvests the oxygen and the cardiovascular system which distributes it for consumption. The two are closely interrelated, the common factor being the *erythrocytes* or red cells of the blood of which there are about 5 million to the cubic millimetre.

Red cells derive their colour from the pigment *haemoglobin* – a combination of iron and protein – the function of which is to accept oxygen in the lungs and to surrender it in the tissues. Maximum contact with the surroundings is achieved at both these points by passing the blood through vessels which are approximately the diameter of individual red cells – these vessels are known as *capillaries*. The extremely delicate nature of their walls allows controlled transference not only of gases but of water and salts or *electrolytes*; this system is most sensitive to oxygen deficiency and it is abnormal capillary permeability which is mainly responsible for the condition of *surgical shock*. This is an important concept – shock in medical terms is not a matter of mental distress; it is a profound biochemical disturbance which, triggered by capillary hypoxia (*see* p. 405), leads to alterations in the distribution of body water and, particularly, of blood volume. Surgical shock is a condition of immense medico-legal importance as it occurs most commonly as a result of trauma; anything which reduces the peripheral blood pressure, particularly haemorrhage or fluid loss due to burning, can precipitate the condition which is self-perpetuating – low peripheral pressure means oxygen starvation which leads to capillary damage, local fluid loss and increasing failure of the blood pressure.

The blood pressure which is generally described in medical reports is measured in the arteries; its maintenance is a function not only of peripheral resistance but also of the pumping action of the heart. The pressure is described in two phases – the *systolic* pressure, which is the maximum achieved as a result of the heart beat, and the *diastolic*, which is the residual pressure maintained while the heart is refilling; in general, it is the diastolic pressure which reflects most accurately the level of strain upon the system.

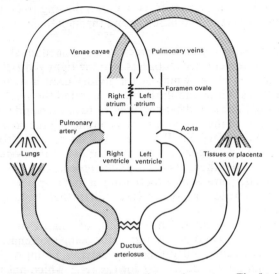

Fig. 2. Diagrammatic illustration of the cardiovascular system. The fetal connections used to bypass the lungs are shown as zigzags.

The *heart* consists of specialized muscle tissue – the *myocardium* – and is enclosed in a fibrous sac, the *pericardium*. Essentially it consists of two separate pumps (*Fig.* 2) – the left and right *ventricles* – which are fed with blood through non-return valves from the left and right *atria*. The size and weight of the heart are largely dictated by the condition of the ventricles which, in turn, depends mainly upon the peripheral resistance to the flow of blood. A ventricle which is coping with increased resistance will grow in bulk or *hypertrophy*; one which is failing to do so will *dilate*. These observations are, therefore, of great importance in assessing matters such as life expectancy in compensation cases. Blood passes from the ventricles to the tissues through *arteries*. The main artery of the body is the *aorta* which branches into vessels of descending calibre until the capillaries are reached. The capillaries then coalesce into tributaries or *veins* which ultimately form two main rivers – the *superior vena cava* coming from the upper part of the body and the *inferior vena cava* from the lower – which return the blood from the *systemic circulation* to the right atrium. All blood vessels have three coats – the *intima*, a normally thin lining which is subject to the degenerative change of atheroma; the *media*, a muscular coat; and the *adventitia* which is a loose covering responsible for the supply of nutriments to the vessel itself and for its stability in the body. Since the arteries are steadily decreasing in size, a considerable pressure must be maintained within them to ensure adequate blood flow; the arteries therefore have thick muscular walls. The situation in the veins, however, is that of a flowing river; the walls are thin and the deoxygenated blood shows through them as a dark purple colour.

The blood returning in the venae cavae has shed much of its oxygen which must be replenished. It passes into the right ventricle and thence to the *pulmonary artery* which again divides until it forms capillaries within the lungs. These capillaries now surround the smallest air pockets – the *alveoli*. The blood here accepts more oxygen and returns via the *pulmonary veins* to the *left atrium* thus completing the *pulmonary circulation*. The pulmonary capillaries are just as sensitive to changes in blood volume and oxygen content as are those of the systemic circulation; fluid loss from them results in *pulmonary oedema* – or water in the lungs – which is, again, self-perpetuating in that displacement of the air in the alveoli by water simply decreases still further the supply of oxygen to the tissues.

The blood thus circulates in something of a figure-of-eight – that in the systemic arteries and pulmonary veins being oxygenated while that in the systemic veins and pulmonary arteries requires regenerating. Such a circulation will be useless for the fetus which has no access to atmospheric air. The lungs of the fetus *in utero* are, therefore, replaced by the *placenta* – a mass of capillaries derived from both the infant and the mother by means of which the former is supplied with oxygen as a 'tissue' of the latter; the pulmonary artery and veins are replaced functionally by the umbilical vessels. The fetal lungs must be bypassed and this is accomplished through two main mechanisms. Firstly, the two atria are allowed to communicate through the *foramen ovale*. Some of the blood therefore passes from the right atrium to the left atrium rather than to the right ventricle and pulmonary artery. Secondly, a connection – the *ductus arteriosus* – is established between the aorta and the pulmonary artery by means of which the great majority of blood pumped from the right ventricle can be diverted to the aorta and, thence, to the placental circulation. The ductus usually closes a few days after birth and the foramen ovale some weeks later. These points are of major medico-legal importance as so much forensic pathology revolves round the fetal and neonatal period and, in particular, the post-mortem diagnosis of a 'separate existence'.

Damage to the heart or blood vessels results in haemorrhage – one of the most constant complications of trauma of all types. Its severity depends on three main factors. Firstly, there is the size of the vessel. In this respect, the heart itself is the most important part of the system; apart from this, the larger the vessel damaged, the more dangerous is the injury to life. Secondly, the type of vessel is all-important – damage to an artery, subject to high internal pressure, will obviously be more dangerous than damage to a vein of comparable size. Thirdly, there are the secondary effects, not only those resulting from oxygen deprivation in specific organs but also those due to occupation of space by extruded blood – thus, haemorrhage into the skull will have very different effects from the same amount of bleeding into the abdomen.

The *haemostatic* mechanism of the body – that is, its ability to control haemorrhage – rests, firstly, on the properties of blood and, secondly, on the capacity of the vessels to contract – a matter of vascular health and size. The properties of the blood derive from two distinct sources – the *coagulation factors* and the *platelets*. The former, designated by Roman numerals, are protein substances circulating in the plasma which, when activated in the presence of calcium, take part in a complicated chain reaction. The result of this reaction is to form *thrombin* which then reacts with the circulating protein *fibrinogen* to form *fibrin* which is, in effect, the scaffolding of a clot. Deficiency of any factor can break the chain and cause one of what are collectively known as *bleeding diatheses*; for practical purposes, Factor II or prothrombin, Factor VIII, Factor IX and Factor I (fibrinogen) are the most important. Prothrombin is formed in the liver; severe liver disease will therefore predispose to a bleeding condition. Deficiency of Factor VIII results in the hereditary disease *haemophilia* (lack of Factor IX is responsible for haemophilia B or Christmas disease). The function of the platelets is twofold. In the first place, they release substances which activate the coagulation mechanism and, secondly, they aggregate to form 'plugs' at the site of injury to a vessel and thus consolidate the fibrin clot. Excessive bleeding is therefore likely if platelets are absent, as happens in disease or poisoning of the bone marrow, or if they are abnormal.

The medico-legal importance of bleeding diatheses lies in several fields. The response to injury will be abnormal – trivial wounds may result in severe haemorrhage or excessive bruising – and this will greatly affect their interpretation as to the time of infliction, the force used and the like. Secondly, the abnormal condition can be remitted by replacement of the deficient substance; it follows that failure to identify and neutralize the abnormal state before a surgical or dental operation might well be construed as negligent practice. Thirdly, the treatment of the excessive bleeding is expensive and wasteful; pugnacious haemophiliacs are doubly antisocial.

Blood coagulation and haemostasis occur normally only at the site of injury. The reverse of haemorrhage is the very dangerous condition of *intravascular coagulation* which occurs either locally in a diseased vessel or as a generalized condition resulting from severe surgical shock. A *thrombus* forms within the vessel; if this breaks off it becomes an *embolus*. The major significance of these abnormal states is discussed in Chapter 7.

Cardiovascular damage may be the result of indirect or direct trauma. The former is largely a matter of accidental injury and is described in Chapter 10. For present purposes, the most important causes of direct injury include stab wounds – when these are fatal, it is generally by virtue of penetrating the heart or a major vessel; incised wounds, when a major vessel presents under the surface as at the wrist or in the neck; and gunshot wounds, in which not only the bullet is likely to do damage but also fragments of bone which act as secondary missiles.

Natural disease of the heart and vessels accounts for some 80 per cent of the sudden deaths reported to the Coroner or Procurator Fiscal. It represents perhaps the major preoccupation of a forensic pathologist and is discussed in detail in Chapter 7.

The Blood
As has already been described (p. 4), the blood consists of two major fractions – the *cellular component* and the *plasma* in which the cells float. If the blood is clotted, the resulting altered fluid component is known as *serum*. Serum is technically easier to work with in certain laboratory examinations and it is common to speak loosely of 'serum substances'; but such substances circulate naturally in the plasma.

The plasma is responsible for transport of carbon dioxide and of the products of the metabolism of ingested fat, proteins and carbohydrates. It contains many of the mineral salts on which the biochemical balance of the body depends and also the hormones. The clotting factors, described above, are also present in the plasma which, normally, constitutes approximately 60 per cent of the blood volume; a relative fall in this proportion leads to a viscous blood and local tissue hypoxia due to stagnation.

The cells of the blood are divided into the red series (*erythrocytes*) and the white series (*leucocytes*); there is also a platelet component (*see above*). The oxygen transport function of the first has already been described. A relative lack of red cells constitutes *anaemia* which may result from haemorrhage or from an inability to form haemoglobin, usually because of a lack of its inorganic component iron. There are other forms of functional anaemia which are of importance from the medico-legal aspect. Firstly, some poisonous substances convert the haemoglobin into forms which are less capable or incapable of accepting oxygen – the most important of these is carbon monoxide but there are other substances, particularly of an industrial nature, which achieve much the same end. Secondly, inherited abnormalities of the haemoglobin occur which are known as *haemoglobinopathies*; the best known of these is *sickle cell anaemia* but it is by no means the only member of the group.[1] The medico-legal significance of these diseases is not inconsiderable. Firstly, sufferers from the condition, which may present in severe or mild form, are hypersensitive to low blood oxygen tensions arising from any cause; they are at some risk in air travel or in conditions of severe oxygen demand, a situation which might raise a valid defence when sudden death occurs during a struggle. Secondly, most of them show a strong ethnic distribution and are a hazard to the unwary surgeon or anaesthetist.

The *leucocytes* are basically of two types – the *polymorphonuclears* and the *mononuclears*. The former constitute the body's tactical defence against acute infection: the latter are more akin to a strategic force which comes into action more slowly but whose influence persists for some time. The mononuclears are particularly responsible for the formation of *antibodies* and for the ability of the body to recognize a foreign intruder; an immediate reaction can thereby be set up should the intrusion be repeated. Certain poisons – and some drugs in excessive amounts – suppress the formation of the white cells and the subject is then left prey to infections which would be repelled easily in normal circumstances.

The blood cells are formed in the *bone marrow* which is found in the centre of virtually all the bones of the body; any poison or ionizing radiation which affects the bone marrow will affect the blood and its function. The bone marrow consists of cellular and fatty elements, the proportion of the latter increasing with age.

Effete blood cells must be removed and their important components preserved. This is mainly the function of the *spleen*, an organ which lies in the left upper abdomen covered by the lower ribs. It is one of those odd organs which are not essential to a normal life and its main medicolegal significance lies in the ease with which it is ruptured in vehicular accidents. Deliberate rupture of the spleen also had a vogue as a method of murder in malarial areas, the organ being particularly fragile in that disease.

The spleen and bone marrow are parts of the *lympho-reticular system* which is completed by the *lymphatic* system of ducts and glands responsible not only for the immune response of the body but also for the circulation of the extracellular fluid which bathes all the cells of the body. The lymphatic and cardiovascular systems are united where the main lymph duct empties itself into the larger veins of the upper thorax.

---

[1] The condition of *thalassaemia* results from the persistence of a fetal type of haemoglobin in the adult.

Cancer cells are readily disseminated in the lymph and set up secondary deposits (*metastases*) when they are filtered in the lymphatic glands.

THE RESPIRATORY SYSTEM

Without oxygen, there is no enzymatic activity and there is cellular death. The requirement is urgent – the urgency depending on the sophistication of the cells concerned. The body as a whole can survive without food for about 10 weeks; the cells of the brain will die if deprived of oxygen for some 10 minutes. The function of the respiratory system is to trap the oxygen which constitutes about one-fifth of the normal atmosphere, to transfer it to the haemoglobin of the blood and to remove the product of combustion – carbon dioxide – which circulates dissolved in the blood plasma.

Air is passed to the lungs from the nose or mouth, through the *larynx* to the windpipe or *trachea*. The larynx is protected by three bones or cartilages – the *hyoid, thyroid* (Adam's Apple) and *cricoid* – which are of very great importance in the post-mortem diagnosis of strangulation (*see* Chapter 13). The trachea splits into a left and a right main *bronchus* which, in turn, divide into *lobar bronchi* – one to each major lobe of the lungs.[2] The bronchi split into *bronchioles* which end in the air sacs or *alveoli* which, as we have seen, are surrounded by the pulmonary capillaries. The lungs are contained in two layers of a fibrous envelope – the *pleura*, which has two main functions; firstly, a negative pressure between the two layers serves to maintain the lungs in a position of expansion and, secondly, the surfaces combine to reduce the friction which would otherwise exist between the lungs and the chest wall; the formation of pleural *adhesions* is a frequent result of pulmonary disease.

Air is drawn into the lungs as the muscles of respiration – the chest muscles and the diaphragm – create a negative pressure. As compared with the heart, which is innervated by the autonomic system only, the lungs are directed by both the autonomic and voluntary nervous systems (*see* p. 16) – we normally do not consciously think about our respiration, but we are able to alter our breathing should we so wish. In the event of conflict, the autonomic innervation will succeed – it is impossible to die from holding one's breath and, ultimately, an irrespirable medium – whether water or poisonous gas – must be inhaled despite conscious resistance. Expiration requires no muscular effort and, in the event of respiratory failure, positive pressure breathing must be applied as when on a ventilator or in mouth-to-mouth resuscitation or the whole chest must be subjected to artificial vacuum as in a respirator.

In essence, the process of respiration is one of equilibrating the ten-

---

[2] The right lung has three lobes, the left only two. The right lung is therefore slightly larger than the left which must make way for the heart which lies in the left thorax.

sions of the various gases in the air and body fluids. If the oxygen tension is high in the alveoli and low in the pulmonary capillary blood, the gas will pass into the plasma and form oxyhaemoglobin in the red cells; if the oxygen tension is high in the capillary peripheral blood and low in the tissue fluids, oxyhaemoglobin will dissociate and the oxygen will be made available to the tissues. Similar principles apply to dissolved carbon dioxide. Tissue respiration is comparable to an engine boiler – the fuel is oxygen which is used to burn the foodstuffs to produce energy; the resultant 'ash' is represented by carbon dioxide. The analogy is elaborated in *Fig.* 3 which also indicates the ways in which oxygen deficiency can occur.

Fig. 3. An illustrative concept of the respiratory system. A man (1) has to move coal (2) through a series of buckets (3) moved by an engine (4) to a stoker (5) who feeds the factory furnace (6) which represents the tissues of the body. Many things may interfere with the transport of the coal (2) which is supplied to the body in the form of *oxygen*:

1. The man may get tired = respiratory paralysis.
3. There may be insufficient buckets (red blood cells) = anaemia.
4. The bucket transporter may break down = heart failure.
5. The stoker may be ill = toxic hypoxia.
7. The factory gates may be closed to coal trucks = mechanical asphyxia.
8. There may be no coal = environmental anoxia.
9. So much dust may accumulate that the man cannot reach the buckets = lung disease.
In the end
6. The furnace goes out = death.
(After Dr B. G. Lucas in: Camps F. E. and Purchase W. B. (1956) *Practical Forensic Medicine*, London, Hutchinson's Medical Publications.)

The lungs are continually attacked by dust particles present in the air and, normally, the specialized lining of the air passages can cope with this hazard efficiently. In certain circumstances, these defence mechanisms may be destroyed and the lungs will then become diseased as a result of exposure to the environment. The most common precipitating causes are smoking and atmospheric pollution. Alternatively, the lungs may be exposed to unreasonable quantities of dust which may, of itself, be dangerous – most of these *pneumoconioses* or dust diseases are industrial in nature and are discussed in Chapter 15.

Injuries to the lungs are generally of obvious type. They may be penetrated by instruments, by foreign bodies – in particular, bullets – or by the ends of broken ribs. Two consequences arise. Firstly, the negative pressure in the pleural space may be broken and the lung collapses – not only does this lead to inefficient oxygenation of the blood but the immobile lung is a nidus for infection. Secondly, haemorrhage is inevitable and its severity depends on the size of the vessel involved. Blunt injury is commonly caused by crushing, as in vehicular accidents. Additionally, the large number of gas/fluid interfaces in the lungs renders them particularly sensitive to the passage of shock waves. Generalized pulmonary trauma is typical of falls from a height or of exposure to an explosive blast. The injuries consist of haemorrhage, laceration and destruction of the walls of the alveoli.

One of the most important medico-legal involvements of the lungs is that type of inflammation known as *hypostatic pneumonia* which is likely to follow enforced bed-rest following any injury. The lungs are inadequately expanded and oedema is common; the situation is ripe for the establishment of widespread infection. The less fit the subject, the more probable is the onset of pneumonia and the less likely is he or she to withstand the assault. The common fatal injuries in elderly persons are not those which are of immediately lethal severity; they are those which entail lengthy periods in bed.

THE NERVOUS SYSTEM

Anatomically, the nervous system is divided into the *central nervous system* (CNS) and the *peripheral nervous system* which involves all those nerves which pass out from the CNS to the remainder of the body. The CNS consists of the *brain* and *spinal cord*, the latter being divided into a number of segments related to the vertebrae of the spinal column; a major efferent or *motor* root and an afferent or *sensory* root passes through the lateral aspects of each vertebra. The motor and sensory nerve pathways pass respectively downwards and upwards in the spinal cord between the brain and the nerve roots appropriate to the area of the body they supply. It follows that damage to the spinal cord will result in functional abnormality of a *regional* distribution, the region affected being that which is supplied by nerve roots situated below the point of damage; thus, severance of the cord at the neck will result in paralysis of all four limbs (*quadriplegia*) while severance in the thoracic region leads to paralysis of the legs (*paraplegia*). Division of a nerve root on the other hand will show itself in a segmental distribution – either anaesthetic or paralytic – while damage to a peripheral nerve will cause similar changes either in a group of muscles (or wide area of skin) or in an individual muscle depending on the size of the nerve affected. One further major difference in response to injury must be noted. While some regrowth and recovery of function is possible in the peripheral nerves (the degree depending to some extent on the surgeon's skill) there is no true regeneration in the CNS;[3] this applies not only to the nerve fibres (akin to electric flex down which the impulses travel) but also to the nerve cells – or batteries – from which derives the ultimate nervous function; a child is born with the maximum number of brain cells it will possess and the decreasing mental capacity of senility is to some extent a measure of how these degenerate during life.

In the event of damage to the spinal cord, some functions can be retained through the medium of spinal reflexes which operate without the control of the brain; following division of the cord some useful reflex actions such as the uncontrolled emptying of the bladder when it is full may be established.

It is convenient to regard the central nervous system as a core running from the head to the 'tail' with nerve fibres carrying information and commands in both directions. The spinal cord forms the lowermost part and, above this, lies the hindbrain consisting of the *medulla* and *pons* where many centres organizing the vital functions of the body – e.g. respiration – are situated; the pons is of very great medico-legal importance owing to the frequency with which it sustains fatal haemorrhage following head injury. There is then a narrow midbrain and, above this, the forebrain of which the central core is the *thalamus* and *hypothalamus* where, as a great simplification, the instinctive or animal processes are organized. Two major, bilaterally symmetrical, masses are connected to the centre core; these are the *cerebellum* which overlies and is part of the hindbrain and the *cerebrum* (covered by the *cerebral cortex*) which forms the major part of the forebrain. These masses are concerned with the more complicated functions of the body. The cerebellum essentially coordinates movements and posture. Anatomically, the cerebrum is divided into four lobes – the frontal concerned mainly with personality but also with the initiation of muscle movements, the parietal which is the area associated with sensation, the occipital concerned with vision and the temporal which is mainly associated with speech, hearing and equilibrium. Special areas within each lobe are related to special areas of the body, the important feature being that head injury can have reasonably predictable results.[4] The highly developed cerebral cortex

---

[3] Clinical recovery of *function* may appear when the effects of haemorrhage, oedema, etc. resolve.

[4] Within the head, cranial nerves are given off to supply the special senses and are analogous to the peripheral nerves of the spinal cord.

acts in many ways as a controller of the instinctive thalamus. Thus, some drugs – and, in particular, alcohol – which appear to be stimulatory in nature are, in fact, depressants; the most highly developed part of the brain is most easily affected and this leads to diminished conscious control of activity.

This concept of conscious control extends also into the peripheral innervation where, in addition to the nerve supply already described, all the organs are subject to nervous control through the *autonomic system*. This consists of two functional moieties – *sympathetic* and *parasympathetic* systems; the vagus nerve forms a major component of the latter. The autonomic system is responsible for all those activities which are subconscious – for example, the beating of the heart, the production of sweat, movement of the bowel, etc. By and large, its two components are antagonistic; thus, it is the function of the sympathetic system to quicken the heart beat while impulses acting through the vagus nerve will slow it. This raises an important concept in forensic pathology – that of death due to cardiac inhibition resulting from vagal activity.[5] Basically, a sudden and, particularly, an unnatural stimulation of the sympathetic nerves will lead to reflex compensatory action of the vagus nerve; this, being equally severe and unnatural may so slow the heart as to paralyse it completely. The mucous membranes contribute a potent source of such dangerous reflexes but pressure on special centres of sympathetic activity – especially the *carotid sinus* in the neck or the *solar plexus* in the abdomen – may lead to a similar result. No pathological proof of this sequence can be shown at autopsy but it is widely accepted as the physiological explanation of sudden deaths of this type.

The coverings of the brain and spinal cord are of great medico-legal importance. From without inwards, the brain is covered, firstly, by the skull and the cord by the component parts of the backbone. These rigid structures, designed to protect the delicate nervous structure from direct external violence, also have obvious disadvantages – there is no room for expansion or displacement of the contained organs and, if fractured, the broken bones themselves become potential lacerating instruments; skilled treatment of injury to the skull and spine is, therefore, a matter of urgency. Within its bony coverings, the CNS is surrounded by a tough membrane known as the *dura mater*. Large blood vessels flow between the bone and the dura; internally, numerous small veins drain into the *dural sinuses*. Head injury can, therefore, result in either *extradural* or *subdural* haemorrhage. The *arachnoid mater* is a thin membrane lying under the dura. A relatively wide space exists be-

---

[5] This is often loosely known as 'vagal inhibition' – an abbreviation of 'vagal inhibition of the heart action'. The shorter term is unfortunate as the physiological principle involved is the direct opposite of that implied.

tween this membrane and the *pia mater* which invests the brain closely and, in this subarachnoid space, are to be found *cerebrospinal fluid*, the main function of which is to give some leeway for expansion and to act as a water cushion, and also the main arteries as they pass from the neck to supply the brain substance; rupture of these vessels due to injury or natural disease results in *subarachnoid haemorrhage*. The thin pia mater invests the brain so closely that there is, effectively, no subpial space – any haemorrhage occurring in this area is of superficial *intracerebral* type. Deep intracerebral haemorrhage is often divisible into two types – petechial (or capillary), which is commonly associated with asphyxial states of all types, and massive, which may be traumatic in origin but is more likely to be due to natural disease. Intracranial haemorrhage is discussed in detail in Chapter 11.

A review of the nervous system is incomplete without consideration of the special senses but such a discussion is beyond the scope of this volume. It is obvious that the loss of a special sense is of particular civil medico-legal importance and that, of these senses, vision is not only the most important but is also, perhaps, the most vulnerable. In addition to penetrating wounds, partial or complete loss of vision due to trauma can result from damage to the outer covering (*corneal abrasion*), to infection due to the presence of foreign bodies, to intraocular haemorrhage and to *retinal* detachment; *sympathetic ophthalmia* is a particularly distressing situation in which the other eye may lose its function 'in sympathy' with one which is damaged. Internally, the *optic nerve* may be damaged in association with fractures of the skull and, finally, blindness may result from damage to the occipital lobe of the cerebral cortex where the centres for vision are located – falls on the back of the head are, therefore, important in regard to vision. The importance of the eyes as a *cause* of death due to accidents – particularly vehicular – requires no emphasis.

GASTRO-INTESTINAL SYSTEM

The function of the gastro-intestinal system is to accept food, digest it, store it, circulate it to the tissues in a form which provides a ready source of energy and to excrete unused residues. The whole process is controlled by a complex system of enzymes (*see below*).

The *alimentary canal* starts at the mouth and leads into the straight *oesophagus* which traverses the length of the thorax. The oesophagus opens into the *stomach* which, in turn, empties into the *duodenum* or first part of the small intestine. The *jejunum* and *ileum* form the second and third parts of the small intestine which is about 20 ft (6 m) in length and closely coiled within the abdomen. The large intestine consists of the *caecum* and its attached *vermiform appendix,* the ascending, transverse, descending and sigmoid *colon* and the *rectum* which opens to the exterior at the *anus*.

The *peritoneum* lines the abdominal cavity and invests the small and large intestines. The envelope of peritoneum which is attached to the posterior abdominal wall and from which the small intestine is suspended is known as the *mesentery* and the major blood vessels lie within this. Tissues which lie posteriorly in the abdomen behind the mesentery are said to be *retroperitoneal* in position.

Constituents of food absorbed from the bowel are passed to the *liver* where they are both processed and stored. The liver is the largest organ in the body and occupies the upper right quadrant in the abdomen. It has numerous functions including the metabolism of carbohydrates, fats and proteins; the storage of a readily available source of energy (glycogen); the processing of waste material derived from breakdown of body tissue; the preparation of many of the substances essential for blood clotting; and the formation of bile which is stored in the *gall bladder* and passed into the intestine where it assists in digestion. Failure to secrete bile or to excrete it into the bowel shows itself as *jaundice*.

Ferments from the *pancreas* are also essential to digestion; this organ lies in the posterior part of the abdomen and empties its secretions into the duodenum.

The forensic importance of the gastro-intestinal system is very great. The majority of poisons which are administered homicidally must be given by mouth; it follows that the primary symptoms of poisoning are commonly gastric or intestinal in nature and the early diagnosis of this form of crime depends greatly on the skill of the family doctor (*see* Chapter 22). The liver itself is also very sensitive to poisonous substances many of which are industrial in nature; jaundice is, therefore, an important sign of poisoning at work. The function of the liver may also be greatly impaired by infection of the organ – when the condition of *hepatitis* is established. A proportion of these cases result from the 'hepatitis B virus' which is transmitted from the blood of infected persons; the significance of the condition in blood transfusion is discussed in Chapter 31.[6]

The results of trauma to the bowel may be very serious. The contents of the bowel may be irritant – as in the stomach – or they may be heavily contaminated by bacteria – as in the large bowel. In either case, rupture of the viscus will result in severe damage to the abdominal cavity and death may follow due to shock (*see* p. 405); stab wounds and gunshot wounds of the abdomen thus require urgent surgical treatment. The hollow organs are also sensitive to explosive blast particularly if this is transmitted through water. The bowel itself is surprisingly resistant to

---

[6] It used also to be transmitted during mass immunization procedures but, nowadays, the reuse of unsterilized needles for this purpose would be unacceptable.

blunt, nonpenetrating trauma, but both the intestine and its mesentery can be ruptured when massive force is applied from outside over a limited area; the single lap-belt type of restraint used in some motor cars and light aircraft is a modern means of transmitting such forces in a crash situation.

The sheer bulk of the liver increases its susceptibility to penetrating injury but it is at its most vulnerable in crushing accidents or in conditions which set up severe vibrations in the body, such as falls from a height.

The pancreas, on the other hand, is well protected and is only occasionally injured. The organ is, however, prone to damage by disease in alcoholics and degenerative changes are found when cold injury occurs in the undernourished.

THE URINARY SYSTEM

When considering the respiratory system, the body was compared to a furnace; following the same analogy, a mechanism for waste disposal or removal of the ashes is essential if the organism is not to be poisoned. Gaseous products of combustion are eliminated in the breath but soluble waste products circulating in the plasma of the blood are excreted in the urine, which is prepared and voided through the urinary system (*Fig.* 4).

Fig. 4. The anatomy of the urinary system. *a*, Macroscopic structure. *b*, Microscopic appearance of a nephron. Note that the blood supplies the tubule after it has passed through the glomerulus.

This consists of a pair of *kidneys*, placed posteriorly in the abdomen with their upper portions covered by the lower ribs, from which pass a pair of tubes, the *ureters*. Each ureter drains into the *bladder*, a muscular reservoir the outflow of which is protected by sphincters. Urine which is stored in the bladder is passed to the outside of the body through a single pipe – the *urethra*. The urethra in the female is short; in the male it is long and assumes a serpentine shape as it passes through the *prostate* gland and the *penis*.

The kidneys play a major part in the regulation of the body's biochemical status and have two further roles in the maintenance of health. Firstly, as indicated above, there is the elimination of waste products. The primary mechanism of clearance is pressure filtration through a vast network of blood capillaries. It follows, secondly, that any disease of the kidneys will have a profound general effect on the cardiovascular system; the most common adverse result is a raised blood pressure – the condition of hypertension. Disturbance of the blood pressure may, indeed, be the cause of death from a primary disease which started in the kidney tissues.

The excretory function with which this section is most concerned is based on the individual excretory units, the *nephrons*, each of which consists of a *glomerulus* and a system of *tubules*. A glomerulus, of which there are approximately 2 million, is essentially a skein of blood capillaries enclosed in a capsule. The wall of the capillary acts as a semipermeable membrane – semipermeable because it will allow the passage of water and small dissolved particles but will retain particles of large molecular size, especially proteins. Filtration pressure, aided, perhaps, by diffusion, results in the appearance within the capsular space of what is effectively protein-free blood plasma. This contains not only waste products but also materials which are of value or even essential to the body, notably glucose and sodium; moreover, the body cannot lose all its water. Some sort of selective concentration is needed.

This is the role of the tubules, which, from the functional aspect, can be divided into proximal and distal portions. The glucose, sodium and much of the essential water are reabsorbed in the former while complex reactions designed to regulate the degree of acidity of the blood take place in the latter. The distal tubules run into collecting tubules which act as tributaries to the ureters. The importance of clearly distinguishing between the glomeruli and the tubules is that the function of the latter is active and requires the use of much energy. They are, therefore, very dependent on an effective blood supply and, since the vessels to the tubules have already supplied the needs of the glomeruli, conditions at tubular level are ripe for the development of an 'energy crisis'; any condition which interferes with the free delivery of oxygen to the tissues will affect the renal tubules with particular severity.

Abnormal conditions which damage the glomeruli differ markedly from those affecting the tubules and, while the former have comparatively little medico-legal significance other than in respect of treatment, they illustrate some important principles of pathology which have widespread implications and might well be considered at this point.

Immunity
The body has a remarkable capacity to recognize strange materials within its substance and, save in exceptional circumstances, will defend itself against invasion. The defence mechanism is referred to as an *immune reaction* and the foreign substance which precipitates it is known as an *antigen*. The immune reaction may be of two types: (*a*) Humoral – this involves the formation of circulating antibodies which react specifically with antigens and can generally be demonstrated to do so in the laboratory; (*b*) Cellular – in which the body musters forces of migrant cells which will actively attack and either destroy or eliminate the intruder.

A major result of antigenic challenge is to stimulate the body's powers of recollection. Thus, the first intrusion causes comparatively gradual recognition followed by reaction. The pattern of the foreign substance is remembered, the templates of antibody production are retained and a second attack can be met by the immediate mobilization of reserves. Repeated stimuli result in increasing immunity. Normally, this system is entirely to the body's advantage – it forms the basis, for example, of vaccination against various infectious diseases. Occasionally, however, the body may fail to distinguish between self and non-self with disastrous consequences; this occurs in two basic ways. The first mechanism is incompletely understood but, possibly because of abnormal position rather than abnormal constitution, the body reacts against its own tissues without any stimulus from outside. This constitutes *auto-immune disease* and need not be considered further. As to the second form, it must be appreciated that antigens are molecular in nature and that any organized biological particle contains a number of antigens; individual antigens may, therefore, be common to substances of dissimilar nature. Once having recognized an antigen, the body will react to it similarly irrespective of its mode of presentation. As an analogy, the body might remember being attacked by a villain armed with a willow bough; it will react violently and defensively to a subsequent friendly offer of a cricket bat.

The immediate application to the urinary system lies in the relationship between the glomerular capsule and a relatively common micro-organism responsible in the main for severe sore throats – the group A *streptococcus*. Whether it be by reason of a common antigen or whether the streptococcus so transforms the glomerulus as to make it appear 'foreign', the body, in reacting to the dangerous organism, may at the same time attack its own kidneys – the disease condition of acute *glomerulonephritis* is set up, the significant feature being that the condition is diffuse with all the glomeruli at equal risk. Fortunately, in the vast majority of cases, a sufficient number of glomeruli survive and clinical recovery is the rule. Occasionally, however, the glomeruli are overwhelmed and, after a variable time, the kidneys cease to function. Medico-legally, the importance is that treatment depends on replacement by machine or transplant and this important subject is discussed later.

Occasionally, the functional integrity of the glomerular filtration membrane is compromised and, as a result, the body protein is lost steadily into the urine – the condition of *nephrosis*. Few of the causes of this condition have forensic interest but it may result from medical treatment – particularly by drugs containing heavy metals.

The Syndrome of Acute Renal Failure[7]

In contrast with conditions affecting the glomeruli, extraglomerular disease of the nephrons is a common complication of unnatural disease and is of special medico-legal interest.

Shock as defined medically is discussed at p. 405. It essentially results in inadequate oxygenation of the tissues. The condition may arise from blood loss which, in turn, may be due either to bleeding or to destruction of the blood (haemolysis) within the body. Haemolysis may result from inherent enzyme deficiency diseases, auto-immune diseases, infection of the blood cells as in malaria or, occasionally, from the inadvertent precipitation of an immune reaction, the most obvious example of which is a mismatched blood transfusion. Oxygen lack may be induced during anaesthesia (*see* Chapter 31). Reduction of the plasma component of the blood may follow burning, severe surgical trauma or unusual conditions such as crushing of the muscles or subatmospheric decompression.

Acute renal failure may accompany any of these conditions. The medico-legal significance of the syndrome is twofold – firstly, nearly all the basic causes of the condition are unnatural and, secondly, the condition is in many cases recoverable provided some mechanism can be substituted for the kidneys during a period of recuperation. This substitution treatment is known as haemodialysis, or 'the artificial kidney', in which the blood is diverted to a man-made membrane simulating the glomerulus. Passage of dissolved substances from the blood across this membrane can be controlled by altering their concentration in the 'bath' fluid which takes the place of the filtrate in the glomerular capsule – in effect an 'osmotic gradient' can be established for any constituent of the plasma.

Sometimes, the kidneys fail to recuperate (treatment is notoriously

---

[7] The condition is often referred to as 'renal tubular necrosis'. Recent research, however, indicates that this may be a misnomer.

difficult when the condition has been precipitated by burning) and hae-modialysis carries hazards of its own including the increasing possibility of blood transfusion reactions and cross-infection between staff and patients – especially by the agent responsible for infective hepatitis. Generally, however, treatment is successful after a finite number of sessions.

By contrast, dialysis used for the treatment of glomerular death must be continued throughout life. This process involves sustained and regular occupation of machines which are unlikely ever to be available in numbers adequate for the needs. It is also expensive in bed space and nursing manpower so that the tendency is to encourage home dialysis treatment despite the attendant difficulties associated with asepsis and like problems. Decisions as to treatment must involve socio-economic considerations and the treatment of chronic renal failure is a good example of the modern doctor's inability to treat many of his patients on purely medical criteria; much must nowadays be a compromise with external factors. Habits and opinions change but, at the time of writing, many physicians would regard haemodialysis for irrecoverable kidney failure as an ideal treatment only while awaiting transplantation (*see* Chapter 12).

Both the glomeruli and the tubules may be involved in inflammation resulting from infection ascending from the bladder; this important subject is referred to later in this section.

Injury to the Urinary System
The kidneys lie posteriorly in the body, and are comparatively well protected by large muscle masses; they also lie in a good shock-absorbing bed of fatty tissue. Laceration by indirect trauma is, therefore, comparatively rare and the kidneys are not often torn in fatal accidents which inflict severe damage to other solid organs such as the liver and spleen. Nonetheless, damage to the kidneys is surprisingly frequent in nonfatal automobile accidents – a situation probably associated with the great vascularity of the organs and consequent severe bleeding as a result of compression.

The kidneys are also prone to injury during violent attack. They are common targets in assaults by kicking – in which case very severe internal injury may be present in the absence of obvious external damage – and they may be involved in knifings. It is fortunate that the body can function perfectly well with only one normal kidney.

The ureters are well protected from external injury but, as they pass into the pelvis, they come close to the female generative organs; they are therefore at risk when the latter are subjected to surgical operation. The error of tying the ureters during gynaecological operations is well known and may occasionally be very difficult to avoid in the presence of widespread chronic inflammation.

The bladder in both male and female is closely associated with the bones of the pelvis. Fracture of the pelvis, which results from a variety of accidents such as those associated with transportation, falls from a height, crushing, etc., is commonly accompanied by rupture of the bladder or of the urethra. Both these injuries are treatable by surgery but often the condition of the casualty dictates a delay in operation. The possibility is then raised of ascending infection of the urinary tract with consequent involvement of the kidneys as discussed below.

Disorders of the Bladder of Medico-legal Importance

The bladder itself is under control of the autonomic nervous system and the muscle is generally in a state of relaxation; distension results in reflex contraction and expulsion of urine. Autonomic urination is prevented by additional control of the external sphincter through the voluntary nervous system.

Since the nerve supply to the bladder sphincter originates in the lower part of the spinal cord, any injuries of the cord are likely to upset the capacity to control the act of micturition – the organ will revert to automatic action. Apart from the social inconvenience, the stage is then set for ascending infection of the urinary tract and it is not uncommon for the life of a paraplegic to terminate years after the spinal injury as a result of inflammatory destruction of the kidneys.

The different shape of the urethra in the male and female has a profound effect on the establishment of infection in the bladder. Thus, in the female, it is not difficult for organisms on the skin of the external genitalia to pass in retrograde fashion to the bladder, while the inherent laxity of the perineum predisposes to prolapse and inefficient emptying of the viscus. Inflammation of that organ (*cystitis*) is, therefore, common in women. The male urethra, by contrast, can protect the bladder from external invasion relatively well but the prostate gland is subject to enlargement of either a benign or cancerous nature. Obstruction to the flow of urine due to prostatism is a common accompaniment of later middle age; the resultant 'back pressure' may have serious effects on the kidneys themselves while the stagnation of urine induced is, as in the female, conducive to the establishment of infection; the process may be accelerated by the need to pass catheters into the distended organ.

Stagnation of urine leads to its prolonged contact with the inner wall of the bladder. Injurious substances which are excreted in the urine might be expected, therefore, to strike selectively at the bladder and this is indeed the case. Some hydrocarbons are active in the production of epithelial cancer (carcinoma) which may arise as a result of occupation (*see* Chapter 22).

Infection of the Kidney

It is convenient to complete this section by returning to the kidneys themselves with a comment on inflammation due to infection. In the end, infection of the kidney probably results in as much glomerular destruction as does primary glomerular disease and, in contrast to the latter, inflammatory disease has considerable direct medico-legal significance. Thus, anything which facilitates the introduction of, or encourages the growth of organisms within, the bladder – including injury, surgery or simple instrumentation – may ultimately lead to severe disability or even to death.

THE REPRODUCTIVE SYSTEM

The male reproductive system consists of the twin *testes* which usually descend into the *scrotum* just before birth. The organs are formed of coiled tubules in which the *spermatozoa* mature. A spermatozoon consists of a head (approximately 4 μm in length), a neck and a tail which is some 50 μm long. When stained, the head shows a typical dark nucleus at its base, an appearance which is quite characteristic even when the tail is lost. Some 400–500 million spermatozoa are shed with a normal ejaculation. The bulk of the seminal fluid is derived from the *epididymis* one of which lies close to each testis; together they drain into the *vas deferens*. The vas deferens on each side opens into the *urethra* at the base of the bladder. Other small glands contribute to the total seminal ejaculate.

The female reproductive organs consist, first, of two *ovaries* which lie on each side of the pelvis. Each ovary has a finite store of *ova* which is greatly in excess of the requirements for the normal single egg which matures each month between the onset of menstruation and the menopause. The ovaries on each side are connected to the *uterus* by the *fallopian tubes* down which the ova pass. There is a potential space between the ovary and the receptor end of the tube; occasionally, ova are fertilized and yet do not reach the uterus, in which case the dangerous condition of *ectopic pregnancy* is established. The outlet of the uterus is a tightly closed canal surrounded by the *cervix* which juts into the *vagina*. The vagina opens through the *vulva*. In the virgin state, the vaginal opening is protected by the *hymen*, a sheet of fibrous tissue with, usually, a small opening which will permit the passage of normal secretions. The size of the hymenal opening varies – it may be large originally or it may be dilated by tampons or masturbation. In general, however, the size is such that the first penetration by the male penis results in laceration which is usually posterior in position; the distinction between the virginal hymen and one showing old or recent rupture is of obvious importance in accusations of rape. The vulva consists, internally, of paired *labia minora* which join anteriorly and posteriorly as commissures, the posterior commissure being known as the *fourchette*; this again is likely to be damaged during forceful intercourse and during childbirth. The *labia majora* lie outermost; they are joined in front at the *mons veneris* but posteriorly dissolve into the tissues of the perineum.

Spermatozoa injected into the vagina make their way into the uterus or tubes where they may meet a mature ovum; the ovum is fertilized by penetration of the spermatozoon. An unfertilized ovum will die in some two days but the fertilized ovum implants itself on the uterine wall and begins to divide. After some three months' development, a *placenta* forms which is attached to the developing fetus by the *umbilical* cord. The fetus is surrounded by a fibrous sac known as the *amnion* and floats in the *amniotic fluid*.

The birth process is started by rupture of the amnion which is followed by contractions of the uterus and dilatation of the cervix. If the placenta becomes detached, the fetus will die and be expelled as a foreign body; it will be similarly rejected should the fetus itself die. Unnatural dilatation of the cervical canal will, of itself, cause the uterus to contract. Any of these situations can be simulated in order to procure abortion (*see* Chapter 19).

THE ENDOCRINE SYSTEM

The body contains a number of glands which discharge 'hormones' into the blood stream. These hormones have specific actions on various parts of the body; overproduction or failure of the 'endocrine' glands can, therefore, result in disease or dysfunction of the target organs.

There are seven different glands secreting some thirty hormones which are commonly likened to an orchestra. The 'conductor' of the orchestra is the *pituitary* gland which lies in the base of the skull. The pituitary stimulates activity in many of the other glands but is itself sensitive to circulating hormones; once sufficient hormones are present in the blood, this servo-mechanism inhibits further stimulation. In addition to its supervisory function over the other glands, the pituitary itself controls growth, the secretion of urine and the contraction of the uterus during childbirth. Damage to the pituitary gland is, therefore, a very serious matter; it is a common result of fracture of base of the skull and the gland may be damaged by the effects of haemorrhage following complicated childbirth.

The remainder of the endocrine glands, while vital to health, are of little medico-legal significance, but, as the names will certainly appear in autopsy reports, a brief description is given.

The *thyroid* gland lies in the neck and is responsible for mental and physical growth in childhood and for the general rate of metabolism in the adult body – deficiency of thyroid hormone leads to cold and apathy, excess results in production of heat and hyperexcitability. The position of the thyroid renders it susceptible to bruising which may be of considerable evidential value in strangulation.

The *parathyroid* glands are small and closely associated anatomically with the thyroid. They control the distribution of calcium as between the bones and the body as a whole.

The *adrenal* glands lie against the kidneys and are of immense importance to the body. Their central parts secrete *adrenalin* which affects the tone of the blood vessels and also the heart rate; its action is similar to that of the sympathetic nervous system. Adrenalin is secreted in response to sudden stress and, in effect, brings the body to a fighting trim in response to alarm. When given therapeutically, it has profound effects on the blood pressure and blood distribution; these must be considered in relation to death associated with surgical operations. The outer parts of the adrenal glands control the salt and water balance of the body, exert an effect on the metabolism of carbohydrates, influence the sex glands and are very much concerned with the response of the body to infection or other conditions resulting in inflammation. Large doses of adrenal hormones are used to suppress the immune response which underlies the rejection of transplanted organs (*see* Chapter 12).

The *pancreas* secretes the hormone *insulin*, absence of which causes the disease *diabetes* in which the storage of carbohydrate is inhibited and the blood contains large amounts of sugar. The converse situation, *hypoglycaemia*, results from an excess of insulin. This is a rare natural condition but is an obvious hazard of the treatment of diabetes; hypoglycaemia can be fatal and insulin has been used as a refined method of homicide. Hypoglycaemia may occur spontaneously in sensitive persons independently of insulin secretion; the syndrome closely simulates alcoholism and was a not uncommonly successful defence to motoring charges prior to the enactment of the Road Safety Act 1967.

The *testes* and the *ovaries* secrete hormones which, in the former, are concerned with the secondary sex characteristics and physique of maleness and, in the latter, with the control of menstruation and pregnancy. Perhaps their main medico-legal connotation is in the use of sex hormones in competitive sport (*see* Chapter 16).

THE MUSCULOSKELETAL SYSTEM

This system consists of the bony skeleton (*Fig.* 5) to which the muscle masses are attached often through the medium of tendons. These muscles, which can be activated at will, are known as *voluntary* muscles (or *striated* muscles, because of their appearance under the microscope). Many organs – for example, the bladder or bowel – are equipped with

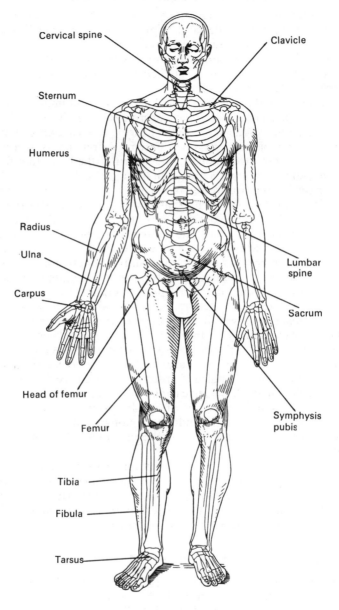

Fig. 5. The major relationships of the human skeleton. (From an original diagram by Professor G. J. Romanes.)

muscle which is not under conscious control and is therefore known as *involuntary* or, on the microscopic appearances, *smooth* muscle; such muscle is, however, an integral part of the system with which it is associated. Where bones articulate with one another in joints, the surfaces are covered with cartilage; cartilage is also formed at bony junctions when some mobility is needed – the prime example being the junctions between the breast bone and the ribs.

The *skull* is divided simply into the vault, which covers the brain, and the base on which the brain rests – on each side the base forms the anterior, middle and posterior *fossae* or cavities in which are accommodated the lobes of the brain (*Fig. 6*). The skull rests on the spine which is formed of a number of individual vertebrae, the uppermost which is known as the *atlas* bone. The atlas and six small vertebrae form the *cervical* spine or neck; below this are twelve *thoracic* vertebrae with which the ribs articulate posteriorly; five large vertebrae lying in the small of the back form the *lumbar* spine and below this are the fused vertebrae of the *sacrum* which makes up the rear wall of the pelvic cavity; the tail of the primates is represented by the small *coccyx*. The sacrum joins the two *pelvic* bones posteriorly; anteriorly the pelves are united by a cartilaginous band known as the *symphysis pubis* which is often split in severe accidents.

Anterior fossa

Pituitary fossa

Middle fossa

Petrous temporal bone

Foramen magnum

Posterior fossa

Fig. 6. Diagram illustrating the inner surface of the base of the skull. The frontal lobes rest in the anterior fossae, the temporal lobes in the middle fossae and the cerebellum lies in the posterior fossae. The spinal cord passes through the foramen magnum.

The front of the chest is protected by the solid breast bone or *sternum* which is, again, a common casualty of accidental trauma. The shoulder girdle is formed by the *scapulae* or shoulder blades posteriorly and the *clavicles* or collar bones anteriorly. The *humerus* articulates with these to form the shoulder joint and, at the elbow, forms a joint with the two bones of the forearm – the *ulna* and the *radius* which is on the thumb side. The bones of the wrist are collectively known as the *carpus*, those of the hand as the *metacarpals* and those of the fingers the *phalanges*; the knuckles may, therefore, be either metacarpophalangeal or interphalangeal joints.

The thigh bone or *femur* has its large circular head embedded in the *acetabulum* of the pelvis. The hips must be wide in order to accommodate the massive leg muscles and the first part of the femur – known as the neck – must therefore adopt a relatively horizontal position before joining the main thigh bone at an obtuse angle which approximates, as will be seen later, to a right angle in the female. The neck of the femur is therefore a mechanically weak point and is of great forensic importance owing to the ease with which it can be accidentally broken in elderly women whose bones are becoming brittle; the condition then requires either prolonged bed-rest or the surgical insertion of a pin before the broken ends will reunite – conditions are ripe for death from hypostatic pneumonia or from pulmonary embolism (*see* pp. 14 and 85).[8] The femur articulates at the knee joints with the large *tibia*, which lies medially in the lower leg, and with the slender *fibula* which lies laterally. Unlike the bones of the forearm, the bones of the lower leg cannot cross over – the foot cannot be peronated or supinated as can the hand. The bones of the ankle are known as the *tarsus* and contain two particularly large individual bones – the *talus* and the *calcaneus*. The foot contains the *metatarsals* and the toes the *phalanges*.

The voluntary muscles are rarely described individually in postmortem reports and need not be detailed at this point. Paralysis of individual muscles may be of great importance in relation to claims for compensation but, in those circumstances, far more information will be needed than could be provided in a book of this size.

The importance of fractures in virtually all aspects of forensic medicine is clear. Apart from their frequency in violence, they are demonstrable and readily presentable by means of X-rays (*see* Chapter 27), they can be 'dated' and many are of specific type; fractures are, therefore, discussed in regard to special situations throughout this book.

Otherwise, the major forensic significance of the skeletal system lies in its relationship to identification of an unknown body.

The bones of the body consist of calcium salts deposited in an organized fashion in a protein medium. Calcification and the laying down of bone in soft connective tissue begin in *centres of ossification* which are demonstrable visually and by X-ray at different times in individual bones. Although there is considerable biological variation, ossification centres are generally established in a regular order and with reasonable

---

[8] The application of the modern operation of total hip replacement to increasingly elderly patients has greatly modified the outcome of such an injury.

constancy so that their assessment can give a fair guide to the age of a fetus or young infant – it is only in these age groups that such early development is progressing.

Centres of ossification in the long bones are generally multiple and at least triple – one centre appearing in the shaft or *diaphysis* and one at each end or *epiphysis*. These must fuse in order to form adult bone and, again, this process is one of some regularity which extends throughout childhood and adolescence.

The individual bones of the skull unite in older age. This feature is, however, extremely variable.

The skeleton also gives considerable evidence as to sex. The bones of the female are, in general, less robust than are those of the male and the ridges formed where muscles and tendons are attached are less massive. Certain bones give particular indications of sex and, amongst these, the pelvis is pre-eminent, being designed to allow the passage of the fetus in the female. Other bones – notably the thigh bone and the skull – show particular sex differences but the appearances are not always easy to interpret; the advice of a skilled anatomist will be found very valuable in all aspects of the identification of skeletal remains.

This is particularly true when estimating stature in life from the findings in one or two bones. The number of formulae which have been devised for this purpose testifies to the difficulties involved – whichever figures are used, allowance must be made for drying of the bone, for the age of the subject and for race.

The application of the principles outlined above is further described in Chapter 3.

BIOCHEMISTRY OF THE BODY*

The cell is the basic unit building block of the body; the human body may consist of up to 5×10^{12} units. In order to maintain its viability each cell must manufacture energy from a series of chemical reactions that take place within the cytoplasm and are controlled by its nucleus. The sum total of these diverse chemical reactions taking place within a cell is known as cell metabolism and biochemistry defines and describes the nature of metabolism. The fuel for the metabolic process comes from ingested food, consisting of proteins, carbohydrates and fats that are themselves composed of varying combinations of molecules of carbon, hydrogen, oxygen with lesser amounts of nitrogen, phosphorus and sulphur. Energy is obtained and stored during the process of breaking down these compounds to carbon dioxide and water. This process requires a constant supply of oxygen (aerobic metabolism) although an alternative pathway (anaerobic metabolism) provides lesser amounts of

* This section on biochemistry is by T. J. Anderson, MB, PhD, MRCPath.

energy for a limited time where oxygen is lacking. The energy thus provided has two main purposes – the maintenance of equilibrium and the manufacture of new material.

The metabolic processes are conducted in a fluid medium which is an aqueous solution containing chemicals that exist as electrically charged particles known as *electrolytes* or *ions*. The most important chemicals, in addition to hydrogen and oxygen, are sodium, potassium, chloride, calcium, phosphate, sulphate and bicarbonate. However, there is a difference in chemical composition between the fluid which is intracellular and that which is extracellular. To function properly, cells must sustain a difference across the membrane of the cell surface such that the fluid inside is more concentrated than that on the outside. This is effected principally by the constant pumping out of water and sodium, with a resultant perpetual requirement for energy. It is also necessary to ensure an environment within and around the cells that is neither acidic nor alkaline but is neutral as valued in units of pH.[9]

The second use for energy is in the acceleration of the chemical reactions of a constructive nature. The cell is in a constant state of turnover and not only must it keep manufacturing new components to replace those lost or broken down, but it may also have a specific function to store and release compounds. Many and complex components are utilized in the formation of the ultrastructure of the cell, for there are numerous membrane-bound organelles – such as *mitochondria* and *lysosomes* – in its cytoplasm. These membranes are composed of proteins, sugars and fats that are assembled together in as yet poorly-understood ways. The most important – and also the simplest – components, which are in fact often attached to these membranes, are *enzymes*. Enzymes are proteins having the property to accelerate chemical reactions and each cell must manufacture enzymes to accelerate the chemical pathways not only essential to maintain viability but also for which it is particularly specialized (or differentiated). Regulation of the specific qualities and quantity of such enzymes is determined by information contained in the genes of the chromosomes. Errors in this information may occur, resulting in faults in or absence of particular enzymes, and these errors may be transmitted to succeeding generations via the chromosomes of the sex cells. Diseases due to such enzyme abnormalities are termed *inborn errors of metabolism*.

It is important to realize that interference in enzyme function within cells is directly responsible for the lethal effects of ingestion or inhalation of many poisons such as cyanide, arsenic and mercury. In the case of cyanide the enzymes of the mitochondria are inactivated with subse-

---

[9] pH is a logarithmic notation of hydrogen ion concentration in a solution, with 7 representing neutrality. Acid solutions have a pH less than 7, and alkaline solutions have a pH greater than 7.

quent blockage of oxygen transfer for metabolic processes.

Other factors which influence the activity of enzymes are temperature, pH and, perhaps most importantly, the presence of specific substances in trace amounts. These latter, termed 'essential *co-factors*', may be simple chemicals such as magnesium or zinc, or may be more complex molecules known as *vitamins*. The vitamins, which are designated alphabetically, are either fat-soluble (A, D, E and K) or water-soluble (B, C) and are essential constituents of the diet.

Whilst it is convenient to consider the biochemistry of the body at a cellular level, it is important to appreciate that an equilibrium must be maintained within and between the body fluid compartments, defined as intracellular, extracellular and vascular. For example, the concentration in the blood of glucose and calcium must be carefully monitored to remain within upper and lower limits. The endocrine system is principally responsible for controlling this balance, and achieves it by the elaboration of specific *hormones* in the cells of this system. These hormones are secreted into the blood to be carried to distant tissues where they affect the functions of specific 'target' cells. The release of these hormones is in turn regulated by the level of the target-cell product in the vascular compartment. This 'feed-back' control situation exists to maintain normal biochemical values. The function of individual hormones has been described above (p. 26).

Another factor in the maintenance of biochemical equilibrium is the requirement to replace the water and electrolyte loss that occurs continuously (and often insensibly) in urine, faeces and perspiration. Situations in which this replacement assumes critical significance arise in the surgical patient who requires intravenous fluid therapy because of inability to receive or retain any food or fluid by mouth over a sustained period. Provision of this balance is further complicated by the change in general body metabolism which takes place in response to trauma, of which surgical intervention represents a more planned form. A distinct alteration in the nature of metabolic processes, to become destructive (catabolic) as opposed to constructive (anabolic), results in loss of important nutriments, electrolytes and water. These changes are hormonally induced and constitute a reaction to stress – the so-called preparation for fight or flight. The observed decrease in body temperature in the period after trauma provides a further index of the profound alteration in body metabolism.

Chapter 2

Comparative Medico-legal Systems

ALL countries have evolved methods of primary inquiry into sudden or unnatural death. The major systems from which these derive can be described in the simplest way as the English, or Coroner, System and the (European) Continental System. The further distribution of these throughout the world largely follows the pattern of early colonial expansion. The Scottish Procurator Fiscal has absorbed points from both these systems; it is therefore convenient to leave discussion of his office until the others have been described.

THE CORONER

The office of Coroner in England and Wales developed from the twelth century at which time the Coroner was largely responsible for supervising the material interests of the Crown in criminal cases. As these could well be affected by the status of the dead person and the precise conditions surrounding the death, the Coroner's office became intimately concerned with the overall investigation of suspicious deaths. Many practices still current evolved at an early date; the identity of the deceased was always fundamental, the Coroner had to view the body – at the locus if possible – and inquests were held with juries. The financial connotations of sudden death gradually relaxed, or were diverted to other offices, and the position of the Coroner declined until it was revived in the Middle Ages. At that time, the Coroner's attention was specifically directed to the establishment or exclusion of criminality, a principle which persisted until the nineteenth century and which still motivates the Procurator Fiscal's office in Scotland.

It was not until 1860 that Coroners could fairly claim that they were free to act independently of outside influences and the election of Coroners was abolished in 1888. The major legislation establishing the present system was the Coroners Act 1887 which stated (s. 3 (1)):

Where a Coroner is informed that the dead body of a person is lying within his jurisdiction, and there is reasonable cause to suspect that such person has died either a violent or an unnatural death, or has died a sudden death of which the cause is unknown, or has died in prison, or in such place or under such circumstances as to require an inquest in pursuance of any Act, the Coroner, whether the cause of death arose in his jurisdiction or not, shall, as soon as practicable, issue his warrant for summoning not less than 12 nor more than 23 good and lawful men to appear before him at a specified time and place, there to inquire as jurors touching the death of such person as aforesaid.

This compulsion to hold an inquiry with a jury was greatly modified by the Coroners (Amendment) Act 1926, which enabled a Coroner to look into certain types of death without recourse to open inquest. The 1926 Act also laid particular stress on the Coroner's function in establishing the causes of sudden natural death and reduced his responsibility for the investigation of homicide. The most recent regulations governing the functions and *modus operandi* of the Coroner are contained in the Coroners Rules 1953, which, among many other details, pay particular attention to the conduct of post-mortem examinations.[1]

Important functional aspects of the Coroner, who must be either medically or legally qualified and be of at least 5 years' standing in his profession, are that he is independent of the government and that he is solely responsible for his actions – only the High Court can give him instructions. He is, however, limited in some ways; he cannot, for example, apportion – or seem to apportion – civil liability. Perhaps one of the most controversial requirements of the office is that Inquiries must be held in public.

His duties are strictly curtailed as to the conduct of inquests in cases of death due to suspected crime, including killing by dangerous driving. In these cases, the Coroner may only open an inquest for burial purposes and must adjourn during the criminal legal procedure. Subsequently, the Coroner will be informed of the verdict and the inquest will be closed. An adjourned inquest is reopened only when no person has been charged with an offence and, in this case, the Coroner's jury has a residual right to indict named persons. This right is now subject to severe criticism and will almost certainly be abolished.[2]

A general duty rests on 'any person about the deceased' to inform the Coroner of circumstances which indicate the need for an Inquiry. Otherwise, there is no statutory obligation on a doctor to report a death directly to the Coroner although, in practice, he commonly does so when he judges it necessary. The duty by regulation to do so is vested primarily in the Registrar of Deaths.[3] In brief, the circumstances in

---

[1] New Coroners Rules are now being drawn up.

[2] Persons so committed do not have the protection of the Criminal Justice Act 1967, which would have prevented publication of the evidence had the proceedings been before the magistrates.

[3] Registration of Births, Deaths and Marriages Regulations 1968, Regulation 51.

which he must refuse to register a death without reference to the
Coroner include:

    a. When no medical certificate of death is available because there
was no doctor in attendance during the last illness.

    b. When the certifying doctor states he has neither seen the body
after death nor attended the deceased within 14 days prior to
death.

    c. If the cause of death is in doubt.

    d. All deaths which were unnatural, were due to or associated with
accident, violence or neglect, were due to any form of poisoning –
which includes alcohol – or which were in any way suspicious.

    e. Deaths occuring during an operation or before recovery from the
effects of an anaesthetic.

    f. Deaths associated with industrial disease or poisoning.

The only statutory duty to report directly to the Coroner is imposed
on Governors of Prisons, Borstals, Detention Centres and other similar
institutions. The Medical Protection Society has drawn up a list of circumstances in which the doctor concerned is advised to inform the
Coroner as soon as possible although there is no compulsion for him to
do so; this is reproduced as Appendix B.

On being informed of a case which he considers to be within his jurisdiction, the Coroner has certain options open to him. He can decide that
no further action is called for; in this case, he notifies the Registrar to
accept the certificate of death granted by the medical practitioner. He
can order a post-mortem dissection and, if he decides as a result of this
that no further investigation is required, he himself may certify the
cause of death as indicated by the autopsy; this Coroner's certificate
invalidates any previous medical certificate as to the cause of death. In
any other circumstances, he may hold an inquest and he must do so
when death was due to any unnatural event. The inquest must be held
with a jury if it is suspected that death:

    a. Was due to murder, manslaughter or infanticide.

    b. Occurred in a prison or in such circumstances as to require an
inquest under any Act other than the Coroners Act 1887.

    c. Was due to an accident, poisoning or disease that must be notified
to any Government department or Inspector or Officer of a
Government department[4] or an Inspector approved under s. 19 of
the Health and Safety at Work, etc., Act 1974.

    d. Resulted from the use of a vehicle on the public highway.

---

[4] Any aircraft accident would, therefore, be included (Civil Aviation Acts 1949 and
1968); a major accident would also be subject to a Jury Inquest under condition (*e*).

  e. Occurred in circumstances, the continuance of which is likely to be prejudicial to the public.

A list of conclusions open to the Coroner's inquest is given as Appendix C. Subsequently, the Coroner provides the registrar with a certificate after inquest which includes the circumstantial as well as the medical causes of death. Statements signed by both the witness and the Coroner are known as depositions and can be used in subsequent legal proceedings provided they were taken in the presence of the person who is accused at any later criminal trial.

The Committee on Death Certification and Coroners headed by Judge Brodrick have made it abundantly clear that, in their judgement, it is accurate certification of the cause of death which has become the most important function of the Coroner. 'Today (1971) the role of the Coroner as an investigator of crimes against the person has become a relatively insignificant one.'[5] Certainly, while very nearly a quarter of all deaths occurring in England and Wales are dealt with by the Coroners Service, natural disease accounts for at least 80 per cent of the cases currently examined by Coroners' pathologists.

THE SYSTEM IN EUROPE

In general, the comparable systems on the European Continent are dominated by the concept of personal property rights in a dead body. Accordingly, the medico-legal systems are almost expressly designed to obviate the need for post-mortem dissection.

Deaths, the cause of which cannot be certified immediately, are reported to the police who will call upon a selected doctor – comparable to the British Police Surgeon – to make an external examination. The purpose of this examination is essentially to exclude the possibility of criminality; further action is improbable once this is achieved.

Should suspicion of criminality be raised, the case is reported to the appropriate legal authority – magistrate, public prosecutor, *juge d'instruction* and the like – who conducts his inquiries initially in private. The legal authority will then appoint a qualified specialist in forensic medicine to make a further external examination and, as a result of this, an internal autopsy may be authorized. The widespread establishment on the Continent of Medico-Legal Institutes very often results in the provision of opinions which are backed by several individuals of high repute.

In general, the magistrate or his equivalent is responsible for certification of the cause of death in those cases falling within his disposal; in criminal cases this function is assumed by the higher court.

---

[5] *Report of the Committee on Death Certification and Coroners* (1971). Cmnd. 4810. London, HMSO, p. 130.

THE MEDICAL EXAMINER

The medico-legal system of many of the United States rests on the office of Medical Examiner. This has much in common with the European system, with the major difference that the investigation of sudden and suspicious deaths is the responsibility of a medical rather than a legal organization. Thus, a single medical man inspects the locus of death, decides the need for internal autopsy and, in many instances, performs the post-mortem dissection himself. Only when his inquiries are complete and these indicate the possibility of criminality does he notify the District Attorney of his findings although, in the meantime, a close liaison has been maintained with the police.

His powers of investigation are wide but his jurisdiction is very limited; two courses are open to him – he can either issue a death certificate or refer the case to the prosecutor.

THE PROCURATOR FISCAL

The origins of the Procurator Fiscal in Scotland are as old as those of the Coroner in England and Wales. Possibly commencing as a collector of dues in the Ecclesiastical Courts, the Fiscal was gradually integrated into the civil jurisdiction, through the Sheriff Courts, in the fifteenth and sixteenth centuries. In 1746, his office was formally recognized as one of service to the Crown and his financial independence from fines collected became assured some 100 years later. Modern Procurators Fiscal are appointed by the Lord Advocate. Their function is to receive reports from the police of all crimes committed in their districts – and to direct the police in their task;[6] additionally, the Fiscal prepares the Crown case in criminal trials committed to the High Court and conducts the prosecution in the Sheriff Court. It follows that the Procurator Fiscal must be a lawyer and is very unlikely to be also medically qualified. For the purposes of this chapter, the main responsibility of the Fiscal is to investigate any sudden, violent, suspicious or accidental deaths or any other death which is reported to him. A list of reportable deaths is given in Appendix D.[7] Although some of the items on this list are clearly associated with Public Health or with the possibility of civil negligence, it remains true that the basic medico-legal function of the Fiscal is to exclude criminality; it is no part of his duty to establish the precise cause of death.

As in England and Wales, the statutory responsibility to report appropriate deaths to the Fiscal rests with the Registrar but, by com-

---

[6] Smith v. H.M.Adv. 1952 J.C. 66. at pp. 71–72.

[7] Registration of Births, Deaths and Marriages (Scotland) Act 1965, s. 28.

mon usage, most of his preliminary information stems from the police, medical practitioners or the next-of-kin, the last two often working through the medium of the first. The Fiscal will then call for a report from the 'sudden deaths' officer (a member of the police force) and from the Police Surgeon who will have examined the body externally; these reports will include information about the medical history of the dead person. If the Fiscal decides that no further inquiry is needed, he will invite the Police Surgeon to grant a death certificate; the system clearly operates very much more smoothly when there is a close working relationship between the Fiscal and his medical adviser.

Should the Fiscal decide, or should he accept the advice of the Police Surgeon, that a post-mortem dissection is required, he will seek the authority of the Sheriff giving one of the following reasons for so doing:

a. that his inquiries cannot be completed unless the cause of death is fully established;
b. that there are circumstances of suspicion;
c. that there are allegations of criminal conduct;
d. that death was associated with anaesthesia in connection with a surgical operation and the fact that all precautions were taken must be established.

The dissection is carried out by two doctors whenever the circumstances give grounds for suspicion or suggest the possibility that criminal proceedings may follow. Following the autopsy, the Fiscal's pathologist may issue a death certificate.

All the Fiscal's inquiries are conducted in private. In the event that further proceedings are likely he has the power to precognosce material witnesses. Precognition implies the private interrogation of witnesses which will amplify their preliminary statements and which will form the basis of the Fiscal's final report to Crown Counsel in whom is vested the ultimate decision as to what proceedings, if any, are to follow upon a death. In passing, it is worth observing that not every death reported to a Fiscal requires to be reported by him to Crown Counsel. Sudden deaths which, in the opinion of the Fiscal, are free from suspicion and certain other difficulties may be cleared by him upon his own responsibility; a list of those conditions which must be reported by him to Crown Counsel is given in Appendix E. Precognitions are informal and the evidence is not usually taken on oath. Whilst the defence have a right to precognosce witnesses, they cannot enforce their attendance and they may have to call upon a witness to take the statement which he is under a duty to give to them. They can, of course, cite an unwilling witness to attend Court at a trial even though he or she failed to attend for precognition.

Outwith criminal proceedings – in which, it will be noted, privacy is maintained until the hearing in the definitive court[8] – the Fiscal's inquiries can be made public by way of the Fatal Accidents and Sudden Deaths Inquiry (Scotland) Act 1976.

Under s.1(1), the Procurator Fiscal for the district with which a death is most closely associated must apply to the Sheriff for the holding of a Public Inquiry under the Act when:

(a) (i) it appears that the death has resulted from an accident occurring in Scotland while the person who has died, being an employee, was in the course of his employment or, being an employer or self-employed, was engaged in his occupation as such; or

(ii) the person who has died was, at the time of his death, in legal custody; or

(b) It appears to the Lord Advocate to be expedient in the public interest that an Inquiry under this Act should be held into the circumstances of the death on the ground that it was sudden, suspicious or unexplained, or has occurred in circumstances such as to give rise to serious public concern.

Public Inquiries are mandatory in respect of deaths detailed in s.1(1)(a) but it is entirely within the discretion of the Lord Advocate whether or not a Public Inquiry is held under subsection (b); serious public concern might, for example, attend cases of alleged negligence in hospital, accidents involving public transport etc. Any person with an interest may make representations to the Lord Advocate that an Inquiry should be held. Such representations will be considered but the Lord Advocate's decision is final. The Sheriff sits without a jury but an expert assessor may be appointed at the request of any properly interested party. No witness can be compelled to answer any question indicating that he is guilty of any crime or offence. The Sheriff determines as to when and where the accident and the death(s) took place, their cause or causes, the reasonable precautions which might have prevented the accident, any defects in the system of working which contributed to the accident and any other relevant facts. The determination of the Sheriff is not admissible in evidence in any judicial proceedings, of whatever nature, arising out of the accidental death. The Act applies to fatal accidents related to North Sea exploration.

---

[8] Up till recently, this contrasted with the procedure in England where much publicity arose as a result of the preliminary Magistrates' hearing. Since the passing of the Criminal Justice Act 1967, the situation has approached more closely to that applying in Scotland.

MEDICO-LEGAL SYSTEMS IN SOME PARTS OF THE COMMONWEALTH

Australia*

In common with the majority of Commonwealth countries, Australia retains the Coroner as the primary medico-legal authority. However, the autonomy of the States is such that, while practices are very similar, there is no absolute uniformity.[9] Medico-legal autopsies are performed at varying rates which extend from the unusually high proportion of 30 per 10 000 population in the Northern Territory, through the fairly steady range of 12–15 which holds in Victoria, New South Wales, Queensland, Western Australia and Tasmania, to 7 per 10 000 population current in South Australia.[10] The comparable rates in the United Kingdom are 25 in England and Wales and 5 per 10 000 population in Scotland.

Australian Coroners are, in general, stipendiary Magistrates having jurisdiction throughout their particular State or Territory, but Justices of the Peace, Clerks of Court or other proper persons (e.g. Medical Practitioners) may be appointed in some States.

As in England and Wales, the Coroner's autopsy is considered part of the ordinary process of certifying the medical cause of death; death is certified on the basis of autopsy as being due to natural causes in approximately 70–80 per cent of Coroners' cases. A minimum of 70 per cent of cases reported to the Coroner are examined by internal dissection.

The Coroners' powers to dispense with Inquest are varied. Such a course is open in most States but, in Victoria, for example, the procedure of certification on the basis of written statements alone, while being effective, is not at present statutory; in Queensland, the Coroner can only recommend to the Justice Department that an Inquest is unnecessary if it would serve no useful purpose. A Coroner may sit with a jury if he thinks it desirable or if he is requested to do so by relatives; in Western Australia, the Coroner must sit with a jury of three in the event of death being due to accident in a factory or mine; there are, however, no Coroners' Juries in Queensland, South Australia and the Territories.

Other than in New South Wales and South Australia, the Coroner

---

* Based on information kindly supplied by Dr J. I. Tonge, Dr V. Pleuckhahn and Dr J. Hilton.

[9] The relevant statutes include: *New South Wales* – Coroners Act 1960–1970; *Victoria* – Coroners Act 1958; *Tasmania* – Coroners Act 1957; *South Australia* – Coroners Act 1975; *Western Australia* – Coroners Act 1920–1960; *Northern Territory* – Coroners Ordinance 1974–1975; *Queensland* – The Coroners Acts 1958–1972; *Australian Capital Territory* – Coroners Ordinance 1956–1974.

[10] The data quoted are taken from Tonge J. I. and Wilkey I. S. (1974) 'Report on forensic medicine in Australia', presented at 19th Annual Meeting, R. Coll. Path. Aust., Auckland, N.Z.

has a power to commit to trial for murder or manslaughter; only in Victoria is this power used with any frequency.

New Zealand*

Primary medico-legal responsibility rests with the Coroner whose function is similar to that of his English counterpart – that is, to decide who died, when and where and from what cause. He has no authority to commit for trial. The relevant statute is the Coroners Act 1951. The Justice Department has recommended that all autopsies for the Coroner should be carried out by specialist pathologists; while usually acceding to this, the Coroner may choose his own pathologist – an option which is generally subject to agreement with the police authority in cases of suspected homicide.

The proportion of autopsies performed on cases referred to the Coroner is similar to the high figure found in England. Public inquests can be dispensed with but the opportunity to do so is generally taken only when death has been shown by autopsy to be from natural causes. The situation in New Zealand therefore approximates very closely to current English practice – there is a firm commitment to establishing the precise cause of sudden death.

Canada†

The Federal Government of Canada has no overriding authority over the medico-legal system, which is established on a Provincial basis.

The Coroners' system operates in Ontario (The Coroners Act 1972) where there are a full-time Provincial Coroner and a Deputy Provincial Coroner who act in a supervisory capacity. Under them are Regional Coroners and each city and district has one or more Coroners; there are 380 Coroners in Ontario, all of whom are appointed. Medical qualification is a prerequisite for the position. The Coroner visits the scene of death and carries out a full investigation of all cases notified; as a result, an autopsy is requested in some 20 per cent of these. Inquests are, in some cases, mandatory – e.g. when death occurred in custody or was due to a mining or railway accident; otherwise, an Inquest may be ordered by the Coroner investigating the case or by the Chief Coroner. Inquests are heard by a jury and the bases for their being called are generally similar to those described under the two Scottish Fatal Accident Acts; the Coroner is generally motivated by a concern for public safety. The jury cannot make any finding of legal responsibility.

Alberta, by contrast, is in the process of creating a Medical Examiners' system. The Chief Medical Examiner will be based in Calgary and

---

* From Cairns, F. J. (1974) 'Concerning forensic services in Australia and New Zealand', presented at 26th Annual Meeting, N.Z. Soc. Path., Auckland, N.Z.

† Based on information kindly supplied by Dr J. A. J. Ferris and Dr Margaret Milton.

the Deputy Chief Examiner in Edmonton. Each Pathologist/Medical Examiner will have a staff of part-time assistants; it is intended that all will be medically qualified and will function somewhat similarly to Coroners. Post-mortem dissections will be carried out either by or on behalf of the Chief Medical Examiners in major hospitals. Inquiries will be held into selected cases before a Provincial Judge. Somewhat similar systems operate in Manitoba and in Nova Scotia.

British Columbia and Saskatchewan still use lay Coroners who are assisted by trained investigators. There seems a probability that these Provinces will shortly alter their medico-legal systems to correspond to those operating either in Ontario or in Alberta.

The system in Quebec is rather less precise but is based on a form of coronial hierarchy served by a Government Medico-Legal Institute to which many of the more serious cases are directed. Understandably, there is an influence from the system which operates in Continental Europe.

The Far East*

Malaysia, Singapore and Hong Kong retain the Coroners' system but this has adapted pragmatically to prevailing circumstances.

The Coroners' system in Singapore can be taken as an example of practice in conditions of exceptionally high density population. The Coroner is legally qualified and, as in England, his duty is to decide who died, when, where and from what cause. He has comparable status to a Magistrate and has power to commit for trial. All sudden, unexpected, unnatural, accidental, violent and cause unknown deaths are reportable to the Coroner; in Singapore some 2200 cases are reported annually. The autopsy rate is 75 per cent giving a medico-legal autopsy rate of 7·5 per 10 000 population. The Coroner can dispense with a post-mortem examination if the cause of death is known to be natural and, in such cases, certification by a doctor is required; post-mortem examination will also often be waived in cases of suicide and in certain accidents of domestic nature where the circumstances are clear. The Coroner can dispense with an Inquest when death is due to natural causes but, in all other cases, a Public Inquiry must be held unless the case is proceeding to the Criminal Court. In these circumstances, there is a reversal of the usual findings in forensic practice – 70 per cent of the autopsied cases disclose death to be due to unnatural causes with only 30 per cent due to natural disease. Although there are various religious and customary objections to post-mortem examination, the Coroner's ruling is final and binding.

Malaysia is, by contrast, a predominantly rural country. The primary medico-legal system operates less precisely and, in general, the decision

---

* Based on information kindly supplied by Dr Chao Tzee Cheng.

as to post-mortem examination rests with the investigating police officers; dissections are not carried out on cadavers of persons of the Muslim faith.

Sri Lanka and India*

The medico-legal system of the Indian subcontinent largely reflects the contents of the original Indian penal code, compiled by Lord Macaulay. The first recorded list of Coroners was published in 1844; the Sri Lankan penal code dates from 1883.

The investigation of sudden death in Sri Lanka centres around an Inquirer (known in the principal towns as a Coroner) who is appointed by the Minister for Justice; Inquirers appointed for the main towns are usually qualified either in law or in medicine. The Inquirer is assisted by the police and, when necessary, by a medical officer. The law requires that anyone who knows of a sudden, unnatural or suspicious death must report it to a police officer; a magistrate must be informed if a person dies in custody or in a mental or leprosy hospital.

The Inquirer may call upon a qualified medical officer (not necessarily a Judicial Medical Officer) to perform an autopsy and may summon witnesses to give evidence upon oath. The Coroner's Court is public but there is no jury. The Inquirer's report is forwarded to a Magistrate or, in case of homicide, to the Director of Public Prosecutions.

In India, the Coroners' System operates in Calcutta and in Bombay; the Coroners' Courts function with a jury. Elsewhere, the inquiry into an accidental or unnatural death is conducted by a Senior Police Officer in the presence of two respected citizens of the area who subsequently sign the report. The report, known as Panchnama, embodies the significant findings at the scene, the external appearances of the body and the apparent cause of death. An autopsy by a medical officer is requested in cases of doubt or suspicion. Deaths in prison or while in police custody are subject to a Magisterial inquiry.

In both Sri Lanka and India, the Medical Officer – who, outwith the large towns, usually undertakes medico-legal duties as part of a more general commitment – may also be called upon to report to the police on nonfatal injuries sustained. He thus combines the roles of Coroner's pathologist and Police Surgeon, the system being very similar to that obtaining in Scotland.

AN ANALYSIS OF THE VARIOUS SYSTEMS

Although the reader will have formed his own opinions, it is not out of place to present a brief review of the advantages and disadvantages of

---

* Based on information kindly provided by Professor N. Kodagoda.

the systems described. Before doing so, a cause of some confusion must be removed. Much unfounded suspicion of the Coroners' system is based on the nature of this office in the United States. In practice, the office of Coroner in the USA has little more than nominal similarity with that in the English system, the Coroner in the United States being generally an elected, political appointee. He is often unqualified either medically or legally and there is considerable basis for distrust of the system; but this is no reason for extrapolating that the English Coroner would be better replaced by a Medical Examiner.

Perhaps the most frequently raised valid criticism of the system in England and Wales relates to the publicity given to many cases which are of no public concern. The increasing use of the dispensation given in the 1926 Act has done much to dispel this objection but, nevertheless, there are instances – of which suicides are the most prominent – in which much unnecessary distress must be given to relatives. Privacy, on the other hand, is dependent on the qualities of those acting within its protective ramparts; all the other systems described will be effective only if there is public confidence in the officials concerned – perhaps this is most evident in the case of the Medical Examiner. At the same time, these systems have an inbuilt protective mechanism in that, unlike the Coroner who is solely responsible for his actions, all other comparable officials are subject to an immediate higher authority. The system whereby two doctors must attest to the autopsy findings in serious cases, which obtains in Scotland, the USA (under the Medical Examiner system) and in many European countries, undoubtedly enhances the quality of the medical evidence and nullifies many of the arguments in favour of publicity.

The true function of the primary medico-legal system is currently receiving much attention. The undoubted trend towards the role of adjusting the records of the Registrar, which is evident in England, leads to a very high autopsy rate with a potential limitation in standards – 20 per cent of deaths in England and Wales were the subject of a Coroner's autopsy in 1972. The rigid interpretation of the Fiscal's function to exclude criminality would, on the other hand, lead to undue constriction of the pathological service and, in practice, a wider spectrum of sudden death is examined by dissection; even after selection by external examination, natural disease accounts for some 55 per cent of deaths in which a Fiscal's autopsy is performed – from about 5 per cent of the total deaths in Scotland. At present, however, it seems that neither system meets ideally its function of eradicating conditions which operate against the public interest. The Coroner's Court has insufficient jurisdiction for any recommendations made to have a great public impact. There is greater scope in Scotland under the 1976 Act but, under the earlier legislation which the Act repeals, this avenue of life-saving propaganda was used comparatively seldom. For example, some 800 road deaths occur annually in Scotland, yet such deaths are rarely the subject of a Public Inquiry in the absence of criminal proceedings.

The writer does not agree with the Brodrick Committee in its attempts to overwhelm the Coroners' service still further with diagnostic autopsies many of which would, if undertaken, be more beneficially routed through academic departments of Morbid Anatomy. The Fiscals' service strikes a good balance between available resources and value to the public although support to community health might be still further improved by greater use of the Public Inquiry; the effect of the 1976 abolition of juries in such cases will need to be evaluated.

Chapter 3

Identification of the Dead and of Remains

THE problem of identification of the dead arises in two ways which require rather different methods of solution. Firstly, there is the identification of the single unknown body. The most difficult situation is provided by the body which is discovered in some place unrelated to habitation – the classic example being the body discovered in a wood or a shallow grave. Such subjects may well have died by criminal means and are commonly decomposed. It is likely that no immediate clues to identity will be available and the problem will therefore be one of deductive identification – fitting a name to a body. If, on the other hand, a body is discovered in a house, there is, at least, a possibility that it is a cadaver of a person associated with that house and, in the initial stages, the identification team can work from that premiss. The problem is then the much simpler one of fitting a body to a name; only when the probable names have been excluded does one have to revert to the random situation.

The second type of identification problem relates to conditions resulting from a major disaster. Even here, the subject is not quite homogeneous – the identification of a large number of victims of a flood is likely to be more difficult than in the case of a train accident which, in turn, may well be more complex than is the air disaster situation in which an accurate list of those presumed killed is generally available. In all such cases, crime is the exception and, other than in aircraft accidents, when extensive mutilation and burning is likely, the bodies will probably be found in a reasonably preserved condition; at least some clues as to likely identity will be to hand and, in particular, circumstantial evidence in the form of clothing, documents, jewellery and the like may well be available. Identification in the mass is a matter of fitting a number of bodies to a number of names known with varying certainty.

These categories will certainly overlap but, for descriptive purposes,

48 FORENSIC MEDICINE FOR LAWYERS

it is convenient to discuss primary characteristics, comparative methods and circumstantial means of identification and to relate these to the random body, to the single body of likely identity and to the mass disaster.

THE PURPOSES OF IDENTIFICATION

Excluding such philosophical concepts as the right of every free-born man to an identity after death, which has been implied from the United Nations Declaration of Human Rights, identification of a dead body is needed, in the first place, in the field of criminal investigation; the chances of apprehending a criminal are greatly increased once the identity of the victim has been established. Secondly, many important procedures in the civil field – e.g. grant of probate, resolving of partnerships and the general administration of estates – depend upon accurate identification; failure in this respect may result in a delay of up to seven years before death can be presumed. In disasters of an explosive nature, the process of identification might well have to be limited to establishing the total number of deaths – this may be the only way in which the standard period required for presumption of death may be acceptably shortened. Thirdly, there are purely social reasons for assigning a correct name to a dead body – many people have an understandable affection for the remains of their next-of-kin and certain religions have strict and conflicting rules as to the disposal of the dead. Finally, accurate identification of the fatal casualties and correlation of their injuries with their environment in transportation accidents – particularly those involving airlines – may greatly assist the accident investigation authorities either in relation to the cause of the accident or as to the prevention of fatal injury in the future.

IDENTIFICATION OF THE SINGLE
UNKNOWN BODY

Proof that the Remains are Human
Surprising as it may seem, mistakes as to the human or animal origin of decomposed or skeletonized remains are not uncommon at first assessment. At least one murder investigation has been mounted because a bear's paw was mistaken for a human hand, and bones are often referred to Forensic Departments suspected as being the remains of human infants which are, in fact, derived from middens. Such errors are, however, generally corrected rapidly; in case of doubt, the opinion of a specialist anatomist should always be sought and be backed, if necessary, by a veterinary or zoological appraisal.

A more difficult situation arises when only soft tissues or unidentifiable bones are available; it may then be necessary to invoke immunological evidence. All tissues of animal species, including humans, contain antigens (*see* p. 21) which are more or less specific to that species.[1] It is possible to prepare artificial antibodies to these antigens which can thereby be identified in the laboratory. The commonest method is to precipitate the antigen/antibody complex and, for this reason, the test is often referred to as a 'precipitin test', the details of which are not needed here. A similar technique is used in the preliminary study of blood and other biological stains (*see* Chapter 18).

Determination of Sex

It may be difficult to establish the sex of a body by cursory superficial examination even in the absence of severe burning or putrefaction. In a case investigated by the author, two hours was allowed for the examination of 114 coffins primarily to establish the total number of dead; despite the observations of three pathologists, it was found that, while the total number was correct when compared with the manifest, the division of males and females was still not accurate. Unisex fashions in hairstyle and clothing contribute to the difficulty and problems may arise from congenital deformities of the genitalia. Such difficulties are, however, unlikely to be serious in single bodies other than in those which are severely damaged.

Early putrefaction and burning short of combustion may actually accentuate secondary sex characters – particularly the size of the breasts. On the other hand, severe burning, putrefaction and the ravages of animals or of insects may destroy the genital region. The sex can then generally be determined by the finding of either a uterus in the female or a prostate gland in the male; these organs are among those most resistant to putrefaction in the body. In the event of complete skeletonization, the sex of the dead person can be derived, with varying degrees of certainty, from a study of the total skeleton or from individual bones. Many bones show *comparative* differences between male and female but the pelvis very often provides definitive indications of sex (*Fig.* 7).

Fig. 7. The pelvic bones of the male (left) and the female (right).

---

[1] There may be some cross-reaction between closely related species but this is of little practical importance in human forensic medicine.

There are many sophisticated measurements which can be made to this end but, for present purposes, only a general summary is needed – the female pelvis is wider and squatter, with a far straighter sacrum, than is found in the male; the dorsal surface of the pubic bone also becomes pitted during childbirth. An accuracy of 95 per cent or more is claimed for the determination of sex from the pelvis. The wide hips of the female dictate a more acute angle between the neck and shaft of the femur than is needed in the male in order to bring the knees together; the thigh bone is perhaps the most valuable of the long bones which may be available for sexing – provided the ethnic origin is known, an accuracy of some 80 per cent can be obtained. Sex differences are also notable in the skull which is one of the bony specimens most frequently presented to forensic departments. The features which are sought include the round orbits and more vertical forehead of the female; the greater surface area of the mastoid process in the male; and the prominent supraorbital or eyebrow ridges which are a feature of masculinity.

Determination of Age

In the presence of putrefaction or burning, a superficial examination can result in gross error as to the age of a cadaver; objective parameters are needed. The condition of any remaining organs may provide these but, again, the skeleton can give very useful clues. The significant findings in the bones depend to a large extent on the age group; it is convenient to consider the fetus and neonate, the adolescent and the adult as separate categories.

The Fetus and Neonate

Objective evidence of age at this stage is to be obtained from the development of the bones and, in particular, from the presence of certain centres of ossification; these have been described at p. 30 and a representative list is given in Appendix F. The most important centres are those which distinguish the legally viable (28-week pregnancy) and the full-term fetus (*see* Chapter 19 for details). Although it is simple to demonstrate these centres at autopsy, the most objective, and permanent, record is obtained by the routine radiological examination of unidentified fetuses. Anomalous appearances occur in individual centres but, at this stage of development, the *overall* picture can produce an accuracy of ± 1 month.

In Childhood and Adolescence

Up to the age of 20, the most useful information as to age is given by the joining of the epiphyses to their shafts (Appendix G). Although such unions generally follow in a definite chronological order, the variations in individuals are wide and, certainly when using a single observation, an accuracy greater than ± 2 years can rarely be claimed. The bracket contracts as the number of observations made increases and numerous attempts have been made to summate these mathematically, allowance being made for 'weighting' the relative accuracy of the individual observations. Such problems are for the anthropologists.

Adult Life
After the age of 20, the ageing of an unknown body becomes progressively more difficult. The sutures of the skull close in adult life but, apart from the interfrontal suture, union does not commence until approximately the age of 35 and, even then, the findings are subject to wide variation. It is extremely doubtful if it is possible to age the skeletal remains of an adult closer than ± one decade.

Other gradual changes associated with use, such as the angle of the jaw bone, occur as part of the natural process of ageing; the presence of disease states either in remaining soft tissues or in the bones may give general indications of age but only within very wide bands.

Ageing from the Teeth
In the experience of nearly all observers, the most valuable indication of age from infancy to adulthood can be obtained from the teeth and it is in this field that the greatest advances have been made. The subject is discussed in detail in the section on Forensic Odontology (Chapter 29).

Determination of Stature
The determination of the stature in life from post-mortem remains is fraught with difficulty. Even if the whole cadaver is available, a direct measurement has its own inaccuracy as the body in life measures some one inch (2·5 cm) less than the body when dead. There is also the complication of age. After the age of 30, the natural processes of senile degeneration are said to result in an average decrease in stature of something of the order of one-fortieth of an inch (0·6 mm) per year.

It follows that mathematical formulae designed to assess the *in-vivo* stature from limited remains must be treated with reserve. Moreover, the exact height of an individual during life is available only rarely – far more likely, only a subjective assessment or, at best, a fairly rough measurement will be forthcoming.

The bones of the lower limb provide the best evidence and the more bones which are examined, the narrower will be the range within which is put the final estimate of living height. Taking everything into consideration it is doubtful if an accuracy of greater than ± 1 inch can ever be achieved by studying individual bones and this may represent considerable overconfidence; the interested reader is referred to specialized monographs.[2] Simple calculations are probably best used in practice. A useful rule of thumb is that the humerus (arm bone) is 20 per cent, the femur (thigh bone) 27 per cent and the tibia (lower leg bone) 22 per cent of the subject's height in life. The spine, if available, is some 35 per cent and the distance between the outstretched fingertips approximates to the total height.

The Use of Comparative Methods
The problem of allotting a body to a probable name is very much simpler because information concerning many characteristics individual to the presumed person is likely to be available. The matter is then one of comparing these with the findings in the cadaver. It is not necessary to discuss here such obvious characteristics as colour of hair or eyes, save to point out that these may alter considerably post mortem. The forensic medical practitioner will, however, be much concerned with the provision of medical information in relation to identity.

Medical Information
Recognizable disease states, evidence of past surgical procedures, deformities and tattoos can be included under this general heading.

The value of the past medical history depends on the nature of the information. Thus, a history of cardiac pain in a missing person is relatively useless as damage to the heart muscle is discovered at post-mortem examination in a very high proportion of persons beyond middle age. A history of gall bladder disease might, on the other hand, be much more significant. A combination of evidence – e.g. severe arthritis of the spine together with disease of the thyroid gland – will provide far greater probability of identification than would be suggested from the sum of the diseases present in the population as single entities.

Similar considerations apply to surgical procedures. A history of removal of the appendix is unhelpful; partial removal of the female genitalia is less common but would certainly be insufficient evidence by itself on which to base an identification. Each case requires individual assessment as to significance and, again, a combination of surgical procedures may provide virtually incontrovertible evidence of identification. The presence of surgical prostheses – particularly if X-ray or other in-life records are available for comparison – may provide evidence which would satisfy even the most sceptical. Old fractures, which can also be compared by X-ray, can be very useful.

Deformities may also be common or rare. They may be congenital –

---

[2] Of which the classic is probably Krogman W. M. (1962) *The Human Skeleton in Forensic Medicine*. Springfield, Ill., Thomas.

that is, present from birth – or acquired. Very often, they provide little more than confirmatory evidence of identification made on other grounds.

Tattoos present some interesting problems in identification. Firstly, it has been pointed out that many tattoos are of standardized pattern and the presence, say, of a heart pierced by an arrow, cannot be regarded as proof of identification. Secondly, the investigator must be wary of descriptions of tattoos; what may be a clear illustration to one party may be quite differently interpreted by another. It is, however, fair to say that so long as an adequate description of tattoos in life is available – particularly in the form of photographs – they may provide excellent evidence of identification. It is of practical importance that, although tattoos may be superficially obscured by the carbonization of burning, scrubbing of the area may reveal an easily identifiable pattern in the deeper tissues (*Plate* 1a).

Personal Identification

Two methods of positive, personal identification are outstanding – finger-printing and dental comparison.

The science of dactylography or finger-printing is one for the expert and is outside the province of this book. Indeed, for present purposes, finger-prints have a limited use in identification in so far as permanent records are available in the United Kingdom only in the case of criminals and merchant seamen. The main value of finger-prints in the identification of a body from the general population depends on the ability to compare the prints from the cadaver with those on the personal possessions of the supposed person. The more personal the possessions, the more certain becomes the identification. The preservation of heel or sole prints in those who are at risk of sudden death with mutilation – e.g. airline crews – is probably of more practical value, and less emotive, than is the taking of finger-prints, as the feet are commonly preserved from burning by boots or shoes.

The importance of dental identification is becoming increasingly recognized, particularly as dental records are available for a very high proportion of a population served by a National Health Service. The methods involved in and the limitations of dental identification are discussed in Chapter 29. It is enough to say here that the method is wholly dependent on the quality of record-keeping by practitioners and that the certainty of identification increases in almost geometrical progression with the number of positive correlations present; ultimately, a comparison of ante- and post-mortem charts may be as personalized a method of identification as is a finger-print. A comparison of X-rays taken before and after death may provide incontrovertible evidence of identification.

IDENTIFICATION IN A MAJOR DISASTER

The identification of a large number of casualties presents problems which are mainly organizational and which are, in other respects, dictated by the nature of the disaster. It may be that the subjects are well preserved but that there is little knowledge of their origin, as may occur in a rail accident; they may be relatively unclothed and severely carbonized, as in a hotel fire. The aircraft accident is, perhaps, the commonest form of mass disaster and, by virtue of its unforeseeable and varied location, is certainly likely to present the most urgent difficulties in identification. The aircraft accident can be taken as a model for mass disaster investigation so long as it is appreciated that there are certain unique features involved. Great differences are likely even within the category of aircraft accident – thus, one accident may present as a problem of disintegration while another may approximate to a mass cremation.

Fig. 8. Diagrammatic representation of the identification commission established for a major disaster. Sources of observations and information are shown. The importance of numbering the bodies – and of maintaining a single set of numbers – is emphasized.

The secret of accurate, rapid identification of mass casualties lies in the organization. The essential is to establish a 'commission of identification' which, on the one hand, is receiving information about missing persons and, on the other, is being advised of observations on the dead bodies from various sources. The scheme is illustrated in *Fig.* 8. Standardized documentation which can be completed easily is essential; the disaster victim identification form introduced by the International Criminal Police Organization has been criticized on many counts, and alternative forms, which have been recommended by the International Civil Aviation Organisation, are used by the Accident Investigation Branch of the United Kingdom Department of Trade.[3] Whatever forms

---

[3] The use of these forms has been well described by Stevens P. J., in: Mant A. K. (ed.) (1973) *Modern Trends in Forensic Medicine – 3*. London, Butterworths.

are used, the process of identification is essentially one of sorting through numerous 'information' files and attempting to 'marry' these to 'observation' files.

The essential difference between identification in the mass and identification of the single unknown body lies in the enforced use in the former of much circumstantial evidence. Thus, a large amount of preliminary or 'primary' identification is done on the basis of documents carried, recognizable jewellery and clothing; jewellery, being fire-resistant, is especially valuable in this context.

The use of such evidence requires much care – it is, for example, essential to ensure that possessions attributed to a given body in the furore of cadaver retrieval were, in fact, incontrovertibly associated with that body. Vagaries such as exchange of tickets and the widespread use of chain-store clothing must be accepted as potential hazards and it is important that any circumstantial evidence should be confirmed by an alternative method, preferably one involving 'personal' identification. Of these, dental evidence is of outstanding importance; medical evidence, particularly if it is of an unusual nature, has a significant part to play.

Visual identification, the standard 'personal' method of many police forces, is highly suspect in the context of a mass disaster. Not only may recognizable peculiarities be erased or mimicked but the observers are often under such emotional stress that they are particularly prone to unwitting error. It is generally far better to present next-of-kin with a maximum of three bodies, ideally already identified by other means, when subjecting them to the ordeal of recognition. In practice, the enforcement of visual identification would be inhumane in the majority of aircraft disasters.

Chapter 4

Post-mortem Changes and the Timing of Death

THE maintenance of life by a machine is a controversial topic which poses very many medico-legal questions. This aspect of death is, therefore, discussed in greater detail elsewhere (Chapter 12). For present purposes, death is defined as irreversible failure of the cardiovascular system and is considered only in the natural situation. Functioning heart and blood vessels are essential for the transport of oxygen without which the body tissues must die; on the other hand, the heart may continue to beat and nourish the tissues despite the presence of irrecoverable damage to the central nervous system – the judicial hangings of the past were examples of such action. For these reasons, the cardiovascular system provides the optimum index of true life or death; the concept of 'brain death' arises only in relation to artificial survival and is considered at p. 144.

The main practical function of the doctor called to the locus of an unexplained death is to decide whether death has taken place or not; other considerations must take second place. This decision may be difficult in the event of grossly diminished cardiac output – as may occur in hypothermia or in drug-induced central depression of the vital functions. But some form of heart activity, even if demonstrable only by special techniques, is always present when death is apparent rather than real.

The changes which occur after death can be deduced from the functions of the cardiovascular system. The cessation of oxygen transfer results in cellular death. Those components of the cell which are most sensitive to hypoxia – for example, the enzyme systems – will be first affected. After a variable period of residual activity, energy production ceases and the body cools. Blood which has been circulating is now stagnant and settles under the influence of gravity. There is a final attempt at metabolism in an environment increasingly deprived of oxygen and waste products accumulate where they are formed; the ground substance of the body degenerates and the individual cells lose

56

cohesiveness. In the absence of a viable blood stream, the body is defenceless and bacteria, whether derived from within or without the corpse, are left to multiply at the expense of the tissues – the process of putrefaction is set in train and may be augmented by the flesh-eating larvae of various flies. The process of skeletonization may be hastened by carnivorous animals and, ultimately, the skeleton itself may crumble to chalky dust. These changes can be used to estimate the time of death.

THE TIMING OF DEATH

The First 24 Hours
It is only within the first 12–18 hours that any reasonable accuracy can be expected as to the time of death. Even then, it is important that basic inaccuracies inherent in any biological phenomenon are appreciated.

The estimate of the time elapsed during the first 12 hours after death is based mainly upon the body temperature. Theoretically, this temperature falls according to a sigmoid curve; numerous attempts have been made to liken the body to an experimental cylinder to which the laws of physics can be applied without reservation. However, no matter how many variables are introduced into a mathematical calculation, accuracy cannot be guaranteed in a practical situation.

Factors which must influence the rate of cooling include:

a. The body *temperature* at the time of death. Conditions which tend to raise the temperature at the time of death – for example, infection or cerebral haemorrhage – will result in an artificially short estimate of the post-mortem interval based on temperature recordings; hypothermic and algid states will produce the opposite effect.

b. Clothing. A naked body loses heat more quickly than does a fully clothed one.

c. Body insulation. A fat body is insulated against heat loss as compared with a lean one while those with a large surface area in relation to the body weight will cool faster than will those of more massive physique; thus, children will always cool faster than will adults.

d. Convection currents. A body will cool faster in the presence of moving air than does one in a closed environment.

e. The *environmental temperature* is a variable which will always affect the rate of cooling.

In order to accommodate all these factors, one needs a complicated formula. But no such formula can take into account variations of which the extent is unknown – e.g. the effects of moving the body before measuring the temperature, changes in environmental temperature and the action of draughts. It is better that a relatively simple approach be adopted and the limitations freely admitted. A method is described by

Knight[1] in which the temperature at death is assumed to be 37° C and the difference between this figure and that recorded by a rectal thermometer is the degree of cooling observed. The degree of cooling is then multiplied by 1, 1¼, 1½, 1¾ or 2, according to an air temperature of 0°, 5°, 10°, 15° or 20° C respectively; the resultant figure is taken as the time in hours elapsed since death. The answer is achieved ignoring many variables and represents no more than an approximate centre point for what Knight calls a 'bracket of probability'. When this centre point lies on that part of the curve representing maximum theoretical rate of heat loss, the bracket can be reduced to its minimum; it is seldom, however, that the doctor at the locus can suggest better than a ± 1 hour time of death and this may well be overambitious. Greater confidence is gained if it is possible to make repeated readings at the scene. It is agreed that once the body temperature has approached to within 85 per cent of the environmental temperature the method loses all semblance of accuracy.

These considerations apply to bodies found on land. As expected, cooling of the body is more rapid in cold water although, here again, much will depend on the quantity and the flow of the medium.

1–3 Days
As the enzymatic processes of the body fail, so too does the elimination of waste products. The tissues of the body become altered in consistency and the most prominent representation of this is the phenomenon of *rigor mortis*. Biochemically, this is associated with a massive increase in the lactic acid content of muscle; clinically, the resultant stiffening and shortening of the muscle fibres presents as a relative fixation of the joints which can be broken down only by force.

Rigor results from reduction in the chemical constituent of the muscles known as adenosine triphosphate. The stiffening of the muscles commences when the level of this substance is reduced to 85 per cent of the normal but the process is not demonstrable clinically until some time has passed. All muscle fibres are affected but stiffening will be demonstrable earliest in those bundles of smallest mass; joints supplied by very large muscle groups will be affected the slowest.

In theory, therefore, one would expect the muscles of the face to be the first to demonstrate rigor. The larger muscles would then become involved, the arms appearing stiff before the knees and hips. In practice, however, this order is not always maintained. The condition is apparent some 5–7 hours after death and is usually established throughout the body in 8–12 hours. The muscles remain in rigor until the processes of degeneration and putrefaction cause secondary laxity. Rigor has been observed to disappear clinically in much the same anatomical order as it

---

[1] Knight B., 2nd ed., (1976) *Legal Aspects of Medical Practice*. Edinburgh, Churchill Livingstone, p.96.

became established but, again, the process is variable. The body is generally free of rigor some 36 hours after death but it is by no means uncommon for the condition to persist for 4 days. Relating the degree of rigidity to the body temperature will help to indicate the phase of the rigor 'cycle'.

Theoretically, the degree of distribution of rigor should give a useful indication of the time elapsed since death but, in practice, a phenomenon which is dependent upon biological processes is inevitably capricious in its presentation. Its onset is accelerated in conditions leading to an antemortem excess of lactic acid in the tissues including, in particular, exercise or a pyrexial illness. It will come on slowly, if at all, in persons whose muscle is degenerate as in those who have suffered wasting illnesses. Children demonstrate the phenomenon far less readily than do adults and it is, to some extent, dependent upon the ambient temperature, being accelerated in the summer months and retarded in the winter. Probably, the best that can be hoped for from a consideration of rigor mortis is a 'time of death' at the centre of a bracket of probability extending over some 6–12 hours – and this only over a very limited total period.

Certain conditions simulate rigor mortis but are easily distinguished. Probably the most common of these is cold stiffening; a body which has been placed in the refrigerator is virtually beyond assessment as to rigor. At the other end of the scale, intense heat will result in shrinkage and stiffening of the muscles; but the effects of the heat will be readily seen on the skin. Cadaveric spasm deserves a mention. This is a contraction of the muscles which is probably mediated by the central nervous system when death occurs in conditions of high emotional tension; it is instantaneous and permanent until putrefaction occurs. The most common manifestation is seen in the hands which may be found grasping some object, particularly one which gives some hope of support (*Plate* 1b). Cadaveric spasm may, occasionally, involve the hand which has held a firearm used suicidally. The medico-legal importance of this is that, while the absence of spasm is of no significance, cadaveric spasm cannot be simulated after death in an attempt to disguise a homicide.

Attempts have been made to improve the timing of death during this difficult period by investigating other biochemical changes which occur in the body after death. For obvious reasons, the parameters must be simple to measure and resistant to putrefaction; effort has, therefore, been primarily concentrated on the changes in the distribution of inorganic salts found in those fluids which classically remain sterile after death – in particular the cerebrospinal fluid and the vitreous humour of the eye. The level of, say, potassium alters with time after death and does so very nearly in mathematical progression in a single individual. The variations between individuals are, however, so wide as to eliminate any real hope of improvement in the accuracy of the timing of death by the routine use of such laboratory investigations. There seems to be no present method of estimating the post-mortem interval in practice which will satisfy the needs of the detective story.

Beyond the 3rd Day – Putrefaction

The process of putrefaction begins with death but only becomes manifest after a few days. Again, many variables have to be considered, particularly the condition of the body before death, the temperature and humidity of the environment and the relative sterility of the area. Thus, the bodies of persons who have died while suffering an acute infection or of those subjected to open injury will decompose faster than the norm; particularly rapid changes occur in dead bodies which are allowed to lie in bed under activated electric blankets.

Generally, there is discolouration of the abdominal skin in 2–3 days and swelling of the tissues with the formation of blisters towards the end of the first week. Gross disfiguration is present in some 3 weeks. Partial liquefaction is commonly evident in the body at the end of a month. It will be seen that an estimate of the time of death in a putrefied body can generally be given only in terms of weeks.

Putrefaction of the body is normally delayed in water unless this be heavily contaminated by sewage. In ordinary circumstances, an immersed body will tend to float after a week to 10 days but this will be greatly modified by clothing and water temperature; in deep cold water a body may not surface for some 3 weeks or, indeed, may never do so. There is a similar retardation of putrefaction in coffins in which bursting of the body, an almost invariable accompaniment of putrefaction in the open, is an uncommon finding.

Some features of putrefaction are of forensic importance. Muscular and, particularly, fibrous tissues are resistant and certain organs – for example, the uterus and the prostate gland – may be recognizable for a considerable time; this is of obvious importance in identification. Vascular walls tend to resist decomposition and evidence of coronary insufficiency can often be discovered when the general appearances would suggest that a search would be unlikely to be rewarding; this will be particularly so if calcification has occurred.

The combination of destruction of the blood and formation of gas may lead to the issue of bloody fluid from the orifices. The appearances may closely simulate those of antemortem haemorrhage and must be interpreted with caution.

Finally, there is the problem of the body which appears to have resisted decomposition to an unusual degree. This may happen as a natural phenomenon in the closed environment of the coffin. Nevertheless, it has been stated that the finding of such a cadaver should raise the suspicion of poisoning by metallic compounds; this association between preservation and poisoning may, however, be little more than folklore.

Two well-known modifications to the normal process of putrefaction require mention. The first of these is mummification where, in the presence of drying conditions and the absence of bacterial contamination, the tissues may become desiccated rather than putrefied. Ultimately, the mummified tissues may be reduced to powder but, in the meantime, the general format of the body may be remarkably preserved. The bodies of infants tend to mummify very readily.

Secondly, there is the formation of adipocere which results in the transformation of the normal fluid fats of the body to solid compounds. This variant of putrefaction may occur in any tissue containing fat if associated with moist conditions; it is therefore prevalent in bodies recovered from the water and in bodies exhumed from coffins. Adipocere adheres to the bone, the result being that, even after the skin has disintegrated, the body may retain recognizable characteristics of importance in identification; injuries to soft tissues may also be preserved. The presence of adipocere almost invariably means that the body has been dead for some weeks if not months.

Stage of Skeletonization
Ultimately all the soft tissues of the body will decompose, the tendons and other highly fibrous tissues remaining most resistant.

The time for complete skeletonization is extremely variable and depends not only on the natural processes of decomposition but also upon predators from the insect and animal worlds – and from fungi and other moulds. The author has seen two bodies reduced to skeletons within their clothing in a light aircraft which remained undiscovered for 2 months in an English summer; it is doubtful if such rapid skeletonization would occur in winter.

Although the time can be much shorter, it is probably fair to estimate a skeleton with which are associated remnants of fibrous tissue as having been dead for approximately 1 year but, from this point, estimates of the interval since death can be assessed in brackets only of years or even decades. The environment is all-important – bones many hundreds of years old have been discovered well-preserved, particularly in dry caves. Numerous scientific techniques, including some of great sophistication – such as the analysis of radioactive carbon – have been introduced for the dating of skeletons but are beyond the scope of this book.

HYPOSTASIS

As the stagnant blood pools under the influence of gravity, its presence becomes apparent on the skin and contrasts vividly with the exsanguinated portions. Similar changes occur in the internal organs where it is important that they are not confused with antemortem haemorrhage, for example in the lungs.

Hypostasis, or lividity, can often be seen within 1–2 hours after death and is generally fully established in 6–12 hours. At this point, although fluid blood itself may be displaced, there is sufficient staining of the tissue to maintain some evidence of hypostasis irrespective of the subsequent position of the body. Sustained pressure prevents pooling of the blood and it is common to find that generalized lividity of the back is notably absent from the buttocks and shoulder blades which take the main weight of the recumbent body.

Hypostasis is of relatively little value as a method of timing the interval since death although, taken in conjunction with other signs, it has some use in this respect during the first 6 hours. Its distribution is, however, a fundamental observation in establishing the position of the body after death and, particularly, whether it has been changed. In the event that the body has been moved, the examining doctor may discover either a dual distribution of lividity or a distribution which is incompatible with the locus as presented to him. Either finding must raise the possibility of outside interference.

There are two conditions which require differentiation from hypostasis. The first of these, bruising, is a relatively simple decision. Apart from the fact that bruises are commonly localized they are, by definition, the result of bleeding into the tissues as opposed to stagnation of blood in the vessels. A rather more difficult situation arises in the distinction between hypostasis and the congestion of an asphyxial death; this has considerable practical significance. Thus, a baby dying in the prone position will show a facial distribution of lividity with pallor over the pressure points – the centre of the forehead, the tip of the nose, the chin and the cheekbones. The contrast between this appearance and that of congestion of the face resulting from an asphyxial death may be difficult to appreciate.

The colour of the lividity also provides evidence as to the mode of death. No great reliance can be placed on the 'blueness' as all deaths are, ultimately, anoxic in type. A lividity of bright-red colour however indicates the presence of fully oxygenated blood which is typical of death in the cold or of exposure to cold after death. Perhaps the most well-known example of this type of observation is the diagnosis of poisoning by carbon monoxide. The cherry-pink colour is usually obvious when sought in a good light.

POST-MORTEM ARTEFACTS

Artefacts resulting from efforts at resuscitation are not uncommon.

Heat, be it in the form of direct application or resulting from electrical stimulation, is the most common form encountered. It is perfectly possible to produce burns in a dead body but these can be characteristically differentiated by the absence of so-called vital reaction – that is, the defensive reaction of the living body to injury. The most immediate vital reaction to a burn is dilatation of the surrounding capillaries which shows as an area of redness diffusing into the normal skin colour. Blisters formed before death contain more protein than do those arising post mortem. Infiltration of the area by white blood cells is evident microscopically in a few hours and, later, there is repair by connective tissue cells (fibroblasts). None of these signs will be present in a burn inflicted after death.

A very frequent series of artefacts results from attempted resuscitation by external cardiac massage. The breast bone is almost invariably bruised if not dislocated and fractures of the ribs are often caused. The difficulty in distinguishing such injuries from those inflicted during life on purely pathological grounds rests on the self-evident fact that *efficient* cardiac massage simulates a functioning circulation. Any bruise or fracture caused by this means will, therefore, closely resemble antemortem injury (*see also* p. 127).

Severe post-mortem injuries may be inflicted by carnivorous animals or crabs on land (*Plate* 2a) and by fish or shellfish in water – the latter may bare exposed parts to the bone in a matter of days. Injuries inflicted by rats may closely mimic those of suicidal or homicidal origin; again, it is the absence of vital reaction and an awareness of the possibilities which simplify the interpretation.

Infestation and accelerated destruction of decomposing tissue by larvae of dipterous flies and of beetles is so common as to deserve special mention. It has forensic significance in that entomology has been used on numerous occasions in an attempt to assess the time interval since death. Thus, the insects present can be correlated with their known preferred feeding habits while the age of the larvae and the number of generations can give further information; methods are, however, still in something of an experimental stage. The assessment is more complicated than would appear theoretically and is certainly a matter for the expert who should, ideally, collect his own specimens in the post-mortem room and at the locus.

Finally, traumatic injuries inflicted on the dead body must be mentioned. A body lying on a roadway may be damaged by vehicles whose drivers are genuinely ignorant of having done so. Post-mortem injuries are outstandingly associated with bodies in the sea where buffeting on rocks by the waves, contact with ships' propellers, grappling in fish nets and the like may result in a confused picture. The important practical point is that the possibility of such sources of injury must be considered in relation to the locus of death.

Chapter 5

Legal Disposal of the Dead

WITH one minor exception,[1] it has been illegal since 1836 in England and Wales to dispose of a body unless the death has been registered. There is a wider relaxation of the general rule in Scotland which was designed to take into account the difficulties of communication which used to exist in parts of the country but, in the event of burial before registration, the person in charge of the cemetery must notify the Registrar of the occurrence. Under neither jurisdiction is there a statutory compulsion that the cause of death is certified but such is the current climate of opinion that, although cases do occur from time to time, very few bodies are disposed of uncertified. The current legislation relating to disposal of the dead in Great Britain is contained in the Births and Deaths Registration Act 1953 and in the Registration of Births, Deaths and Marriages (Scotland) Act 1965. In either case, legal disposal begins with medical certification.

MEDICAL CERTIFICATION OF THE CAUSE OF DEATH

Although the general layout of the certificate conforms in each case to the international system of certification of the cause of death, there are some important differences of practice in England and Wales and in Scotland.

In England and Wales, there is a statutory duty laid upon the doctor who attended the deceased during the terminal illness to issue a medical certificate of the cause of death. This obligation does not cease simply because the case is one reportable to the Coroner. If this be so, the correct procedure is for the doctor to issue the certificate, personally report the case to the Coroner and initial the box printed on the reverse of the certificate to indicate that he has done so. The practice of reporting the death to the Coroner and taking no further action is commonly adopted

---

[1] A Registrar in England and Wales may issue a certificate for disposal before registering the death if he has received written notice of the death from a qualified informant and has received a medical certificate of the cause of death – provided the death was not one which should have been reported to the Coroner.

but has no foundation in law; on the other hand, there is no absolute obligation on the doctor to inform the Coroner – to pre-empt the Registrar in this duty is only a most desirable way of saving valuable time.

The English medical certificate requires the certifying doctor to state the date on which he last saw the deceased alive and, in common with the Scottish certificate, to indicate whether or not the body was seen after death and, if so, by whom. The certifying doctor does not have to view the body after death but, in the absence of such precaution, the Registrar must refer the case to the Coroner if the remainder of the certificate indicates that the doctor had not seen his patient during the last 14 days of the latter's life.[2] The doctor in England and Wales further certifies that he was in medical attendance during the deceased's last illness; if no one can so certify – a situation which often obtains in holiday periods – there can be no medical certificate and, *ipso facto*, the case is referred to the Coroner.

A 'Notice to Informant' is attached to the English certificate and the doctor is required to furnish this forthwith. The medical certificate may be sent without delay to the Registrar but, since the death cannot be registered in its absence, it is often handed to the informant together with the notice.

The most important respect in which the Scottish process of medical certification varies from that in England is that, in Scotland, there is no requirement upon the certifying doctor to have been in attendance during the last illness. Under Section 24 of the 1965 Act, it is proper for any doctor who is able to complete the certificate 'to the best of his knowledge and belief' to do so. While this has the great merit of removing a large number of manifestly natural deaths from the intricacies of the medico-legal system, it carries some disadvantages; many doctors are unwilling to certify a cause of death of which they are not quite certain while, on the other hand, the Procurator Fiscal has no wish to accept the English Coroner's responsibilities as to the accuracy of the mortality statistics. There is, therefore, a tendency for certificates to be couched in such terms as 'death from natural causes, probably . . .', which is regarded as a generally satisfactory compromise. There is nothing in the certificate relating to the last time the deceased was seen alive; it follows that there is no obligation on the Registrar to refer a case to the Fiscal for reasons similar to the English '14-day rule'.

There is no space on the Scottish certificate for indicating that the Fiscal has been informed of the death; this is done in the great majority of cases by the doctor himself on a relatively informal basis – once the case has been referred, the certification of the cause of death is generally taken over by the Police Surgeon. Nor is there a 'Notice to Informant'.

---

[2] These regulations will almost certainly be strengthened as a result of the findings of the Brodrick Committee.

The certificate as to the cause of death must be transmitted to the Registrar within 7 days; in practice, it is nearly always given to the informant for transfer to the Registrar.

THE INFORMANT

Persons qualified and liable to act as informants in England and Wales include a relation of the deceased present at the death, in attendance during the last illness or residing in the subdistrict where death occurred; a person present at the death; the 'occupier' of the house or any inmate of the house if either knew of the happening of the death; or a person causing the disposal of the body. If death occurred outside a house, informants may include any relative of the deceased having knowledge of the necessary particulars; any person present at the death; any person who found the body, who is in charge of the body or who is causing the disposal of the body.

In Scotland, the duty to give information of particulars of death devolves, in succession, upon any relative of the deceased; any person present at the death; the deceased's executor; the occupier of the premises where the death took place; or any other person having knowledge of the details to be registered. If the deceased's home is unknown, any person finding the body, including the police involved in the investigation, has a duty to inform the Registrar but all such deaths are then reportable to the Fiscal.

REGISTRATION

The importance of registration of a death is often inadequately emphasized. The Registrar must be informed even in the unusual situation of a body being buried without registration; cremation without registration is not permitted (*see below*). As stated above, it is fundamentally the duty of the Registrar to report certain deaths to the Coroner or to the Fiscal. The process of registration provides an essential back-up service in the detection of secret homicide.

Informants must attend personally at the Registry and provide the necessary information within 5 days of the death in England and within 8 days in Scotland. The Registrar will then issue a disposal certificate or certificate of registration.

BURIAL

Almost incredibly, there is no general statute which requires any individual to dispose of a body and there is nothing which says that a body must be buried or cremated. The local authority may have to take the responsibility when no other arrangements have been made[3] but, otherwise, only the general health laws govern the method of disposal; thus, the burial or cremation of a body may be ordered by a magistrate should its retention above ground be considered a danger to health.[4] Equally surprisingly, there is no national law as to the place of burial but most local authorities have imposed their own rules. Burial outside the United Kingdom requires the authority of the Coroner or of the Procurator Fiscal.

Following burial, a notification that the body has been disposed of must be delivered to the Registrar within 4 days of the event. Failing such advice, the Registrar must report the matter to the appropriate Community Physician (or Specialist in Community Medicine) of the Area Health Authority or Board.

EXHUMATION

Exhumation is an unpleasant procedure, particularly if the body has been buried only recently, and is one which engenders considerable emotion. Although the practice is, as a result, very strictly controlled, there are occasions when the re-examination of a body already buried may be of overriding importance either to the State, as in the case of suspected criminality, to insurance companies or to individuals when civil actions for damages are contemplated or when identification is disputed.

If a Coroner in England and Wales considers it necessary to hold an inquest on a body already buried, he can, himself, authorize exhumation. In all other cases, permission must be sought from the Home Secretary.[5] Only 20 medico-legal exhumations were carried out in England and Wales during the period 1959–68; 18 of these were ordered by Coroners and 2 were authorized by the Home Secretary.

In Scotland, the person requiring the exhumation, whether it be the Procurator Fiscal or a member of the public, petitions the Sheriff to that effect. The Sheriff must notify the next-of-kin of the deceased who are given the opportunity to make objections at a hearing. If the petition is granted, the Sheriff will issue a warrant for exhumation.

Presumptive identification is made by the superintendent of the graveyard consulting his records and by the undertaker's recognition of the coffin and of the internal wrappings. Whenever possible, relatives

---

[3] National Assistance Act 1948, s. 50, as amended.

[4] Public Health Act 1936, s. 162; Public Health (Scotland) Act 1897, s. 69.

[5] Burial Act 1857. These limitations do not apply when a body must be moved to another burial ground as a matter of public need. The bishop of the diocese can then grant a faculty to do so; local authorities also have powers of removal and reinterment of remains (e.g. Town and Country Planning Act 1971, s. 128).

should be asked to confirm the name on the identifying plaque.

Many exhumations authorized for the purpose of establishing the precise cause of death are concerned with suspected poisoning. It is then incumbent upon the pathologist in charge of the operation to obtain a full series of control specimens which can be analysed for the poison along with the tissues from the body. These include earth from above, around and below the coffin, the wood of and fluid from inside the coffin, and portions of the burial robes. It is also advisable to collect further control specimens of soil from a distant area of the cemetery. Parallel analyses will provide valuable evidence as to the possibility of any poison having entered the body from outside after burial rather than having been ingested before death.

There is considerable onus on the pathologist to make a particularly thorough examination of exhumed bodies – they certainly constitute cases which justify a full-body X-ray survey as a routine; so far as is known, no request for a second exhumation has ever been granted.

CREMATION

As a reflection of its finality, cremation as a method of disposal of the dead is carefully regulated.[6] Cremation is the ultimate method of concealing a crime; on the other hand, it has certain advantages over burial as a legal method of disposal of the dead.[7] Moreover, the Brodrick Committee has pointed out that the modern operation of the Coroners' (and Fiscals') system has greatly reduced the opportunity for the concealment of homicide. Any regulations must, therefore, be so designed as to permit without undue hindrance a process which is in the public interest and, yet, at the same time, safeguard that interest in respect of criminality. The Cremation Act 1902 and the regulations made thereunder in 1930, 1952 and 1965 constitute the law in both England and Wales and in Scotland although the regulations are currently subject to governmental review. The process of cremation can be described conveniently in relation to the Forms which must be completed:

Form A. This constitutes an application for cremation which sets out, *inter alia*, the relationship of the applicant to the deceased, the wishes of the next-of-kin, the details of the death, an affirmation to the effect that there is no reason to suspect foul play or the need for further examination of the body and a statement concerning those who have

---

[6] In contrast to the surprisingly lax attitude to burial, the Cremation Regulations 1930 prohibit the burning of human remains in any place other than a recognized crematorium.

[7] The early objections to cremation voiced by the Roman Catholic Church have now been withdrawn in Great Britain and, while burial is still the preferred method of disposal, priests may conduct services at the crematorium. Some 11 000 Roman Catholics are cremated annually in Great Britain.

been in medical charge of the deceased. The application must be countersigned by a householder who knows the applicant.

Form B. This is the certificate of the medical attendant who has 18 questions to answer relating to the mode and cause of death, the scope of his attendance on the deceased, operative treatment and nursing care in the recent past. The doctor must certify that he has no reason to suppose that further inquiry is needed and he must also affirm that he is not related to nor has he a pecuniary interest in the death of the deceased.

Despite its comprehensiveness, Form B does not replace the medical certificate as to cause of death; the latter is essential for the registration of the death whereas Form B is related only to the process of cremation.

Form C. This is a confirmatory medical certificate which must be completed by a practitioner of at least 5 years standing who has no family or professional relationship with the practitioner signing Form B. He must state whether he has seen the body and whether he has made a careful external examination. There is no requirement for him to have done so but a negative answer might well result in the rejection of the certificate. There is provision for stating whether or not he has performed a post-mortem dissection. There are 5 questions relating to his having questioned various categories of person as to the circumstances of the death; there must be a positive reply to at least one of these. Finally, the certifying doctor must affirm that he is satisfied as to the cause of death.

Form F. This form is completed by the Medical Referee (a medical officer nominated by the Crematorium and approved by the Home Secretary or Secretary of State). The signature confirms that the Referee is satisfied that the regulations have been complied with, that the cause of death has been established and that no further examination is required; cremation of the remains is authorized.

The Cremation Act gives very wide powers to the Referee. He can complete Form C himself; he can withhold Form F without giving reasons and can make any inquiries he thinks fit; he can report the case to the Coroner or Procurator Fiscal; he can also invite a pathologist to perform a post-mortem examination or make such an examination himself. In the last circumstance, the person performing the autopsy completes *Form D* which will then replace Form C and will also override Form B. In the event that the case has been reported to the Coroner or Procurator Fiscal, the certificate of those officials, *Form E*, replaces Forms B and C and clears the case for the Medical Referee. Form E may be issued before the conclusion of the medico-legal enquiries but, in England and Wales, it does not state the cause of death; it does not replace either the Coroner's death certificate (Pink Form B) or Certificate after

Inquest. The version of Form E provided by the Procurator Fiscal does indicate the cause of death but, notwithstanding, a normal certificate must be provided by his medical adviser.

It is re-emphasized that the discretionary powers under which a body can be buried without certification as to the cause of death and prior to registration of the death do not apply to cremation.

THE ANATOMY ACTS 1832 AND 1871

These Acts govern the retention of a body for the purposes of use in an Anatomy School. The Human Tissue Act 1961 extends the scope of, but does not repeal, the Anatomy Acts; the 1961 Act raises issues of far more general application and is discussed in detail in Chapter 12.

In general, the disposal of a body through the dissecting room is subject to the dissection being conducted only by a licensed person in a notified establishment. The person in lawful possession of the body can give permission for the examination provided no relative has objected; in this instance, the 'person in lawful possession' means the hospital authority or the management of a similar institution in which the death occurs.[8] The body cannot be disposed of without a valid certificate of the cause of death and it must not be removed for anatomical dissection until 48 hours after life has been pronounced extinct. The receipt of the body must be acknowledged within 24 hours by supplying the local Inspector of Anatomy with details as to the source of the body and of the date and place of death, the sex and, if known, the name of the deceased; the certificate of cause of death is attached to these details. The body must be disposed of by interment in a proper cemetery or by cremation within 2 years and the Inspector must be so informed.[9]

One medico-legal distinction between the Anatomy Acts and Section 1(1) of the Human Tissue Act is that, whereas the former is specially designed for the provision of teaching material to medical schools, dissections under the latter must be carried out by registered medical practitioners. It would seem that, even if a person has expressly bequeathed his body to a medical school, the Inspector of Anatomy would not be able to proceed in the event of objection from a near relative.[10]

---

[8] R. v. Feist [1858] Dears & Bell 590. It has been pointed out that this very old case, referring to conditions in a nineteenth century workhouse, is not immediately relevant to the present day; nevertheless, it is frequently quoted (*see* Chapter 12 for further discussion).

[9] The sole purpose of the 1871 Act was to allow flexibility in the provision of such information.

[10] It is probable that public opinion would support this; there is an emotional difference between study in the dissecting room and the use of cadaver organs to save other lives (*see* Chapter 12).

THE DISPOSAL OF STILLBIRTHS

A stillbirth is defined as a child which issued from the mother after the 28th week of pregnancy and which did not at any time after being expelled from its mother breathe or show any sign of life.

The pathological distinction between stillbirth and perinatal death is discussed in Chapter 19. We are concerned here only with the regulations surrounding the actual disposal of the body; these are governed in England and Wales by the Births and Deaths Registration Act 1953 (s. 11) and in Scotland by the Registration of Births, Deaths and Marriages (Scotland) Act 1965 (s. 21). The process is essentially similar under both statutes.

The body of a stillbirth cannot be disposed of without a valid medical certificate of stillbirth which, throughout Great Britain, can be completed by virtue of the certifier either having been present at the birth or having examined the body following information as to its birth. The certificate may be signed by a registered medical practitioner or by a certified midwife. In the event of the Registrar being in any doubt as to whether the child was born alive, the case must be reported to the Coroner or to the Procurator Fiscal; in practice, many cases are reported direct when the certifier thinks it necessary. There is provision under both jurisdictions for a declaration by the informant that the child was stillborn when, for some reason, there is no professional person available to provide a certificate.

A stillbirth is, technically, a birth rather than a death. The informant therefore has 42 days in England and 21 days in Scotland to register the event. Stillbirths do not come within the compass of the Human Tissue Act and, in the present state of the law, must be buried or cremated. There is no requirement for the superintendent of the place of disposal to notify the Registrar of disposal of a stillbirth – as there is in the ordinary case of death – unless the body has been buried without a certificate of registration. It scarcely needs mention that, if a child has survived birth for even a fleeting time, certificates both of birth and death are required – the normal medical certificate as to cause of death is then used.

THE DISPOSAL OF FETUSES

There is no law as to the disposal of a fetus which is expelled from the mother dead before the 28th week of pregnancy. There is no requirement for registration and the method of disposal must simply comply with current standards of proper public behaviour and with the various Public Health Acts. Fetuses of this type are not subject to the restrictions of the Human Tissue Act and may be retained for scientific purposes, but there are serious ethical problems. The Advisory Group[11] have proposed that fetuses weighing less than 300 g are previable and may be suitable for research purposes. The same group, in attempting to distinguish between the viable and nonviable, has proposed that the dividing line should be at 20 weeks gestation when the fetus is obtained as a result of hysterotomy. The problem is bound up with the working of the Abortion Act 1967. The original Abortion (Amendment) Bill proposed that experiments of any kind on a human fetus or fetal material which had become available as a result of the termination of a pregnancy would only be legal if carried out on a dead fetus weighing less than 300 g. This Bill never reached the Statute Book and the Bill currently under discussion contains no similar clauses.

DISPOSAL OF BODIES RETURNED FROM OUTSIDE UNITED KINGDOM

Although the procedure is not quite uniform – any differences depending upon the actual country in which death has occurred – it follows generally similar principles.

The death is certified according to the regulations of the country in which it occurred and, usually, the death certificate is accompanied by further certificates as to freedom from infection and to embalming. The papers are notarized by the Consul who may also add his own certificate.

In the event of burial in the United Kingdom, all the documents are referred to the Registrar of the area where the body is to be interred; the Registrar then issues a Certificate of Non-liability. If the next-of-kin wish for a cremation, an application must be made on Form A which is sent, with all the relevant documents, to the Home Office or the Home and Health Department whence a licence to cremate is provided. The matter is then passed to the local Registrar of Cremations who will, again, issue a Certificate of Non-liability.

---

[11] Department of Health and Social Security (1972) *Use of Fetuses and Fetal Material for Research*. London, HMSO.

Chapter 6

The Spread of Communicable Disease:
Some Aspects of Public Health

EPIDEMIOLOGY is the study of the determinants and mode of distribution of disease. All natural disease is to some extent subject to outside influences but communicable disease is that type which can most obviously be controlled by legislation.[1] Community health is, therefore, a part of the general spectrum of forensic medicine and virtually all the early university chairs in Forensic Medicine combined Medical Jurisprudence with Public Health; at the present time, certain categories of death reportable to the Fiscal (Appendix D) are there by virtue of their importance to the health of the community. Actions for tort or delict may well be based on transference of preventable disease, an aspect of forensic medicine which has come to greater prominence with the availability of cheap, world-wide travel facilities. Some understanding of the spread of communicable disease should be available to the lawyer concerned with medical aspects of the law; it is the purpose of this chapter to present this in outline.

ORGANISMS RESPONSIBLE FOR INFECTIOUS DISEASE

Organisms capable of causing human disease vary greatly in habit and in size. Ascending from the smallest, the groups which are of greatest concern include the following.

The Viruses
The characteristic of these minute organisms is that they are incapable of a free existence and must live as true parasites within living tissue. As a corollary, viruses can only be grown in the laboratory in cultures of live tissues. Examples of virus disease include smallpox and measles.[2]

---

[1] Examples of attempted legal control of noncommunicable diseases include that of disease associated with cigarette smoking, through regulations as to packaging and advertising.

[2] Slightly larger viruses, known as *Rickettsiae*, cause typhus fever.

The Bacteria

These unicellular organisms of great simplicity are omnipresent. Those that cause disease are described as *pathogenic* and those which produce a purulent reaction are *pyogenic*. Bacteria come in various shapes – the round *cocci* which, *inter alia,* cause sore throats, boils and pneumonia; the *bacilli*, which include the organisms responsible for typhoid fever and tuberculosis; the curved *vibrios*, which are responsible for cholera; and the coiled *spirochaetes*, which cause several diseases additional to syphilis. The *anaerobic bacteria* form a group which is of special importance in forensic medicine; they will only grow in the relative absence of oxygen and proliferate particularly well in wounds, causing tetanus and gas gangrene.

The Protozoa

These are relatively sophisticated unicellular organisms which cause many diseases of world-wide economic importance including malaria, sleeping sickness and the bowel disease amoebic dysentery.

The Fungi

These are branching organisms of simple type which are increasing in importance as they may flourish in severely ill patients, particularly those on antibacterial treatment.

The Helminths or Worms

These take many forms and vary from those which are scarcely visible to the naked eye to others which are several metres long. They are often of considerable medico-legal importance due to their close association with food and its preparation. Many have no more than a nuisance value but others – for example, one tapeworm of dogs which causes hydatid disease in man – are potentially dangerous to life; the pork tapeworm may cause an intractable form of epilepsy.

THE SPREAD OF COMMUNICABLE DISEASE *(Fig.* 9)

If a disease is to spread, the responsible organism must be passed from person to person. The simplest way in which this can be done is by *direct contact* in which case the organism must be either in the skin or in secretions which are passed directly from person to person. The most obvious examples of such contact diseases are those which are sexually transmitted and the infectious skin diseases.

Otherwise, human-to-human transfer of disease depends upon excretion of organisms and this can take several routes – particularly via the sputum, the urine and the faeces. Sputum does not mean necessarily the tangible mass of phlegm seen in sufferers from bronchitis but rather the invisible spray known as *droplets* which is spread each time a person

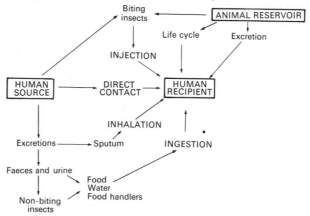

Fig. 9. Schematic representation of the spread of disease due to microbiological organisms.

coughs; in so far as this can be directly inhaled by others, droplet infection is a matter of *proximity contact* and is fostered by conditions of overcrowding with inadequate ventilation. Urine is a vehicle for surprisingly few communicable diseases – typhoid fever is of the most immediate concern but, on a world-wide basis, the condition of schistosomiasis, due to a worm, is a far more important source of morbidity. By contrast, the faeces may contain large numbers of pathogenic organisms – not only those associated with the many infectious bowel diseases but also those which become pathogenic when displaced – for example, when contaminating wounds.

There can be several results when an excretion is passed. It may remain on the hands and any organisms can then be transferred to the utensils or food of others – the role of the food handler in the transmission of disease is, therefore, of great importance. Alternatively, the excretion may be passed into the water supply – either localized, as into a well, or generalized, as into a stream or river; sporadic disease in the local community or explosive epidemic disease involving a whole distant community may then arise. It is probable that the major contribution of the public authorities to the health of the people depends upon the provision of an efficient system of sewage disposal. Otherwise, the excretions may dry and become incorporated in dust; control of those pathogenic organisms which are resistant to desiccation is a major problem within institutions – it is the standard route of cross-infection of patients in hospital. Finally, infected excretions may be transferred to foodstuffs by insects, of which the house fly is the most important.

In many communicable diseases, the responsible organism is not excreted but remains in the blood. Transfer from case to case must then depend upon blood-sucking insects[3] – the importance of *insect-borne disease* is vast in the world as a whole but slight in temperate climates. Pandemics of arthropod-borne disease, amongst which are included yellow fever, typhus, plague, malaria and sleeping sickness, have changed the course of history, and it is only an efficient public health system which prevents their recurrence or limits their effects. Certain arthropod-borne diseases are essentially human in distribution – louse-borne typhus fever, which is associated with overcrowding in conditions of poor personal hygiene, is the outstanding example. Others are, however, dependent upon an animal reservoir – the most historic example being the rat as a source of bubonic plague. Human diseases which are animal-dependent are known as *zoonoses*. Zoonoses may also persist by means of a direct association between man and animals. Some are industrial in nature – for example, the infective jaundice of sewer workers or hydatid worm disease of sheep farmers – but the most urgent contact zoonosis is undoubtedly rabies – a disease of particular appositeness to the theme of this chapter because its control in Great Britain rests almost entirely on legislation.

THE CONTROL OF COMMUNICABLE DISEASE

The general methods for control of infectious disease are clear from the foregoing paragraphs. Firstly, one can attempt to eliminate – or, in human instances, isolate – the source of infection; secondly, knowing the mode of spread, an effort can be made to break the chain at some vital point; thirdly, one can use artificial means to promote immunity in the population.

Statutory powers to achieve these ends are contained in the many Acts and regulations pertaining to public health; the main United Kingdom legislation is contained in the Public Health Act 1936 and the Public Health (Scotland) Acts 1897–1945. Many of the powers are wide and far beyond the ambit of the individual – they include adequate supervision of housing, the control of sewage, drainage and water supplies, the whole range of inspection and control of foodstuffs, the control of imported biological goods likely to be infected such as animal bones or skins and the quarantining of animals.

Much current attention is focused on what are described as exotic diseases – that is, diseases which are imported from abroad. They may be of little or no public concern – if a visitor becomes ill with malaria it will

---

[3] Used in a colloquial sense. Ticks and mites which also transmit disease are not, zoologically speaking, insects; a better general term is 'arthropod-borne disease'.

not be communicable in Britain because the insect carrier, the anopheles mosquito, has been so reduced in number as to be ineffective, this, in turn, being the result of efficient public health measures;[4] they may be of relatively severe consequence – a person with typhoid fever, for instance, could infect a number of contacts before discovery; on the other end of the scale, they could be catastrophic – a classical example would be the importation of yellow fever into an area where the mosquito vector was present in sufficient numbers to start an epidemic. Even in parts of Britain it would be a matter of very great concern if a human or animal case of plague were introduced into an area where rats and fleas abounded.[5] The control of exotic disease is largely a matter of port health control; while the control of shipping has been practised successfully for very many years, the problems are accentuated by the widespread use of air travel – aircraft can transport infected insects, persons incubating disease will reach their destination before becoming overtly ill and there is a rare possibility of infecting a high proportion of the passengers through one ill-prepared meal obtained *en route*.[6] Special regulations[7] are applied to aircraft and, in those parts of the world at special risk, control is exercised on an international basis.[8] Other contact zoonoses are controlled either by prohibition of imported animals or compulsory quarantining – measures which are available only to an island State.

These major concerns are of little interest in the present context. Of greater immediate importance is the fact that certain control measures impinge upon the rights of the individual and also on the doctor/patient relationship.

Notification of Infectious Disease

As indicated above, human infectious disease can be effectively controlled by isolation of infective cases; moreover, the original source of a

---

[4] Most exotic diseases are specifically treatable and diagnosable in the laboratory. It has been suggested that it would be negligent to fail to take the necessary steps to make a diagnosis despite the infrequency of the disease and many practitioners and hospitals adopt a routine in questioning patients as to recent travel. The problem is discussed by Stamm W. P. (1969) Medico-legal aspects of exotic diseases, in: Camps F. E. (ed.) *Recent Advances in Forensic Pathology*, London, Churchill. Extensive damages have, in fact, been awarded for just such a mistake (*see Br. Med. J.* (1975) **4**, 474)

[5] All ships must be in possession of either a Deratting Certificate or a Deratting Exemption Certificate; certificates are valid for six months (International Health Regulations (1969), Art. 54).

[6] See *Br. Med. J.* (1973) Vibrio food-poisoning on an aeroplane. **4**, 117.

[7] Public Health (Aircraft) Regulations 1966; Public Health (Aircraft) (Scotland) Amendment Regulations 1974.

[8] The International Health Regulations (1969, amended 1973), drawn up by the World Health Organization, cover cholera, plague, smallpox and yellow fever.

disease can often be traced through a knowledge of those thereby infected. Both these public health control measures depend primarily upon notification of cases.

A number of diseases are statutorily notifiable[9] to the local Community Physician (or Specialist in Community Medicine) by the practitioner in charge of the case (Appendix H). The general list of some 29 diseases is not exhaustive as the Area Health Authority or Board has the power to add to the printed list when local conditions indicate the need or desirability.[10] There can, therefore, be no question of a binding confidentiality between doctor and patient in this respect (*see* Chapter 30); this statutory type of breach of confidence illustrates two important points of principle in medical ethics – firstly, the 'need to know' quality of the person to whom confidential information is disclosed and, secondly, the precedent which is thus established of the overriding importance of the public need when it is in conflict with that of the individual.

But statutory powers go deeper than this. The two major Acts make it an offence for a person knowing he has an infectious disease to expose himself to others or to carry on with his occupation. In the absence of consent, a Justice or a Sheriff may order a healthy person from a building in which he is considered at risk, he can make a hospital order and he can, further, require a person to be detained in hospital if housing conditions are unlikely to be satisfactory upon discharge; clearly, however, such an order may be difficult to enforce. Perhaps the quickest preventive measure lies in the authority to order a medical examination of a person thought to be suffering from or to be the carrier of a notifiable disease[11] if it is considered to be in the interest of the person himself, his family or the public in general. Control of the carrier state is most important. In this condition, a person feels perfectly well, yet is excreting pathogenic organisms – the state may be a hangover from an overt attack of the disease but, equally commonly, the carrier will never have been aware of being infected. He may, therefore, resent compulsory medical treatment, but the devastation which could be caused by a typhoid carrier who persistently polluted a water supply or who was engaged in food handling of any sort needs no emphasis. Carrier states are notoriously difficult to treat and, in the event of failure, the Local Health Authorities are empowered to arrange a person's occupation so that he will be a minimal danger to the public.

---

[9] Under the Public Health (Infectious Diseases) Regulations 1968.

[10] National Health Service (Scotland) Act 1972, s. 53; Health Services and Public Health Act 1968, s. 52 (which does not apply in Scotland).

[11] Public Health Act 1961, s. 38; Health Services and Public Health Act 1968, s. 54 and s. 72. Section 53 of the latter Act amends s. 38 of the former.

Immunization

There can be no doubt as to the efficacy of mass immunization as a method of controlling infectious disease. At the same time, no immunity procedure is entirely without risk and the controversy which has recently received parliamentary attention[12] centres on the right balance being struck between, on the one hand, the effectiveness and the risk of vaccination against a particular disease and, on the other, the chance of contracting that disease and its short- and long-term effects both on the individual and on the public. A good illustration is provided by smallpox. This very severe disease could have wreaked havoc if introduced into Britain and, consequently, preventive vaccination was at one time compulsory; the procedure had, however, a recognizable mortality and morbidity of its own. By the middle of this century, other control measures had become so effective that the risks of vaccination were considered to outweigh the dangers of contracting the disease and compulsion was abandoned; there has been no increase in the indigenous disease as a result. Nevertheless, a voluntary immunization programme is still an essential part of the control of many infectious diseases; within the United Kingdom, immunization is recommended as a routine against diphtheria, tetanus, whooping cough, poliomyelitis, measles, tuberculosis and German measles.[13]

Immunization is of two types – active and passive. In the former, the body is presented with either an attenuated (made safe) live strain of the wild pathogenic organism or with a killed form. This vaccine acts as an antigen which stimulates the formation of antibodies which are then ready to repel the antigen when it presents in its natural disease-provoking form; antibody production can be boosted by repeated doses of the vaccine and is, therefore, long lasting. In passive immunity, the body is supplied with preformed antibodies; the action is short and is designed only to combat the actual or supposed entry of a dangerous organism before it can take hold in the body.

Active immunization – that type of inoculation or vaccination which is performed in childhood or before travelling to an infected area – has a number of hazards, many of which are now only theoretical. The recipient may have a completely unforeseeable idiosyncrasy to the injection and may sustain a severe allergic shock. More commonly, the organisms in the vaccine may reactivate an abnormal condition present in the recipient – classic examples are skin eczema following vaccination against smallpox and convulsions after whooping cough immunization.

---

[12] *See*, for example, the Parliamentary Notes in *Br. Med. J.* (1974) **1**, 293 and **2**, 395.

[13] Standing Medical Advisory Committee for the Central Health Services Council (1972) *Immunization against Infectious Diseases*. London, Department of Health and Social Security.

The vaccine may cause a modified form of the disease it is intended to prevent – some children, for instance, go through what is apparently a mild attack of measles following inoculation. In the case of live virus vaccines, the growth may not be pure – yellow fever vaccines which are grown on eggs may contain viruses which have been infecting the eggs themselves. This is of little consequence – it is virtually eliminated in modern manufacture. Of far greater importance is the possibility that antibodies may be provoked not only to the desired antigen but also to the medium in which it is prepared. Thus, the original form of anti-rabies vaccine is grown in nervous tissue; when it is used, there is a possibility that anti-nervous tissue antibody will be formed in the recipient with disastrous results within his own brain.[14] Perhaps the major danger, however, lies in the potential effects on pregnancy. This seems to be a hazard almost specific to those vaccines composed of living viruses; these may cause abortion or, more seriously, may damage the growing fetus if given within the first three months of intra-uterine life. This last possibility is particularly evident in immunization against German measles, a fairly predictable chance in that the only purpose in immunizing is to prevent a true attack of the disease during childbearing. The likelihood of damage to the fetus is such that a guarantee of contraception for at least 60 days is generally required of a woman before she can be immunized against German measles.

Formidable though this list may seem, the risks of immunization must be contrasted with the dangers of inadequate control of the relevant diseases; looked at in this way, the hazards as a whole are very slight indeed.[15] Nevertheless, occasional individual tragedies do occur and, in such cases, the possibility of an action for medical negligence must arise. The whole concept of professional negligence is discussed in Chapter 30. For the present, it is sufficient to say that negligence would only be shown if the doctor had failed to follow accepted practice – for example, it might be suggested as being negligent to immunize against whooping cough a child who was known to suffer from convulsions or to continue with a course of vaccination when the first dose had precipitated a convulsion. Even this might be arguable[16] and there is no doubt

---

[14] Research has now developed methods for preparing the vaccine in duck embryos (which is currently available) or in human diploid cells (which may be generally available soon).

[15] Although, clearly, the balance need not necessarily be the same. Diphtheria immunization is, for example, virtually without risk while the disease is extremely dangerous; vaccination against cholera is again without risk but its protective value is very slight; smallpox vaccination has a hazard, although slight, but the chances of contracting the disease in Britain are negligible.

[16] The hazard of whooping cough is greater than that associated with immunization (*Br. Med. J.* (1975.) **3**, 687). Even so, these problems are not always easily solved (*see* Vaccine damage, *Lancet* (1977) **1**, 645).

that the vast majority of postvaccination complications would not constitute a tort or delict. There is a strong lobby to the effect that such cases should attract a form of 'no-fault' compensation, a view which would seem to be most commendable.

Persons travelling abroad present a special problem. There are two types of active immunization involved – those procedures undertaken for the obvious benefit of the individual, of which immunization against poliomyelitis and typhoid fever are good examples, and those which are required by the Health Authorities of the Countries to be visited before entry is permitted. The former category poses little difficulty. If a woman is pregnant or has an infant child and wishes to travel to an area in which an immunity state would be desirable but, at the same time, involves an injection which might present an above-average risk to her fetus or child, she should be warned of the dangers both of immunization and of nonimmune travel and should be given appropriate advice including that of postponing her travel. The choice is then up to the patient within the terms of 'informed consent' as discussed in Chapter 30. Travel to countries which insist on certain vaccinations poses difficulty if it is necessary during high-risk periods. In certain circumstances – such as travel from an area known to be free of a particular disease – a certificate giving a valid reason for nonvaccination may be acceptable; in other cases – for example, in travel from an area where yellow fever actually exists to one where it could be introduced – a period of quarantine on arrival may have to be accepted. In practice, a real problem probably exists only in regard to a pregnant woman travelling to an area where smallpox presents as a serious disease hazard; fears of the effects of other relevant viral vaccines, in particular yellow fever, on pregnancy have probably been exaggerated.

The dangers of passive immunization are of a different type but are very real. Antibodies are produced in the blood of animals. Therefore, when an antibody is injected, foreign antigens derived from the animal are also introduced and an immune reaction of varying severity may be established. This is of wide forensic importance due to the frequency with which anti-tetanus antibodies are required to be given following wounds of all sorts. In many cases it might be at least arguable that the dangers of passive immunization were greater than the likelihood of contracting tetanus; but in the event of misjudgment it would be difficult to defend an accusation of negligence in the light of previous decisions.[17] Such dilemmas should, in practice, become very much rarer if the official policy of active immunization against tetanus in childhood

---

[17] For example, Coles v. Reading and District Hospital Management Committee and Another, (1963) 107 S.J.115. See also the case discussion in Taylor J. L. (1970) *The Doctor and the Law*. London, Pitman, p. 113. (There were additional features in both cases.)

is widely followed – the correct procedure in a wounded person who has been previously immunized is to boost the active immunity with a fresh dose of antigen; this carries no risk of an untoward reaction.

Chapter 7

Sudden Natural Death

SOME 80 per cent of the cases coming to autopsy at the hands of the English Coroner's pathologist are found to have died from natural causes. Even in Scotland, where a high proportion of such deaths are certified without dissection, the majority of medico-legal post-mortem examinations fail to disclose anything unnatural. The proportions differ very much from city to city and, particularly, as between city and rural areas; in Edinburgh, in 1974, a diagnosis of death due to natural disease was made in just over half of the Fiscal's cases which were examined internally. These cases therefore form an essential part of forensic medicine both in their own right and also because it is impossible to appreciate properly the medico-legal interactions between trauma – particularly that due to accidents – and incapacitating disease without a knowledge of the mechanisms underlying the latter.

For present purposes, 'sudden death' is defined as unexpected death following so rapidly from the onset of symptoms that the cause of death could not be certified with confidence by a medical practitioner unfamiliar with the patient – the type of death which is likely to disguise a 'secret homicide'. Sudden death of this sort is almost entirely a matter of disease of the cardiovascular system and will be discussed as such, firstly, in relation to the immediateness of death and, secondly, as to the age of those affected.

In order of increasing suddenness, death may be due to haemorrhage from vessels, to peripheral blockage of vessels or to inhibition of the heart's action (*Fig. 10*).

The mode of death due to *haemorrhage* depends on two factors – on the size of the vessel which bleeds and, when internal, on the ability of the cavity involved to accommodate the blood shed and of the contained organs to continue to function normally. The effects of bleeding from a small vessel should be less than from a larger one but, given the same size of small vessels in the cranial cavity and in the abdomen, the effect in the latter may be slight while, in the former, it may be lethal because of the concurrent effects on brain function.

The effect of *blockage of a peripheral vessel* is determined by the nature of the part deprived of blood, by the size of the vessel blocked and by the method of occlusion. The primary effect on an organ or area is to deprive it of oxygen; the secondary effect on the body as a whole

Fig. 10.   Factors involved in sudden natural death related to the cardiovascular system.

depends on the function of that organ. Thus, a man can well survive a portion of his spleen being deprived of blood, but closure of a vessel supplying the respiratory centre in the brain will cause immediate death. The effect of the size of vessel is obvious – one might be able to withstand the sudden elimination of a lobule of lung but sudden obstruction of a main pulmonary artery would be almost inevitably fatal. Three main processes lead to blockage of an artery. The slowest in effect is restriction of the lumen due to thickening of the wall. This process is one for which the body is often able to compensate by the development of new vessels – known as a collateral circulation. An urgent need for extra oxygen in the organ supplied by the vessel or a very rapid exacerbation of the restrictive thickening may result in sudden incompetence; the subject is discussed later in the context of coronary disease. A faster method of preventing blood flow is provided by local *thrombosis* – that is, abnormal clotting of the blood within a vessel.[1] Generalized intravascular coagulation occurs in surgical shock and in other conditions but the common presentation considered here is that of a single clot forming round a localized area of damage to the vessel lining. Clots of this type may arise in arteries or in veins. Unless a vitally important vessel, such as a cerebral artery, is involved, the main danger of thrombosis is to provoke a third and most rapid form of blockage which is known as *embolism*. In this condition, fragments of preformed clot break off. If this occurs in an artery, the particles are forced into vessels of decreasing size until they lodge and cause a sudden deprivation of blood to the parts beyond, the process being known as *infarction* – death of a particularly sudden type will occur if a cerebral vessel is embolized. If the clot which disintegrates is located in a vein, it passes to the right side of the heart where, if large enough, it will occlude the main pulmonary artery but, if

---

[1] The important word is 'abnormal'. Thrombosis is a 'normal' part of the process of limiting haemorrhage from a vessel, the wall of which is broken (*see* Chapter 1).

smaller, will pass into the lung until it can go no further; this is the condition of pulmonary embolism which is such a common cause of death in persons whose blood tends to clot in the leg veins as a result of enforced immobilization in bed.[2]

Inhibition of the heart action may result from any of these processes. The heart itself may perforate, in which case the blood held within the pericardial sac inhibits the normal heart action mechanically – this condition is known as *cardiac tamponade*. There can be blockage of the coronary vessels, which supply the heart muscle, either by thickening of the walls, by thrombosis or by embolism. The feature distinguishing such occlusions from those occurring in peripheral vessels of comparable size is that sudden deprivation of oxygen in even a small area of heart tissue which is vital to its rhythmic function inhibits its action; the tissues throughout the body are immediately deprived of oxygen. Additionally, any disease of the heart muscle – whether it be inflammatory, toxic or simply due to excessive loads imposed – may, at a particular moment in time, reach just sufficient severity to stop the heart beat and to cause sudden death. Finally, inhibition of the heart through abnormal stimulation of its regulatory nerves must be mentioned; the concept of vagal inhibition of the heart, which was introduced on p. 16, is referred to at many points in this text.

These various processes are likely to present at different times in life; the underlying causes of sudden death must be related to age if their forensic significance is to be appreciated.

SUDDEN DEATH IN INFANCY AND EARLY CHILDHOOD

Death in this age group is discussed in detail in Chapter 20. Many sudden infant deaths are associated with congenital cardiovascular malformations; the presence of these will have been known previously and death will not be unexpected – they are, therefore, beyond the definition of sudden death which is adopted here. This age group, in which the important group of so-called 'cot deaths' occurs, provides the exception to the rule that sudden unexpected death is almost entirely associated with the cardiovascular system. Although it has been suggested that some 'cot deaths' may be due to primary disease of the heart, this is plainly not the common cause. A proportion of these baffling cases may be due to fulminating viral infection and, certainly, many sudden deaths in

---

[2] Strictly speaking, this type of embolism should be referred to as thrombotic embolism. Embolism by itself is a generic term for the process whereby vessels are blocked by particles of any sort. Thus we have conditions such as fat embolism, air embolism or embolism due to particles injected into veins, etc., but the origins in each instance are quite distinct.

early childhood do result unequivocally from infection – either of the brain (meningitis), the lungs (pneumonia) or the bowel (enteritis); such disease states can progress with very great speed and it is seldom that allegations of negligence on the part of the doctor – which are not uncommon in the emotional atmosphere surrounding the death of a child – can be shown to have any substance.

SUDDEN NATURAL DEATH IN THE YOUNG ADULT

Bleeding in the form of *subarachnoid haemorrhage* is the most important process under this heading; since subarachnoid haemorrhage is also a frequent result of injury (Chapter 11), the cases are of particular medico-legal importance.

The common form of naturally-occurring subarachnoid haemorrhage is of congenital origin. As a result of malformation of the muscle wall, balloon-like swellings – known as 'berry aneurysms' – form in the cerebral arteries at the base of the brain, most frequently at one of the comparatively abrupt, geometric junctions in the area. The wall of the aneurysm is thin and is liable to rupture – particularly when the blood pressure is raised. The resulting pressure effect of the extruded blood is particularly concentrated on the vital centres of the brain and can cause sudden unexpected death. Generally, it is the death rather than the symptoms which is sudden – the fairly slow leak of blood may cause a headache for several hours but such premonitory signs are often overlooked.

The distinction between natural disease and injury as a cause of subarachnoid haemorrhage is not always a simple matter. Trauma may rupture even normal cerebral vessels; although there is some difference of opinion among various researchers as to the true cause-and-effect relationship, it is logical to suppose that abnormally weak arteries could be damaged by abnormally slight force and, should the two present together, the precise allocation of responsibility for death might be difficult to make.

The inclusion of the condition in this section does not imply that it does not also occur in older age groups; it most certainly does and, in fact, modern studies draw attention to the increasing average age at which spontaneous subarachnoid bleeding occurs.[3] The incidence in older persons is swelled by rupture occurring in cerebral vessels damaged by the degenerative disease, atheroma. Death seems to be surprisingly often associated with straining on the lavatory pan.

Intracerebral haemorrhage is rare in young persons. When it occurs, it

---

[3] A very useful recent review of the condition is given by Crompton M. R. (1975) The Coroner's cerebral aneurysm: a changing animal. *J. Forensic Sci. Soc.* **15**, 57.

is likely to be due to bleeding into a tumour of the brain which, in turn, may be derived from a primary tumour of the genital system. Haemorrhage into tumours is a more common cause of death in elderly persons, secondary deposits from the stomach and lung being the most common findings.

Acute haemorrhagic deaths in young women may result from bleeding due to growth of the fetus in an abnormal position – the so called *ectopic gestation* which results from the ovum 'losing its way' or being 'held up' in its passage to the cavity of the uterus. Such catastrophes have been largely eliminated by modern antenatal care but it is still probably true that, from the medico-legal point of view, sudden death in a young woman should be suspected of being associated with pregnancy until proved otherwise.

Apart from such relatively obvious causes, the diagnosis of natural sudden death in young persons may present considerable difficulty. In some instances, the deaths appear to be due to one of a group of primary diseases of the heart muscle collectively known as cardiomyopathies. Occasionally, a toxic origin may be shown for such diseases – alcoholic cardiomyopathy is a good example; more often there is an abnormality of growth, one side of the heart being greatly enlarged. This condition is known as asymmetric hypertrophic cardiomyopathy (*Plate* 2b); one possible mechanism of death is that an enlarged left ventricle occludes the outlets into the great vessels but, alternatively, the increasing bulk of muscle may outstrip the available capacity of the coronary arteries, a concept which is discussed further below. On other occasions, 'inflammation' of the heart muscle – so-called 'myocarditis' – has been invoked as a cause of obscure deaths. The condition may be due to true infection, usually of viral type, to an allergic reaction or to disorders of the endocrine system – e.g. overactivity of the thyroid gland. All these conditions have it in common that they can be diagnosed only by a microscopic examination and are characterized by collections of white blood cells in the muscle of the heart. While such a finding may satisfy some observers, others are sceptical of their true significance; the distinction between findings which are causative of death and those which are purely incidental is discussed in Chapter 10.

The mention of scepticism draws attention to 'status lymphaticus' as a cause of sudden death in young persons. This diagnosis, based on the finding of an enlarged thymus gland, often with associated enlargement of the lymph nodes, is an example of a conclusion forced by the absence of recognized fatal pathology despite a thorough post-mortem examination. It has long been discarded, but its memory is a monument to the fact that sudden death in young adults may be as obscure as are cot deaths in infants; the resultant diagnoses may have to be based on equally tenuous findings.

SUDDEN NATURAL DEATH IN LATER YEARS

Sudden death in late middle age is dominated by degenerative changes in the vessels of the cardiovascular system.

The main degenerative change is atheroma, in which the wall of the vessel is replaced by fatty material which, breaking down, leaves a greatly weakened structure. In the absence of surrounding support, the tendency is for such a diseased vessel to dilate – an aneurysm is formed. The commonest site is in the abdominal aorta – rupture is progressive but death is eventually very rapid as the blood intended for the lower limbs is poured into the abdominal cavity. Almost instantaneous death may result from a rather similar process – known as 'dissecting aneurysm' because the blood passes within the wall of the vessel – which occurs predominantly at the origin of the aorta; the blood may sometimes be forced back into the pericardial sac and sudden death is due to cardiac tamponade. Deep vessels in the brain may be weakened by atheroma and, in the event of rupture, will cause intracerebral haemorrhage while massive haemorrhage into the stomach may follow erosion of a vessel at the base of an ulcer in the stomach or duodenum; such deaths are seldom entirely unheralded.

Rupture of vessels is more likely in the present of a raised blood pressure – hypertensive heart disease is a potent cause of sudden death in this age group. Apart from the peripheral catastrophes which may occur, the heart itself, which enlarges in order to perform more work, may 'outgrow its strength' and suddenly fail, a mechanism which is discussed below. High blood pressure is not, however, the only cause of steady enlargement of the heart; disease of the heart valves, in particular narrowing or stenosis of the aortic valve, may provoke the same effects.

CORONARY HEART DISEASE

The subject of coronary heart disease has been left till last because its ability to kill is almost all-embracing in its age span – deaths from this cause have been reported in young men aged 19 and, indeed, the younger the subject, the more likely is the first 'coronary attack' to be fatal. Death from coronary heart disease is, however, most frequent in the period of life from age 45 onwards and, from that point, becomes the commonest single cause of death in most industrialized countries. It is by far the most important cause of sudden death and is almost the only cause of instantaneous death. Inevitably, a high proportion of such cases are reported to the Coroner or the Fiscal. Some understanding of the disease process is essential to the lawyer because of its frequent appearance in pathology reports; the disease also has important associations with accidents – particularly of industrial or vehicular type – and many insurance companies attach much significance to coronary artery disease in relation to life expectation and compensation.

The heart, like any other muscle, depends on an efficient blood supply to provide it with energy. But, whereas most muscles have a comparatively simple action, the heart must contract constantly and rhythmically. This sophisticated action is controlled by aggregations of nerve tissue known as 'nodes', from which extend 'bundles' of conducting tissue; if any of these specialized areas are deprived of oxygen, the muscle as a whole will beat in an arrhythmic fashion – the condition of ventricular fibrillation is established and efficient pumping action ceases. It follows that localized ischaemia of the heart muscle may cause instantaneous death. Deprivation of oxygen in other than an essential area will cause localized ischaemic death of muscle but, very often, this dead area can be repaired by the process of fibrosis or scar formation. A 'coronary attack' has been survived, but the heart wall may be thinned and dangerously short of blood – a pathological process which has struck once is likely to do so again; a person in this situation is, therefore, a bad risk in respect of certain occupations. Oxygen deprivation of a large area of muscle is likely to be fatal because insufficient useful tissue remains; death in such circumstances may be less instantaneous than when a vital area is involved.

The blood supply to the heart is carried by the left and right coronary arteries which normally are of adequate bore. But, for reasons which are not entirely understood, most persons' coronary arteries silt up as a natural process of ageing – the condition is that of progressive coronary atheroma (*Plate* 3a). The process is something like the furring of hot-water pipes but, in the case of the arteries, the atheromatous material is laid down within the lining of the vessel. The body's main defence against the process lies in the establishment of a collateral circulation (*see* p. 85) which is effective so long as the occlusive process is slow. But this may not always be so. The thick atheromatous plaques require a blood supply of their own and, not infrequently, the walls of the minute vessels will give way – the condition of *intramural haemorrhage* is established and the bore or lumen of the vessel is *suddenly* occluded. Very often, the plaques degenerate without haemorrhage and a necrotic 'abscess' forms which, itself, may rupture leading to sudden *atheromatous restriction* of the lumen; in each case, bursting results in *disruption of the intima* which may form a valve-like obstruction to the flow of blood. Finally, the blood in contact with a diseased area tends to clot in situ and the process of *coronary thrombosis* is superimposed on coronary atheroma. The significance of thrombosis in sudden cardiac death is to some extent controversial. Although it is common lay practice to speak of coronary occlusion as thrombosis, the two conditions do not necessarily go hand in hand. It has been stated that thrombi are found less commonly in cases reported to the Coroner or Fiscal than in those dying in hospital, but the degree of disparity depends on such variables as pre-selection of cases for dissection. Thrombosis is, however, not *essential* to the post-mortem diagnosis of a coronary death – many of these are physiological in nature and may be due to localized spasm of the arteries. Similarly, the result of ischaemia of the muscle – infarction – is not always seen at autopsy; death due to ventricular fibrillation may have been too rapid for the formation of visible changes.

The above description refers to acute coronary insufficiency arising at a specific point in the arterial tree. An equally common situation is that in which a sudden increase in cardiac effort is demanded – due either to a physical or to an emotional stimulus – and in which the dis-eased circulation is unable to expand so as to satisfy the immediate need for increased oxygen. Inadequacy of this type is particularly prevalent in those in whom the atheromatous process has advanced to calcifica-tion, with consequent rigidity of the arterial walls, and in those whose arteries have been severely affected by heavy smoking. These cases pose a difficulty in pathological interpretation – death is due to a failure of response and the circulation will have the same appearance after death as it would have done had it been possible to examine it in life; much of the diagnosis must rest, therefore, on the circumstantial evidence or, if none is available, on the absence of any other cause of death.

This physiological type of coronary death relates in the main to inad-equate arteries supplying a heart of normal size. Much the same situ-ation will obtain if normal-sized arteries are required to maintain a heart of abnormally increased bulk. Potential examples of this have already been noted – the heart in hypertension, the effects of valvular disease or enlargement due to cardiomyopathy. Persons so affected are living dangerously because a sudden requirement for oxygen may be beyond the immediate capacity of the relatively small vessels. Sudden death can result but, again, the findings at autopsy will need careful in-terpretation.

Many of the natural sudden deaths described thus far are precipi-tated by the need for increased cardiac output. Major forensic signifi-cance therefore attaches to the conditions leading to that demand because these must be regarded as the basic cause of dying. Thus, the association of disease and death at work is of far reaching importance in relation to benefits under the Social Security Act; this is discussed in Chapter 15. Disease may also cause vehicular accidents which are dis-cussed in Chapter 10, but falls in the house, drowning and many other types of violent death may be precipitated by natural disease. Natural disease is clearly of importance in the evaluation of homicide. Severe disease discovered in a man dying during a fracas may provide grounds for a plea to reduce a charge of murder to one of culpable homicide or manslaughter. It may, contrariwise, aggravate an offence. In a case seen by the author, a man seated in a locked parked car was threatened by a passerby – he died suddenly and autopsy revealed extensive coronary disease with fibrosis of the heart muscle; although there had been no physical contact, the assailant was convicted of culpable homicide.

If the foregoing represents the normal sequence of events, it might be asked, 'Why do so many coronary deaths occur during sleep?' The answer is unclear. It has been suggested that lowering of the blood pressure, which occurs during the early stages of sleep, may predispose to the formation of thrombi (or clots) within diseased and narrowed vessels. But it has also been shown that the blood pressure rises erratically during sleep – possibly associated with dreams – and the effect is a subconscious demand for increased oxygen supply.[4] Such cases do not invalidate the general hypothesis.

CAUSES OF SUDDEN DEATH IN ADULTS OTHER THAN CARDIOVASCULAR

In practice, only two conditions merit space under this heading.

Asthma can undoubtedly cause sudden death. Severely affected persons may enter a condition of grave respiratory difficulty known as *status asthmaticus*. This may occur but it is not essential to the valid attribution of death to asthma as sufferers seem to be unduly susceptible to sudden collapse. It has been suggested that these deaths may, in fact, be due to the general use of potent drug therapy and certainly this is an aspect which should be investigated whenever such a case presents.

Epilepsy is in a rather similar category. *Status epilepticus* – a long-sustained epileptic attack – is a well-known cause of death but, again, epileptics are subject to sudden death in the absence of such obvious symptoms.

---

[4] An example of modern research is given by Snyder F. et al. (1964) Changes in respiration, heart rate and systolic blood pressure in human sleep. *J. Appl. Physiol.* **19**, 417.

Chapter 8

Wounding

FROM the purely medical aspect, anything which damages the body tissues can be described as a wound, but it is more colloquial to speak of an accidental wound – or any wound caused other than by an instrument – as an injury. Medically speaking, wounds and injuries are a single pathological entity. A division of injuries on legal grounds is to some extent artificial and, since the basic problem in the pathology of violence is to distinguish between accident, suicide and homicide, it is almost impossible to discuss one category to the exclusion of the other two. For the purpose of this chapter, wounds are defined as injuries arising from an assault. So far as is possible, suicide and accidents will be discussed only in relation to differential diagnosis; some overlap is, however, inevitable.

The law on wounding in England differs from that in Scotland. In the former, it is governed by the Offences Against the Person Act 1861 which itemizes various offences.

Actions causing or tending to cause either danger to life or grievous bodily harm, including the use of firearms, are considered in s. 18 while s. 20 describes the offence of maliciously wounding or inflicting grievous bodily harm either with or without any weapon or instrument; assault occasioning actual bodily harm and common assault are the subject of s. 47. The nature of a wound is not defined, but there is case law[1] to indicate that a wound must involve a break in the whole skin; Simpson, however, believes that this plainly cannot hold.[2] The point is relatively unimportant as the alternative charges of causing actual or grievous bodily harm will cover bruising or more serious injuries such as may result in fracture without skin damage.[3]

In Scotland, an attack on the person of another is an assault for which punishment is not specified in any rule. An assault is, however, aggravated, for example, by the use of firearms or by throwing corrosive substances. An assault which causes injury is likely to be more severely

---

[1] R. v. M'Loughlin (1838) 8C. & P. 635.

[2] In *Forensic Medicine*, 7th ed. (1974). London, Edward Arnold, p. 48.

[3] Polson C. J. and Gee D. J. (1973) *Essentials of Forensic Medicine*. Oxford, Pergamon, p. 97.

punished than is óne which does not. Assault 'to severe injury' may be libelled – i.e. specified in the indictment – and it is a very severe aggravation to assault 'to the danger of life'.[4]

Murder – the ultimate in wounding – is defined in England as the unlawful killing of a reasonable creature in being with malice aforethought, either express or implied, the death following within a year and a day. In Scotland, voluntary murder is not so confined and is simply murder committed intentionally. The English concept of 'constructive malice', that is, unintentional killing while committing some other offence, has been abolished[5] and the offence is now that of manslaughter. In Scotland, the difference between involuntary murder – that is murder committed without the intention to kill – and culpable homicide is blurred; it would seem that the former must be accompanied by 'wicked recklessness'[6] – unintentional killing short of this is culpable homicide. This chapter is concerned, however, not so much with the law on homicidal wounding as with the general, nonspecific, body responses and pathological evidence which may follow wounding or injury; specialized injuries – such as those due to heat or gunshot – are discussed separately.

BRUISES

Even though the skin is not broken, the subcutaneous tissues – those beneath the skin – may be damaged by blunt violence; the resulting extravasation of blood from broken vessels constitutes a bruise.

Bruising is a matter of bleeding into the tissues. A clean cut with a knife seldom causes a bruise as the blood escapes through vessels which are damaged only on the edges of the cut. Bruising can, however, surround a laceration of the skin if that breach has been caused by a blunt object; in that case, there may be damage to the vessels internal to the cut surface and blood will escape in both directions. The extent of bruising is, in general, inversely proportional to the sharpness of the object inflicting a wound.

The appearances of bruising without laceration of the skin are not uniform and depend on several factors. Firstly, the part involved is important – the more lax the tissue, the easier it is for the blood to spread; the tissues around the eye will bruise far more readily than will the firm tissues of the back. Secondly, there is the age of the person – blow for

---

[4] Gordon G. H. (1967) *The Criminal Law of Scotland*. Edinburgh, W. Green & Son, p. 761.

[5] Homicide Act 1957, s. 1.

[6] Gordon suggests that killing during the course of a robbery is likely to be regarded as involuntary murder, quoting H.M.Adv. v. Miller and Denovan, 1960 Criminal Appeal Court, unreported.

blow, children and old people bruise more easily than do the young or middle-aged; an assessment of the force involved must take these factors into consideration. Thirdly, extravasated blood will move along the tissue lines of least resistance under the influence of either pressure or gravity; the shape of a bruise may thus have – and probably will have – little relation to the agent causing it and its shape may change with time.

Not only the shape but the external evidence of bruising may alter; it is often most valuable to re-examine the victim of an alleged assault some 24 hours after an inspection made shortly after the event – bruises which were indistinct or even invisible may, by then, have become quite defined. Some bruises may not appear on the surface – this is particularly true over flat bones such as the skull when, should the head strike or be struck by a relatively soft structure, maximum damage to the vessels may be effected against the hard underlying bone and bleeding will be internal rather than visible; the extent of a head injury must not be assumed on the basis of an external examination alone.

The degree of bruising is further influenced by the physical state of the injured person irrespective of age. The physiological limit to a bruise is set by the body's capacity to plug the injured vessels and to clot the escaping blood. Persons with inborn coagulation factor deficiencies, of which haemophilia – itself rare – is the best-known form, or with a diminished number of platelets, with abnormalities of the small blood vessels or with liver disease will bleed more readily than normal and may give a false impression of the severity of injury.

Capillary blood is dark-red; recent bruises will be purple in colour. The tint darkens and browns as oxygen is removed and, soon, the enzymes of the body begin to change the haemoglobin into bile pigments; as a consequence, the bruise of a few days' age takes on a greenish hue which, as it disperses, changes to yellow. It is often stated that the cycle takes about one week but this is so dependent upon the size of the extravasation and upon the factors discussed above that accurate 'dating' of a single bruise is by no means a simple matter. The medical witness will be able to provide far more valuable evidence as to timing when this is of a comparative nature – it is often perfectly possible to state that a given bruise or set of bruises is older than another. This is of obvious importance in cases of alleged assault in which it is important to eliminate those injuries which are of no immediate concern; it is probable that such comparative evidence reaches its apotheosis in the analysis of injured children (see Chapter 20). A feature of the natural elimination of bruises is that some free iron is commonly left in the area and this is readily demonstrable under the microscope. Thus, a more objective method of ageing bruises – and wounds of all types involving haemorrhage – is theoretically available following post-mortem dissection. Unfortunately, the appearances are, again, variable and it is scarcely possible to do more than generalize – 'it is probably safe to say that it is not usual to find iron-containing pigment in less than 12 to 24 hours'.[7] The method is of some value in distinguishing cerebral haemorrhage which is the result of an accident from natural haemorrhage – which could have been accruing for some time and which may have caused the accident.

Bruises occurring in the subcutaneous tissue seldom cause significant damage unless they become infected. Bruising may, however, affect the deeper tissue. Thus, a bruise within the eyeball may cause permanent blindness and the possible fibrous reaction to bruises of vital organs – say, for example, bruising involving the coronary circulation of the heart – may cause physical effects some time after the original injury; the significance of such lesions is discussed in Chapter 10. Deep bruises which, by virtue of the size of the vessels involved, amount to frank haemorrhage may have severe immediate and long-term effects which are also influenced by the function of the structure involved – bleeding into the brain, for example, may cause irrecoverable damage to the nerve cells.

All authorities are agreed that bruises can be produced after death. It is likely that such bruises will be of small size and, in the event of doubt, microscopic studies, designed to demonstrate the persistence or absence of enzymatic processes may on occasion distinguish ante- from post-mortem lesions. It is often only possible to say that such bruising occurred 'at or about the time of death'.

ABRASIONS

An abrasion occurs when the outer skin is damaged but the deeper layers remain intact. Although little harm is caused to the body as a whole, rupture of vessels of minute size may result in permanent and relatively faithful reproduction of the object causing the abrasion; it follows that such injuries are of major diagnostic importance.[8]

Abrasions may be due to a frictional movement between the skin and an object or to simple pressure on the skin; in either case, the damage may be ante mortem or post mortem.

Moving abrasions will not replicate the pattern of the offending object but will give evidence, firstly, of the direction of the abrasive force. Thus, by visualizing the 'pile-up' of epidermis on the far end of an abrasion, the pathologist can give evidence as to the direction on a blow or of contact with the ground in, say, a pedestrian street accident. Parallel,

---

[7] In: Simpson K. (ed.) *Taylor's Principles and Practice of Medical Jurisprudence*, 12th ed (1965). London, Churchill, vol. I, p. 189.

[8] Even in the absence of skin damage, antemortem 'blushing' of the vessels beneath a pressure point may leave a distinct pattern – e.g. following a slap.

linear abrasions are suggestive of having been caused by finger-nails; they may confirm the fact of an assault, they may give evidence as to the relative positions of attacker and attacked and they may serve to identify or exclude a suspect by demonstrating finger span or abnormalities of the fingers or finger-nails.

Impact abrasions, without relative movement, often reproduce closely the object causing the injury. Examples include the imprints of weapons, boots or parts of an automobile; even if clothing intervenes and makes its own imprint, the shape of the abrasion may indicate its cause (*Plate* 3b). An outline of a contact object will appear when skin having loose underlying connective tissue is struck; the abrasion is then caused, in effect, by the differential movement of the skin at the edges of the instrument.

Abrasions inflicted coincidentally with or after death merit special mention. They are devoid of vital reaction and take on the appearance and texture of parchment; wide areas of 'parchmenting' may result from contact with a flat object. Such post-mortem 'pressure' abrasions are very common in vehicular accidents and are found in bodies recovered from the sea which have been pounded on the rocks. They must be distinguished from the rather similar appearance produced by the post-mortem application of heat or other forms of localized desiccation.

LACERATIONS

Strictly speaking, any breach in the whole skin thickness is a laceration. It is customary, however, to confine the term to a breach of the skin caused by direct blunt injury or by tearing or shearing forces; a laceration caused by a sharp object is an incised wound or a stab wound (*q.v.*).

Lacerations resulting from blunt force must involve crushing of the skin as a prelude to splitting. They generally occur over a bone which lies close to the skin with little intervening soft tissue – e.g. in the scalp. A blow over the cheek bone may result in a laceration; an identical blow 1 inch below on the cheek itself might well cause no more than a bruise. Perhaps the classic laceration due to blunt injury is the boxer's 'cut eye' which is found in the eyebrow area.

The essential features which define a laceration due to blunt injury are the presence of associated bruising, the irregularity of the split and the manifest crushing or tearing damage to structures *within* the split – an incised wound will merely divide them neatly. A laceration cannot, therefore, give as much evidence as to the shape of the causative instrument as can an abrasion; the two may, however, frequently co-exist. The presence of multiple lacerations of generally similar type, particularly if they are closely grouped but not identical in direction, must raise the suspicion of foul play (*Plate* 4a). Lacerations as here defined can seldom be suicidal unless they result from a fall; remarkable motivation would be needed to produce self-inflicted lacerations by the use of blunt instruments.

Lacerations due to kicking are generally multiple and are concentrated around the ear and side of the neck. Other elective sites for kicking – such as the abdomen – may well not show skin breaks. Whatever the site, the characteristic feature is the unusual extent of associated deep bruising.

Lacerations due to tearing or shearing are characteristic of vehicular accidents. They are often accompanied by severe damage to the underlying muscle or even bone. The extreme example is the very frequent spiral laceration of the leg involving all the tissues which is caused by savage twisting of the limb held firm while the torso is free to move.

INCISED WOUNDS

Incised wounds result from the use of a knife-edge of any type including, for example, glass. The danger of such a wound depends upon the position and its depth; a deep incision of the buttock may cause little more than discomfort while a comparatively superficial cut in the wrist may prove fatal due to division of a major artery.

Incised wounds may be accidental but, as such, are seldom serious. Cutting injuries self-inflicted with suicidal intent are, by contrast, almost always deep and dangerous.[9] A most common problem is to distinguish these from injuries inflicted during the course of an aggravated assault. The major points of distinction include:

> a. The position of the incision. The neck is the most common site for both homicidal and suicidal incisions. Those in the wrist are, however, almost diagnostic of suicide.
> b. Suicidal injuries to the neck are nearly always multiple and show evidence of altering determination, some incisions being superficial while one, or perhaps two, are deep and lethal. True, a suicide may be resolute at first attempt but the murderer is unlikely to be tentative; homicidal incised wounds are, therefore, commonly both severe and of similar depths.

Incised wounds are not infrequently inflicted for the purpose of maiming or disfiguring rather than killing. Intended as punishment, they are nearly always made on the face; deep self-inflicted wounds in

---

[9] Self-inflicted abrasions – made by the finger-nails, gem stones in rings, pointed instruments, etc. – are not uncommon expressions of emotions often associated with sexual relationships. They are seen most usually on the arms or breasts but the face may also be injured superficially (*Plate* 4b).

this location are very rare save in the presence of severe mental derangement or as a form of ritual disfigurement. A specific incised wound of
different type may be found on the fingers or palm of the hand; such injuries, often irregular in distribution and depth, commonly represent attempts at self-defence and strongly indicate that other wounds on the
body are homicidal in nature.

Pathological findings designed to demonstrate the direction of the cut
are often difficult to interpret. The 'exit' portion is almost bound to be
shelving; the 'entry' wound may well be precipitously deep in homicide
or shelving towards the centre when self-inflicted but the appearances
must be very variable and will also be modified by the shape of the part
which is cut.

PENETRATING WOUNDS

A wound can be described as penetrating if its depth exceeds its width.
When the superficial characteristics of such an injury are those of an
incised wound, it is a stab wound; it is customary to restrict the term
to injuries inflicted by pointed instruments, e.g. a needle, a knife or a
bayonet.

Accidental stab wounds are invariably single unless the offending
instrument has multiple penetrating points; an accidental fall on to the
points of a garden fork or a spiked railing could provide multiple stab
wounds of symmetrical pattern, identical direction and equal depth. It
may be difficult to distinguish accident from suicide or homicide when
there is evidence of only a single thrust. Much will depend upon the
findings at the locus of death and on the position and direction of the
wound. The site of a suicidal stab wound must have been accessible to
the dead person and, in practice, the great majority of single suicidal
stab wounds are in an elective site, occasionally deep in the neck but
more commonly following the path of the classic Japanese method of
self-immolation running upwards from below the ribs to penetrate the
heart. Single homicidal stab wounds are comparitively rare as most
wounds leave the victim capable of resistance for a measurable time
during which the blow is repeated; single homicidal wounds are, therefore, often associated with a drugged, drunk or sleeping victim and are
almost always aimed at the heart. Occasionally, single homicidal
wounds may cause difficulty by reason of their unusualness. In a case
seen by the author, a man's body was picked up from his front garden
and treated as a supposed sudden natural death; it was not until the
body was being undressed in the mortuary that a single stab wound was
noted in the right loin – very rapid death had resulted from transfixion
of the aorta. It may be reasonable in such atypical cases to question the

intention to kill and to accept them as instances of involuntary murder or culpable homicide.

Multiple stab wounds are very strongly suggestive of voluntary murder. When a suicide inflicts several wounds upon himself, the earlier wounds are likely to be shallow – a close grouping of the injuries is likely unless the suicide results from religious frenzy or other mental imbalance. Multiple murderous stab wounds show, by contrast, a more uniform degree of force, several being potentially lethal – they are often widely spaced and of different directions unless the repeated stab wounds have been inflicted on an unconscious body (*Plate* 5).

Evidence will be drawn from the pathologist as to the nature and shape of the weapon either to assist in the search for, or for purposes of comparison with, a suspect article. As with all wounds, the sharper the instrument, the less tissue damage and bruising will be found. A stab by a knife will produce a clean incised wound which, by virtue of the elasticity of the skin, will stretch into an ellipse. A double-edged weapon will normally produce a symmetrical surface pattern whereas one with a single edge may show relative blunting, or 'fish-tailing', of one end of the entry slit; all authorities are agreed, however, that differential contraction of the skin and subcutaneous tissue may, on occasion, give a misleading impression. The maximum diameter of the wounds must be measured with the edges opposed. In general, the weapon – and, in particular, a knife – cannot be wider than this so long as the natural taper of the point is taken into consideration and the width is related to the depth of the wound; rocking or twisting the knife obviously may produce a wound which is larger than its maximum width. Similarly, the depth of the wound is unlikely to be longer than the full length of the weapon; a false indication of length may be obtained if the body surface has been compressed by the hilt, as may particularly be the case in wounds of the abdomen. Despite the obvious need for caution, the accurate measurement of a number of stab wounds in a single body may enable the pathologist to give a reasonably accurate description of the likely size and shape of the blade of the weapon used, especially if it was a knife (*Fig.* 11); different measurements may indicate that there was more than one assailant.

These measurements, together with an assessment of the direction of multiple stab wounds, may also enable the pathologist to establish how the knife was held and to gauge the strength with which the blows were struck. The question of the 'force used' is often difficult to evaluate and an opinion must take into account the clothing of the victim. To find that the wounds penetrated 'up to the hilt' is to assess the results of force rather than its degree. Deep penetration of the tissue by a sharp pointed instrument is suprisingly easy and it would be within the power of practically any adult male or female to inflict a lethal wound using the usual pattern of sheath knife which is freely saleable to persons of all ages.[10]

Fig. 11. The shape of a knife assessed from the appearance of three stab wounds of different depth. The actual knife was of remarkable similar shape although the point was curved.

THE MODE AND CAUSE OF DEATH FOLLOWING WOUNDING

Rapid death resulting from incised or stab wounds is usually due either to haemorrhage or to damage to a structure which is vital to life; death may occasionally be caused by air entering a broken vein.

Haemorrhage is by far the most common of these and will be much more severe if an artery is penetrated than if only veins are affected; the speed of death will depend upon the size of the vessel involved and on the secondary effects of the accumulation of blood. It is difficult to inflict a stabbing injury of 6 in. (15 cm) depth without lacerating an artery of at least moderate calibre and the direction of most homicidal stab wounds results in their frequent termination in the heart, aorta or major pulmonary vessels. Death is often very rapid, but it pays to be cautious in interpretation as some remarkable periods of survival have been recorded. Haemorrhage from nonpenetrating incised wounds need not be severe unless a major artery lies superficially at the site of in-

[10] 'Flick knives' may not be so sold – nor, indeed, dealt in in any way (Restriction of Offensive Weapons Acts 1959 and 1961).

jury – the most obvious example of such an area is on the inner surface of the wrist which, accordingly, is a favourite site for suicidal incision.

Rapid death due to interference with the function of structures other than blood vessels is rare and is confined to special situations. Thus, stab wounds at the nape of the neck may result in near instantaneous death, with minimal haemorrhage, due to destruction of the vital centres in the medulla of the brain stem. Incised wounds of the trachea or larynx may lead to collapse of the neck structures with valve-like obstruction of the main airway; more probably, the airway will be blocked by blood or impacted tissues. Incised wounds of the neck may, in fact, result in many modes of death – vagal inhibition of the heart, airway obstruction, air embolism, venous bleeding from the jugular veins or arterial bleeding from the carotid arteries; the length of the agonal period may, as a consequence, be particularly difficult to assess.

Death attributable to wounds or injuries occurring some time after the event presents no special features. Among other complications, those of prolonged immobilization – pneumonia or pulmonary embolism – or of reduction in blood volume – in particular acute renal failure – may arise and must be regarded as logical sequences of the original assault in the absence of proof of intervening medical negligence.

Chapter 9

Injury and Death due to Firearms and Explosives

THE law relating to firearms is statutory throughout Great Britain and is contained in the Firearms Act 1968.[1] A firearm is defined in s. 57(1) of the Act as any lethal barrelled weapon of any description from which any shot, bullet or other missile can be discharged. Excluding air weapons, personal firearms are of two categories – the smooth-bore weapon, or shotgun, and rifled weapons which include revolvers, 'automatic' pistols and rifles. The former were devised primarily for the sport of killing small animals including birds; the latter, while being used in some forms of sport hunting – e.g. deer stalking – were mainly perfected for the killing of man. The regulations governing the possession and use of rifled weapons are, accordingly, far more strict than apply in the case of shotguns. Section 1 defines, by exclusion, those weapons which it is unlawful to possess without simultaneously holding a firearm certificate.

No one under the age of 14 may acquire or use any firearm or ammunition unless as a member of a recognized club or when in a shooting gallery using miniature rifles or air weapons; but an airgun can be used under supervision by an adult over 21 in a private place. Persons over 14 may be given or lent an airgun, or a 'Section 1' firearm subject to the possession of a firearms certificate, but purchase is prohibited below the age of 17; the possession of an assembled shotgun under the age of 15 is subject to supervision by an adult. The carriage of an airgun in a public place by a person under the age of 17 is prohibited unless the gun is securely covered.

Certificates to possess and use an airgun are not required provided the user is over 14 years old; in addition to it being illegal to sell such a gun to anyone under the age of 17, it is also unlawful to present a young person under the age of 14 with an airgun for his possession. These relaxed regulations do not apply to 'specially dangerous air weapons' – defined as pump action air rifles having a kinetic energy greater than 12 ft lb (16 J) or 6 ft lb (8 J) in the case of pistols – which are

---

[1] The use of other offensive weapons of discharge type – e.g. ammonia guns – is dealt with, additionally, under the Prevention of Crime Act 1953.

103

classified as 'Section 1' firearms. Smooth-bore guns having a barrel not less than 24 in. long are not Section 1 firearms and their possession is regulated by the issue of shotgun certificates which are obtained from the local police; there are no further restrictions on the acquisition of shotguns by persons over the age of 17 and, in certain circumstances, shotguns can be used without a certificate being held – the most important of these being when the gun is borrowed from a person with a certificate and is used on his private property. It is an offence to shorten the barrel of a shotgun to less than 24 in.; the resultant 'sawn-off shotgun' would be a Section 1 weapon and its possession restricted to the granting of a firearm certificate.

Whereas it is generally only necessary to be 'of good character' to qualify for the issue of a shotgun licence, a person seeking a firearm certificate must not be of intemperate habits, of unsound mind or for any reason unfitted to be entrusted with firearms. The Chief Constable must be satisfied that the applicant has a good reason for acquiring a firearm and that its acquisition would not be prejudicial to public safety or to peace. Very few categories of person are exempt from the firearm certificate requirements – the commonest are members of approved rifle clubs and cadet corps and race starters at athletic meetings: persons in the service of the Crown or in the Police are exempt although subject to rigid regulation by their parent authorities. The possession of certain weapons – e.g. automatic repeating rifles or weapons discharging a harmful liquid or gas – is prohibited without the specific authority of the Home Office or Scottish Home and Health Department in addition to the possession of a firearm certificate.

Shotguns are, therefore, widely distributed and despite the regulations, legally held firearms are responsible for a substantial number of deaths; the illegal possession of firearms – including the retention of 'war souvenirs' – is fairly widespread. A number of specific offences relating to the use of firearms are created by the Firearms Act. These include:

a. the possession of a firearm or ammunition with intent to injure a person or to damage property;
b. using a real or imitation firearm to resist arrest or with intent to commit a crime;
c. trespassing with a firearm;
d. carrying without reasonable excuse a loaded shotgun or any other firearm whether it be loaded or not together with appropriate ammunition.

To wound or cause grievous bodily harm with intent to do so by any means – which includes shooting – is a statutory offence in England and

Wales.[2] In Scotland, wounding by shooting is a serious aggravation of an assault.[3]

Gunshot injuries are of major pathological interest in that they can be interpreted with considerable objectivity; the pathologist can often give opinions which are very well-based and which are of particular value both to the police and the lawyer.

AIRGUN INJURIES

Unless the pellet penetrates some vital spot, such as the eye or the brain, severe injuries from the normal airgun or air pistol are unlikely. The same is not true of the powerful air weapons described as especially dangerous, the effect of which may be comparable to a small bullet from a rifled firearm. Injuries due to air weapons do not merit a separate description.

SHOTGUN INJURIES

Shotguns may be single or double barrelled. The barrel of the former or one barrel of the latter may be tapered towards the muzzle – a manufacturing process known as *choking* which serves to lengthen the period during which the shot is restrained in a compact mass. The calibre of shotguns is expressed in unusual terms. When the diameter of the barrel is less than half an inch, the calibre is given by that diameter – e.g. 'fourten' means a barrel diameter of 0·410 inches;[4] guns larger than this are measured by 'bore' – or the number of spherical lead balls exactly fitting the barrel which go to make 1 lb. An 8-bore is therefore a larger and more powerful gun than is the common 12-bore.

The shotgun cartridge consists of a cardboard cylinder attached to a brass plate which contains the primer. The main powder charge is separated from the shot by a wad or washer. The shot is maintained in the cartridge by a distal wad. When fired, the shot – which consists of a large number of pellets of a size chosen for the particular sporting purpose intended – is propelled in a solid mass which begins to fan out as the compression by the wads is released. The propellant continues burning as the shot passes down the barrel and some powder always remains unburnt. The effective range of a sporting shotgun is approximately

---

[2] Offences Against the Person Act 1861, s. 18 as amended by the Criminal Law Act 1967, Schedule 3, Part III.

[3] See also the little-used Criminal Law (Scotland) Act 1829, s. 2. which defines the assault of shooting, or presenting, pointing or levelling any kind of loaded firearm and attempting to discharge it.

[4] The Metrication Board probably have by now devised an alternative means of expression.

50 yards (or metres) and the shot is rapidly halted within the tissues of the target.

The pathological evidence as to the distance from which the shot has been fired can be deduced from these principles although it cannot be overstated that some variations occur in practice. A contact injury will, firstly, show bruising due to the recoil of the gun and a perfect representation of the single or twin barrels may be formed on the skin; the shot will enter the body as a solid mass so that the entry wound will approximate to the bore of the barrel; however, explosive gases will also enter the wound so that the external wound may be ragged or the skull, for example, may be literally blown apart; an exit wound may be seen, except in the very thick torso, because the shot in a contact wound is in a solid mass. Shot in its diffuse form – as fired from a distance – has little penetrating power; exit wounds are, therefore, a rare feature of shotgun injuries other than in the contact situation. At very short range, the appearances described above will be modified by the differing effects of the gases of combustion – these will not be forced into the wound but may still cause some irregularity of the entry hole. Unburnt powder will be discharged into the surrounding skin leading to what is known as 'tattooing'; soot is likely to be deposited. The hot gases will burn the skin or clothing either of which may be charred; in both contact and close range wounds, any carbon monoxide contained in the gases of combustion may form local carboxyhaemoglobin which can be recognized by its pink colour.

These effects diminish as the distance from muzzle to wound increases. The critical distance is at about 2 yards (or metres) as, at this distance, tattooing is scarcely visible and the wads fail to penetrate the wound. The shot now begins to fan out and creates a pattern of entry in the clothing and on the skin. Although the inclination of the body to the line of flight of the shot will alter the appearances, ideally the pattern will be circular. The size of this circle depends to some extent on the degree of 'choking' of the gun but the appearances are sufficiently standard to permit the use of a simple rule – the diameter of the shot pattern in inches is equivalent to the muzzle distance from the wound in yards (or the spread in centimetres is some 2·5–3·0 × the distance in metres);[5] estimates derived in this way must be checked by test firing whenever possible. Fatal 12-bore shotgun injuries are unlikely at a range of over 20 yards.

The majority of shotgun injuries are sustained at close range. The internal injuries are therefore due either to the violent expansion of gas within the body or to the penetrating effect of what is, essentially, a solid mass of lead more than half an inch in diameter; the former effect is well

---

[5] Attempts to improve the accuracy of this estimation by complicating the formula probably fail in their purpose and merely make the matter harder for juries to understand.

seen in the head and the latter in the heart which can be torn apart by a shot fired from within a range of 2 yards. Otherwise, the effects of a shotgun injury are variable and depend upon the ability of individual pellets to penetrate either the heart or individual blood vessels or other organs liable to severe bleeding; the surgery of such an injury may present a formidable problem.

RIFLED WEAPONS

The main diagnostic difference between wounds due to shotguns and rifled weapons rests on the fact that, whereas shot will certainly be found in the body, a bullet is likely to have exited; entry and exit wounds are, therefore, a feature of the latter.

Contact and close range entry wounds due to rifle bullets will have much the same characteristics as those of a shotgun injury – bruising, blast effects, soot deposition and tattooing will be present, the last being found up to a range of some 3–4 ft.

If the range has not been so short as to cause explosive damage to the tissues, the characteristics of the entry wound will be governed by the gyroscopic stability of the bullet. In the early phase of its flight – up to some 50 yards or metres for a pistol or 150 yards for a rifle – and towards the end of its effective range – of the order of 500 yards (460 m) for a pistol and $1\frac{1}{2}$ miles (2·4 km) for a rifle – there is considerable 'tail wag' which results in a relatively large and ragged entry wound. In the most efficient phase of flight, the bullet will enter the body neatly nose on and leave a regular, small hole which, because of the elasticity of the skin, may well not correspond exactly to the diameter of the missile. The entry wound will always show inverted edges and is likely to demonstrate 'soiling' – that is, contamination of its edge by the grease covering the bullet which is wiped off either by the clothing or by the skin.

As the bullet traverses the body, it may become deflected, it may be deformed and it may take with it fragments of tissue – particularly bone – to act as secondary missiles. The exit wound is, therefore, likely to be irregular, its edge will be everted and there will be no soiling – it cannot be smaller than the entry wound save at extremes of range. The modern, very high-velocity rifle presents something of an exception. This weapon kills by virtue of the massive internal damage which results from the dissipation of large amounts of kinetic energy; the entry and exit wounds are, however, small and of very similar size. The common tendency for the wound to enlarge from entry to exit is well shown in bone, particularly the bones of the skull in which the penetrating wound bevels outwards to be of larger diameter on the exit side; this difference in size is useful in distinguishing a bullet wound from a surgical burr-hole in a skeletonized skull or fragment of skull bone presented for examination.

As compared with shotgun injuries, the pathologist is likely to be able to give a very good opinion as to the direction of an injury from a rifled weapon but has less evidence on which to base an estimate of range. The recovery of a bullet from the body is, of course, of great importance to the investigation as every weapon leaves a characteristic pattern of scorings on the surface of the bullet; test firing of suspected weapons may then result in a convincing identification by comparison. Equally good – if not better – comparative evidence can be derived from spent cartridges recovered at the scene of a shooting – marks of an individual nature are made by the firing pin and hammer, the ejection mechanism and during extraction; such methods of weapon identification are also open in the case of shotguns but lie in the province of the ballistics expert.

Bullets may kill by virtue of penetrating the heart, a major vessel or a vital centre of the brain. By far the greatest damage is, however, caused by 'cavitation' in the track of the missile and by the discharge of energy which can tear vital tissues associated with, but removed from, the actual path of the bullet; widespread destruction may result from fragments of tissue which form 'secondary missiles'. Delayed death is likely if a solid organ with a large blood supply, such as the liver, is damaged; death from septic shock or simple sepsis may follow penetrating injuries of the bowel.

THE NATURE OF THE WOUNDING

The immediate need in any case of fatal firearm wounding is to distinguish between accident, suicide and homicide. The forensic doctor will often be able to give sound evidence as to the probability of suicide; the distinction between accident and homicide, is, however, a far more difficult problem. The medical evidence will rest, firstly, upon an examination of the locus and, secondly, on the post-mortem findings.

The scene of death will provide much evidence in relation to suicide. Firstly, the weapon must be within reach and almost always will either be retained in the grasp or lie close to the hand of the dead person. A murderer may attempt to simulate suicide and it is most important that the doctor, called in to pronounce life extinct, takes full notes of the precise conditions. The presence of the rare cadaveric spasm is of importance; this is one post-mortem condition which cannot be artificially produced (*see* Chapter 4). Homicide is clearly indicated if the gun is found at the scene and is beyond reach of the deceased (*Plate* 6); the main exception rests in the possibility of a suicidal or accidental shot which is not immediately fatal – in which case, there may well be evidence of movement in the form of blood splashing and the like. Mention is generally made of suicide accomplished by means of a remote firing mechanism such as a pulley attached to the trigger; such contraptions are set for deep-seated psychological reasons and not for the purpose of confusing the investigating officers – they rarely cause difficulty although, again, the possibility of an artefact rigged by an assailant has to be eliminated. The examining doctor should always confer with the police officer in charge as to the presence of spent cartridges; the firing of more than one shot is very uncommon in suicide.

The post-mortem findings indicating suicide can be deduced from the previous pages. Findings indicative of a range within one yard – in particular, the appearance of tattooing – are clearly consistent with suicide as this is the maximum distance it is possible to hold a pistol from the body; similarly, the absence of close-range characteristics in a shotgun or rifle wound will strongly militate against suicide as the barrel length of the gun approximates to that of the arm. In practice, it is extremely uncommon for suicidal wounds to be other than of a contact nature. They will also almost always be in a 'site of election'; these vary according to the weapon. A suicidal pistol wound is generally inflicted in the right temple (whether right-handed or not)[6] and an exit wound is usual close to the opposite temple; an alternative is the centre of the forehead – the precise symmetry is classical and of diagnostic importance – while the roof of the mouth may be chosen. Rifle wounds are, again, common in the centre of the forehead and in the mouth; in either case, massive tissue damage may result. The rifle suicide may lean on the gun with the muzzle on the brow or over the heart, a situation which is not unusual with shotguns. The commonest suicidal shotgun wounds are, however, those in the roof of the mouth or in the centre of the forehead, just above the bridge of the nose; in either case, the head is torn asunder often, again, in a characteristic symmetrical fashion. The important general features of successful suicidal firearm wounds are that they are always so placed as to eliminate the possibility of failure and that the entry point must be accessible. Other evidence of close contact with the gun, such as discolouration of the thighs where the barrel has been steadied, may also be present.

Accidental gunshot injuries may be 'self-inflicted' – as in the classic 'cleaning the gun' situation – or involve a second party as when a moving fellow hunter is mistaken for game. The former situation may closely simulate suicide, the essential differentiation being the asymmetry inherent in a random occurrence. The latter type of accidental injury, showing no more than the effect of a relatively long range

[6] The author is indebted to Professor C. K. Simpson for this expression of his wide experience.

discharge, is indistinguishable from homicide on purely pathological grounds.

Certain features are strongly indicative of homicide – a single wound of contact of very close range type in an inaccessible position is an obvious example, the back, the nape of the neck or behind the ear being the commonest sites; similarly, the existence of more than one fatal injury will be very strong evidence against both suicide and accident – in circumstances of high emotional tension, such as marital brawls, a mixture of both nonfatal and fatal wounds may be found (*Plate* 7). The suspicion of homicide may, however, rest on the exclusion of suicide by the pathologist coupled with the circumstantial evidence obtained by the police officers.

EXAMINATION OF SUSPECTS

There is little or no valuable evidence which the forensic doctor can derive from the general medical examination of a suspected firearm assailant. The doctor may, however, provide specimens for analysis in the forensic science laboratory.

The older relevant tests are based on the assumption that residues of propellant will settle on the firing hand. Both gunpowder and modern smokeless powders contain nitrates which are readily detectable when present. It was the habit to remove skin surface contaminants with paraffin and the test thus became incorrectly known as 'the paraffin test'. The identification of nitrates has since been regarded as nonspecific and, in 1964, Interpol 'did not consider the traditional paraffin test to be of any value'.[7]

Later work has concentrated on the identification on the hands of metallic residues derived from the primer contained in the percussion cap of the cartridge; mercury, antimony, barium and lead can be quantified in this 'dermal residue' test. The residues are removed by swabbing with moistened filter paper. Current work in Belgium has indicated certain drawbacks to a promising approach – for example, the 'natural' residue is strongly dependent on occupation and a negative result, even under experimental conditions, does not necessarily exclude the possibility of a firearm having been used; moreover, the residues are easily removed by washing. Tests of this type must be regarded as still subject to critical appraisal; it is to be hoped that what may be a useful indicative test will not become discredited due to the exaggeration of improbable alternative interpretations.

---

[7] First International Criminal Police Organization Seminar (1964), *Int. Crim. Police Rev.* **174**, 28. Quoted by Cornelis R. and Timperman J. (1974) *Med. Sci. Law* **14**, 98, where an interesting review of the current position is given.

INJURIES AND DEATH DUE TO EXPLOSION

Injury and death due to explosion may occur industrially or in the home as, for example, when gas filling a room is ignited. The resulting injuries will be due, firstly, to the air blast itself and, secondly, to random impacts as the body is hurled against other solid objects. If the blast is due to a bomb, there will be added damage from the splintered casing.

The effects of blast are due to a combination of positive pressure, the blast wave itself and the subsequent negative pressure. The effects, which are exaggerated in an enclosed space, are seen particularly in those organs capable of elastic recoil and containing multiple gas/fluid or fluid/solid interfaces. Thus, the lungs in particular are the subject of much disruption and haemorrhage; the eardrums are also most sensitive to pressure changes. Blast effects are well transmitted in water; the hollow viscera are particularly vulnerable to underwater explosions and, since there are no injuries due to secondary impacts, the persons killed in these circumstances often present with little external but massive internal damage.

Bomb injuries[8] may approximate to disintegration of the body; short of this, the wounds are characterized by their multiplicity and by their association with foreign particles not all of which necessarily derive from the bomb itself – many fragments of glass, brick dust or even pieces of furniture will contaminate the wounds and will give a distinctive pattern of 'peppering' of the body.

As in all types of wounding, death due to bomb blast may be accidental, suicidal or homicidal. Accidental cases are of legitimate and illegitimate type. The former are confined to members of bomb disposal squads and to workers in authorized armouries – for example, in the armed forces. When the device involved is a small one, the track of metallic fragments can often be traced in the body so as to define the reconstruction of events with considerable accuracy. Accidental bomb injuries of an illegal character – e.g. occurring in those manufacturing bombs – are likely to be far more severe. Suicidal bomb injuries might occasionally be used as a form of political exhibitionism but are probably now relegated in history to the more bizarre aspects of the Second World War. Suicidal actions may be differentiated pathologically by the concentration of massive injuries in the abdominal region; the victims of random bomb attacks commonly show maximal injury in the legs. Homicidal bombing in a civilian context is a comparatively recent form of outrage; despite the fact that the conditions in which it occurs are so diverse, the pattern of injuries is surprisingly reproducible.[9]

---

[8] The offence of causing an explosion likely to endanger life or property is defined in the Explosive Substances Act 1883, s. 2.
[9] See Marshall T. K. (1978) Major Civil Disturbance, in: Mason J. K. (ed.) *The Pathology of Violent Injury,* London, Edward Arnold.

Burns associated with bombs are of two types – the 'flash burn' affecting persons close to the explosion from which clothing provides good protection, and ordinary thermal burns resulting either from the clothes or from the building catching fire.

The pathological diagnosis of bomb explosion is never in doubt unless associated with, say, an aircraft (*see below*). The important evidence to be obtained from post-mortem dissection lies in the recovered fragments of bomb casing from which information of value to law enforcement can be derived, much as in the case of firearm wounds; the importance of X-ray study as a means of localizing such fragments cannot be overemphasized.

The deliberate destruction of commercial aircraft in flight introduces a currently interesting variation on the theme of homicidal bombing; the diagnosis of this crime – which occurs on a world-wide basis between once and twice a year on average – has civil medico-legal as well as criminal implications.[10] The nature of the event often results in extensive destruction of the aircraft due to the high forces sustained in the resultant crash while the whole wreckage may be lost should the catastrophe occur over the sea; much may, therefore, depend upon the pathological evidence.[11] This rests upon observations which derive from a full examination of all the human wreckage recovered. The pattern of injuries throughout the dead may indicate an abnormal accident situation; search must be made for the 'target' who may present as an 'odd man out' by reason either of his position relative to the other passengers or of his injuries. Radiological examination of all human tissue is essential – and must nowadays be undertaken in all unexplained accidents until a credible alternative to sabotage is agreed; finally, any metallic fragments other than those which are clearly part of the aircraft structure must be subjected to expert examination. The investigation of such a case is, inevitably, time-consuming and extremely costly.[12] The perpetrators of this form of mass murder have been found to be of various types – political motivation may be present but possibly the commonest reason in the past has been pecuniary and related to life insurance policies; suicides have been suspected and instances have been traced to motives of almost incredible frivolity, such as the removal of an

---

[10] In the event of sabotage being shown as the cause of an aircraft accident responsibility for insurance passes from the 'All Risks' insurers to those underwriting 'War Risks'.

[11] In fact, there is a trend towards an increase in the number of cases of attempted sabotage with a decrease in the proportion of aircraft completely destroyed thereby. The saboteurs appear to be less professional than was once the case.

[12] Two examples of the medical investigation of such cases are: (*a*) Dille J. R. and Hasbrook A. H. (1966) Injuries due to explosion, decompression and impact of a jet transport. *Aerospace Med.* **37**, 5; and (*b*) Mason J. K. and Tarlton S. W. (1969) Medical investigation of the loss of the Comet 4B aircraft, 1967. *Lancet* **1**, 431.

unwanted girlfriend. A main difficulty facing the investigators is to distinguish sabotage from explosive decompression due to structural failure of the airframe in flight.[13]

---

[13] Compare, for example, the case described in footnote (12) above with the loss of the Comet aircraft in 1954 (Armstrong J. A. et al. (1955) Interpretation of injuries in the Comet aircraft disasters. *Lancet* **1**, 1135).

Chapter 10

Accidental Injury and Death due to Deceleration and Acceleration

ACCIDENTS may occur in the home, at work or at play and some of these situations are covered elsewhere in this book. Transportation accidents are, however, not only the commonest single source of severe traumatic injury and death in the United Kingdom but they are also those which are most likely to lead to litigation. The majority of significant injuries sustained in road traffic accidents are of a decelerative or accelerative nature and the forces involved are applied in the horizontal plane.[1] Injuries sustained in accidental falls essentially result from vertical deceleration. Aircraft accidents link these two conditions in that the injurious forces are a varying combination of the horizontal and the vertical. It is with these three categories of accident that this chapter is concerned.

As discussed in Chapter 8, accidental injuries are similar in character to wounds. Although a large proportion of injuries may appear non-specific, many abrasions and some bruises may be remarkably distinctive in both appearance and distribution and may provide important evidence in accident reconstruction – this is particularly well shown in the pedestrian road traffic death.

The source of abrasions discovered on killed pedestrians may be obvious. Examples include the pattern imprinted by radiator grilles or by tyres; on occasion, this may be so individual as to provide corroboration of a cause and effect relationship with a particular vehicle. The importance of scaled photography of such abrasions – particularly in the hit-and-run type of accident – cannot be overemphasized as a means of preserving valuable evidence.

Useful pathological information can often be derived from an assessment of the sequence in which the injuries were sustained. The time intervals are usually extremely short and an evaluation through appraisal of the degree of bruising or of vital reaction is often impossible. Nevertheless, an attempt to distinguish direct contact wounds from those due to abrading, and a division of the latter into those caused by sliding over the structures of the vehicle or along the ground – as shown

---

[1] 'Deceleration' to the physiologists is a substitute term for 'negative acceleration'. But the word is used colloquially and it is in this sense that it is introduced here.

by contained glass, paint or earth – may be of value both to the police and to other interested investigators; whenever possible, the autopsy should include an examination of the clothing in situ – the correlation of clothing damage and bodily injury is one of the most useful examinations in the vehicular accident.

Abrasions in the occupants of cars who are killed in an accident are of particular importance not only in indicating the identity of the driver (*Plate* 3b) but also in relation to the use of seat belt restraint. This has important practical applications; an increasing number of insurance companies are tying the amount of indemnity to the use of or failure to use restraining harnesses while judgments for damages for injuries sustained now take this factor into account.[2] It is clear that, in future, a plaintiff's (or pursuer's) damages will be reduced in part-proportion to the extent that his injuries were caused or aggravated by failure to use a seat belt – generally assessed as 20–25 per cent – and that this will apply even when the plaintiff is entirely blameless.[3] The pathologist may therefore properly be asked for evidence on this point. Although there will often be no residual evidence even though the equipment was used, bruising may be found in accidents involving relatively low force; the shape may be specific to the belt but any fine pattern will be that of the clothing closest to the skin. In accidents of severer type, the abrasion is more likely to be of the parchmented pressure type without pattern or vital reaction. The reflection of belt restraint in more serious injuries of internal type is discussed on p. 119.

Lacerations may have a 'general' specificity. Thus, notes should be available of damage to the legs of pedestrians which are characteristically caused by car bumpers and which may provide excellent evidence as to the positional relationship at the time of impact; very similar injuries are common in pedal cyclists knocked down by motor cars. Multiple lacerations due to fragmented glass are common in killed car occupants, particularly those in the front passenger seat; the distinction between those who have been so injured because they were not restrained by a belt and those who suffered injury when their belts failed can often be made by a simultaneous appraisal of abrasions in the harness area. On the other hand, lacerations may be very specific and diagnostic as to causation – this applies in both automobiles and light aircraft. *Plate* 8 shows an example of how two lacerations, which might well have been annotated as no more than 'multiple external injuries', indicated the cause of a light aircraft accident. This incident underlines

---

[2] For an interesting review of the early cases see *Br. Med. J.* (1974) Seat belts and damages. **2,** 454.

[3] Froom v. Butcher [1975] 3 All E.R.520. The case and its interpretation are discussed in *Br. Med. J.* (1975) Seat belts and negligence. **3,** 315. The importance of the merits of the individual case are emphasized in Owens v. Brimell [1976] 3 All E.R.765.

the importance of photography in the accident autopsy; the significance
of the lacerations shown was not appreciated until some time after the
post-mortem dissection.

INTERNAL INJURY WITHOUT EXTERNAL EVIDENCE

Severe or fatal deceleration injury may be transmitted to the internal
organs without corresponding visible external damage. The two common circumstances àre compression of the chest or abdomen and
accelerative displacement of the viscera.

Compression of the chest may result from impaction against some
object – such as the steering wheel of a car; superficial abrasive evidence
may then be found and the breast bone (sternum) and ribs can be
bruised or fractured. Alternatively, compression may be due simply to
forceful flexion of the upper torso – the head and knees being thrown
towards each other. This often occurs in motor cars when, the abdomen
being restrained by a belt, the legs and arms are flung forward with the
body compressed into a shallow C-shape; the condition is even more apparent in aircraft accidents when the severe vertical component of force
exaggerates the deformity. The heart may burst like a blown-up paper
bag if it is crushed between the breast bone and the spine. The weakest
areas lie in the atria, especially at the entry points of the great veins,[4]
but, often, the compression is such as to lacerate the muscular walls of
the ventricles. There may be important residua if the forces have been
severe yet insufficient to rupture the heart at the time of impact. A
lowering of the arterial blood pressure is an almost inevitable immediate physiological reaction to severe injury; areas of the heart which have
been damaged in the accident may be unable to withstand the increase
in pressure which accompanies the phase of recovery and delayed rupture of the heart may occur within minutes or hours. Additionally, the
process of rupture, which often runs from within the heart to the outside, may cause laceration of only a partial thickness of the muscle; the
wall in the area where the inner lining is thus damaged is weakened and
may rupture some considerable time after the event; a cause-and-effect
relationship may then be difficult to establish.

The heart will be displaced downwards if the major compression between the sternum and spine occurs just above its base (or upper
border); the aorta is, however, tethered to the tissues surrounding the
spine and is unable to move. As a result, the heart is torn from its major
blood vessel much as one squeezes a cherry from its stalk; the effect is
similar to rupture of the heart itself. This sequence is even more probable if the heart is, itself, displaced downwards under the influence of a

---

[4] Damage at these points may also be due to sudden increase in pressure in the venous
system due to compression of the legs or abdomen.

vertical force as occurs in falls or in aircraft accidents. The injury is common in both situations and, again, an incomplete laceration may result in delayed full thickness rupture (*Fig.* 12).

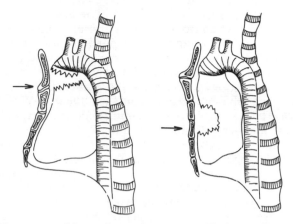

Fig. 12. Major rupture of the cardiovascular system. a, The heart will be torn from the aorta if the pressure on the breast bone is high. b, If the point of pressure is lower, the heart will burst like a paper bag.

Injuries of broadly similar type may be inflicted on the organs in the abdomen. These, by virtue of the organs' functions, may be of less catastrophic nature and prompt surgical intervention may be life-saving.

The great bulk of the liver renders it particularly susceptible to blunt injury. It is easily ruptured by bending and stretching of the upper surface during severe body flexion while its solid structure is particularly vulnerable to the high-frequency oscillations which are set up in a severe accident situation. Hepatic damage may well be fatal because bleeding from the organ is hard to stop and the liver, being essential to life, cannot be removed *in toto*. The almost equally common rupture of the spleen – which is a disposable organ as far as the body is concerned – or of one of the paired kidneys can be treated by removal of the damaged part; the important feature is awareness of the possibility that such injuries can be present despite the absence of external damage. Although rupture of the bowel itself is comparatively rare, compressive damage to its nutrient blood vessels as they traverse the mesentery is not uncommon in car accidents and occurs frequently in aircraft accidents; it may result from violent flexion alone but is more likely when this is combined with sudden and severe pressure on a simple lap belt.

The spine is under considerable strain in those conditions which produce sudden body flexion and, in practice, fracture of the thoracic spine is very common in both car and aircraft accidents. There are two primarily vulnerable points, firstly, in the upper spine if the torso is restrained by a full harness – in which case the forces are likely to be beyond the tolerance of the body as a whole – and, secondly, at the mid-point due to flexion over a lap belt. If severe vertical force is applied to the buttocks – as in a fall, an aircraft accident or, occasionally, in the unusual situation of ejection from a military aircraft – the spine is weakest at the junction of thoracic and lumbar portions. Very severe vertical force will cause fracture of the pelvis. The pelvis is also especially liable to damage from a direct lateral blow and fracture is common in pedestrian or cycling victims of road traffic accidents.

If the spine or pelvis are severely damaged, the sum of bodily injury may well have been sufficient to cause immediate death. Should there be recovery, the long-term disability resulting from fracture of the spine may be no more than stiffness and spasmodic pain of varying severity. If, however, the spinal cord is irrevocably injured, the extent of the resulting paralysis is related to the 'height' of the injury site in the spine; the common lower thoracic fracture is associated with paraplegia – that is, paralysis of the legs and bladder. Apart from the extremely severe disability, there is an increased danger of death due to infection, particularly infection of the urinary tract. The additional disability related to childbirth which may result from fracture of the pelvis in women also requires special consideration as to compensation accruing from an accident.

THE CONDITION OF FAT EMBOLISM

Fat embolism is a form of death, nearly always associated with accidents, which is of sufficient medico-legal interest to deserve individual consideration. It is closely correlated with fractures of the long bones, spine or chest cage though, theoretically at least, it may result from severe injury to fatty tissue of any sort. Following fracture, there is a release of fat from the marrow cavity; this fat is passed into the venous system where, being particulate, it is caught up in the sieve of the pulmonary capillaries – the condition of pulmonary fat embolism is established. Pulmonary fat embolism is of no clinical significance except in the aged with incipient heart failure; its main importance as a post-mortem finding is that it may be indicative of the time of survival between fracture and death (see p. 127). But in a proportion of fracture cases, the fat appears to pass through the lungs and lodges in the capillaries of the brain and kidneys; the potentially fatal condition of systemic fat embolism is established.[5] Some 24 hours after injury the patient's temperature rises and, in severe cases, fatal coma supervenes; treatment of the

---

[5] Precisely how often this occurs is difficult to assess. *Significant* systemic embolism occurs in perhaps as many as 1 per cent of fracture cases.

established condition is unsatisfactory. It is only fair to say that this précis is a gross oversimplification and the development of the clinical syndrome of systematic fat embolism probably depends on many inter-related factors including, particularly, the presence of surgical shock. Whatever the precise mechanism may be, two considerations are unaffected. Firstly, the condition is associated with injury in all but a handful of very unusual conditions and, as a result, it always has medico-legal connotations. Secondly, despite a tendency to an association with manipulation of fractures under anaesthesia, fat embolism is an unfortunate but natural complication of injury. These deaths are in no way associated with medical negligence.

PATHOLOGICAL APPRAISAL OF SAFETY EQUIPMENT

A correlation between the pathological findings and the safety equipment provided – whether the fatal accident results from the use of a vehicle or is of industrial type – is important for several reasons. Firstly, there is the problem of the assessment of damages in car accidents which has been discussed above. Secondly, dependants of an employee killed at work are entitled to any evidence which indicates failure on the part of the management to provide an adequate safety environment; the employer must also be provided with any evidence which might limit his liability as to civil damages. Thirdly, this aspect of his work must be of major professional interest to the pathologist in that the function of any doctor is to save lives; the autopsy following an accidental death provides an almost unique opportunity for the forensic pathologist in this respect – by applying his findings so as to convert fatal accidents to those of non-fatal type, he is practising good preventive medicine. This is a main function of a Coroner's Inquest or of an inquiry under the Fatal Accidents and Sudden Deaths Inquiry (Scotland) Act 1976.

Pathological evidence on this score should be available both when safety equipment was provided and when it was not.

In the former case, the pathologist is certainly not the best person to evaluate the equipment as, by definition, he is dealing with a case in which it has failed to preserve life. The question often arises, however, as to whether the equipment actually contributed to death; an objective assessment, taking all the circumstances into account, is then essential. A number of road traffic accident investigations describe 'seat belt syndromes' and there is no doubt that the seat belt – especially of the lap-strap-only type – can cause rupture of the mesentery, bowel or even major solid viscera. But the alternative to such a syndrome may well be death – and an operable rupture of the bowel is a small price to pay for a life saved. If the accident results in death from multiple injuries, the presence of lesions attributable to seat belts is no more than a part of the pattern of nonsurvivable loads on the body; but an isolated fatal injury positively associated with an intended safety device is of major concern. Thus, a number of fatalities have occurred in light aircraft due to the subject 'submarining' through the harness and sustaining injuries similar to those of the old judicial hanging – such accidents clearly indicate the need for incorporation of a crutch strap; it seems at least possible that the *combination* in a car of a diagonal torso harness *and* a markedly reclined driving seat might produce the same effect.

The pathologist should be able to answer the closely related problem of whether safety equipment which failed to save life could be so modified as to be of greater value in similar circumstances in the future. One example of such research, again stemming from light aircraft accidents, showed that approximately one-third of fatal head injuries discovered at post-mortem were in such a position as not to be preventable by the standard form of 'crash helmet' but the incorporation of an efficient visor skeleton would probably improve the survival rate appreciably.[6]

It should be emphasized that no item of personal safety equipment can be expected to be effective in all possible circumstances. Its design is a matter of compromise – 'child-proof' door locks on cars are, for example, potentially life-saving in ordinary travel but may be positively detrimental to survival in the event of fire after a crash; it is a matter of calculating the risks involved and providing accordingly, the important feature being that a positive assessment has been made and a reasonable decision taken. Escape by traditional means from an aircraft in flight provides another good example of the dilemma – the provision of a bulky dinghy pack must complicate easy egress but, without a dinghy, survival following a descent into water is compromised; the decision to provide a dinghy would, therefore, depend upon whether the aircraft was operating predominantly over land or over water.

In the event that death occurred when no equipment was provided, the pathologist can only surmise as to the likely effect of the omission; an attempt must be made because important questions relating to liability may be raised. In cases in which the material was lost or damaged, it would also be proper to seek pathological evidence as to whether equipment which had been provided was, in fact, used.

THE INTERRELATIONSHIP OF DISEASE AND ACCIDENTS

Natural disease may cause varying degrees of incapacitation in the operator of a vehicle and may, thus, precipitate an accident; such dis-

---

[6] *See* Cullen S. A. (1973), In: Mason J. K. and Reals W. J. (ed.) *Aerospace Pathology*, Chicago, College of American Pathologists Foundation.

ability is likely to be of more serious consequence in pilots than it is in drivers.[7] Further, the driver or pilot may actually die from sudden natural causes while at the controls and it is at least theoretically possible that a passenger might die in the same way while under the stress of an impending catastrophe. The precise relationship between discovered disease and a fatal accident is of medico-legal importance on two main counts – firstly, a suspicion of negligence may be raised either on the part of the operator, in that he was driving or piloting while he knew himself to be unfit, or on the part of those scheduling the task without apparently ensuring adequate medical supervision; secondly, questions may be raised as to the entitlement to indemnity under an insurance policy against accidental death in the event of actual natural death being followed by multiple injuries.

Disease of any sort discovered following an accident may be causative of, contributory to, or merely incidental to that accident. The distinction is often difficult to make; this is for two main reasons which are particularly well illustrated by coronary disease (*see* p. 90). Firstly, there is the simple 'population' problem illustrated in *Table I*; a random search of persons killed accidentally will demonstrate a high proportion with potentially lethal disease of the coronary arteries yet in few, if any, of the cases could there have been more than an incidental association. Secondly, there is the technical problem arising from the fact that the disease process may need to do no more than cause symptoms for it to precipitate a crash; death is then due to injuries and the pathologist is confronted with appearances in the heart which stop short of those which are seen in natural death – the interpretation of events then rests on an opinion as to cause and effect which has to be given with what must sometimes seem to be undue reservation. There is often less difficulty in automobile cases in which the findings may be those which are normally accepted as good evidence of a coronary 'heart attack' but these may then have to be distinguished from appearances resulting from injury to the heart – a problem which is also relevant to aircraft accidents.

In making his assessment, the pathologist must consider, on the one hand, the special quality of his autopsy findings which might distinguish significant from asymptomatic disease[8] and, on the other, the circumstantial details of the accident. He must also know the extent of the disease in the particular group of persons – e.g. drivers or pilots – concerned. Having all this information, he can ascribe the accident to

---

[7] Mason J. K. (1974) Comparative medical requirements for drivers and pilots. *J. Traffic Med.* **2**, 58.

[8] These include evidence of previous damage to the heart muscle (fibrosis), calcification of the coronary vessels and evidence of activity of the disease in the form of infiltration of the vessel's coat by white blood cells (adventitial lymphocytosis).

disease in the operator on a basis of probability running from, say, + (a significant association just possible) to ++++ (a very probable association) but it is doubtful if he should often be more definite. An account of how these problems of interpretation can be argued was given at the inquiry into the accident at Staines involving a Trident aircraft in 1972.[9] A further interesting fatal aircraft accident was reported in which a faulty instrument was discovered coincidentally with inflammation of the pilot's heart. The division of responsibility between the airline and the instrument manufacturers was of obvious significance; in the event, the case was decided out of court.[10]

Table I. OCCURRENCE OF CORONARY ARTERY DISEASE IN
UNITED KINGDOM AVIATORS

Grade of disease	Military		Civilian		Total	
	No.	% of group	No.	% of group	No.	% of group
0	114	40	38	34	152	38
1	103	36	48	43	151	38
2	46	16	16	14	62	15·5
3	23	8	10	9	33	8·5
Mean age	27·6		34·9		29·7	

In the United Kingdom, almost a quarter of persons subjected to relatively strict medical surveillance show occlusion of a main coronary vessel of 50 per cent or more without accompanying symptoms. (Grades 2 and 3.)

TOXICOLOGICAL FACTORS IN VEHICULAR ACCIDENTS

Toxic substances contributing to vehicular accidents may be deliberately ingested or accidentally inhaled. Alcohol is the outstanding example of first category and is discussed in detail in Chapter 25. Other drugs do play a part, the extent of which is at present undetermined. To be significant in accident causation, a drug must be readily available, it must be used generally for the treatment of common ailments and it must have a deleterious effect on concentration and performance; the antihistamines – widely used as cold cures – outstandingly fulfil this specification. Few of these drugs are subject to control by prescription (see p. 287) but when sold, the label must indicate that they may cause drowsiness. Amphetamines used to be a potential cause of accidents particularly when used to excess while night driving or when taken as weight controllers without appreciation of their effect on function; the group is now controlled under the Misuse of Drugs Act 1971. Other

[9] Report of the Public Inquiry into the Causes and Circumstances of the Accident near Staines on 18 June 1972. Civil Aircraft Accident Rep. 4/73 London, HMSO.
[10] For details, see Stevens P. J. (1970) Fatal Civil Aircraft Accidents. Bristol, Wright, p. 19.

commonly prescribed drugs – say, of the tranquillizer groups – may cause accidents by virtue of the taker being unaware of their intrinsic effect on driving or, more commonly, of the potentiating effect of combinations of drugs, particularly those which include alcohol. There are two major difficulties in assessing the role of such drugs in accident causation. Firstly, there is the technological problem of searching post mortem for the presence of virtually unknown substances in near therapeutic concentrations; to do so is generally beyond the laboratory's resources in manpower and finance. Secondly, there is, again, the problem of interpretation. Who, for example, is to say that a light aircraft pilot is any less safe when on a recognized dose of antinauseants than is the same pilot suffering from air sickness? And if traces of the drug are found at post-mortem, how is one to distinguish with certainty between a cause of and an incidental association with the accident?

Barbiturates, which are so commonly the cause of accidental poisoning in the home, are not thought to be a potent cause of vehicular accidents. Together with other drugs, they may, however, be a significant indicator of psychiatric or other nervous disease which is not demonstrable by standard post-mortem techniques – the prime example being epilepsy. Regulations are in force to prevent epileptics obtaining either an unrestricted driving licence or a pilot's licence but it is not difficult in present conditions for these to be bypassed. A search for barbiturates or anticonvulsants may, therefore, yield useful clues in indicating the basic cause of an apparently inexplicable accident.

Of the gaseous toxic factors in vehicular accident causation, only carbon monoxide deserves emphasis. Being a natural product of the internal combustion engine, it may leak into the cabin of the car through a faulty exhaust system or into an aircraft cockpit via a defective cockpit heater; carbon monoxide may also be drawn in from the exhausts of other cars if a car heater fan is connected in heavy traffic conditions.

Fatal levels of carbon monoxide in the blood are unlikely to be discovered in accidental deaths involving cars or aeroplanes; only a level sufficient to cause lack of concentration is required to cause an accident. Levels of 20–30 per cent carboxyhaemoglobin[11] are commonly associated with symptoms of dizziness and headache but there are two reasons why even lower levels may be of significance in drivers and pilots. Firstly, fine judgement is certainly affected at much lower levels. Secondly, a synergistic effect may result from the interaction of carbon monoxide, alcohol, fatigue or hunger while, in aviation, the effect of even slight oxygen lack due to altitude may be compounded to produce a most dangerous situation.

True intoxication of the operator is not the only possible cause of a

---

[11] That is to say, that 20–30 per cent of the normal respiratory haemoglobin of the blood is combined with carbon monoxide and is not available for the transport of oxygen.

raised carbon monoxide level discovered in the blood following a fatal vehicular accident. Survival in a fire after the crash is by far the commonest cause (see p. 165). Low levels, particularly in aircraft, may indicate an engine defect rather than an effect on the pilot while the 'natural background' of carboxyhaemoglobin – which may reach 8 per cent in heavy smokers – must be considered in the interpretation of results.

An analysis for carboxyhaemoglobin should be an integral part of the investigation of any vehicular death but, since levels of less than 20 per cent saturation may be of significance in the accident situation, the methodology must be adequate for the' purpose. The methodology should, indeed, be considered whenever a scientific result is obtained for medico-legal purposes. The technical method used must be shown to be adequate as to sensitivity and specificity at the range of the levels required and it must also be related both to the quantity of the specimen and to its quality – a method useful for examining good samples of blood taken from a living person may be quite inadequate when applied to a partially decomposed post-mortem specimen. The laboratory must be able to state its range of normal values when these factors are taken into consideration.

ACCIDENTS AS A CAUSE OF DISEASE

Although discussion has thus far centred on disease as a cause of accidents, the converse proposition is also of medico-legal importance.

Much of the debate on this subject has centred on the induction of cancer by injury; there is no doubt that this can occur, the most obvious example being the growth of a tumour in scar tissue – especially in scars resulting from burning. Skin cancer is relatively obvious and its topographical associations are clear. The attribution of cancer of the deep tissues to previous trauma is a far less certain matter due, in the main, to the time lapse between any precipitating injury and the clinical recognition of the tumour. Most interest has lain in the possible association of tumours of the brain with head injury although cancer of other tissues – for example, the breast – might well be related to injury. But accidental injury, albeit slight, to the head is commonplace while brain tumours are rare; moreover, even were it suggested that all such tumours were precipitated by injury – and it most certainly is not – the time interval would be such as to make it very difficult to decide which particular traumatic incident during that time represented the trigger mechanism. In an attempt to reconcile these difficulties, a set of rules, commonly known as 'Ewing's postulates', has been evolved. These lay down that, before a tumour can be reasonably attributed to injury:

   a. there must be evidence of previous normality of the part;

b. the injury must have been substantial;
c. the interval during which the tumour matured must have been of reasonable length;
d. the tumour must have developed at the site of injury;
e. the nature of the tumour must be scientifically proven.

Even accepting these premises, the attribution of a tumour to a previous traumatic incident is a matter of probability and there may be room for real divergence of expert opinion.

Similar reasoning can be applied to other types of disease which may be associated with trauma. Very often, there is little ground for disagreement. Thus, it would not be disputed that acute inflammation can be set up in a broken bone if virulent bacteria are present in the blood stream at the time of injury. Or, if a man's pelvis were fractured in a car accident and his bladder was repeatedly catheterized, subsequent damage to the kidneys due to ascending infection would clearly bear a cause-and-effect relationship with the accident.

More difficulty arises in relation to the repair of injury – scar tissue is inherently weak and the effect of its substitution for normal connective or muscle tissue in an organ may appear only some considerable time after the original incident. It has been noted above that the inner lining and associated muscle of the heart may be lacerated during a severe fall or vehicular accident; in the event of survival, such areas must be permanently weakened and liable to rupture. Similarly, bruising and local damage to the muscle fibres of the heart may be caused by direct injury to the chest wall – the area when repaired is likely to be of less than normal strength. The same type of blunt injury causes haemorrhage into the wall of, or into the tissues surrounding, the coronary arteries. In either case, the reparative fibrosis may cause restriction of the blood flow and a coronary 'heart attack' at an unpredictable point in the future. Relationships of this type are very much open to argument though few would deny the possibility of such a sequence of events occurring; as a consequence, expert opinions are likely to be very guarded.

SIMULTANEOUS DEATH

Prior to the late nineteenth century, the establishment of the precise order of death in relation to the disposal of estates seldom gave rise to difficulty. The advent of the steamship, the train and the increasing risk of major conflagrations then exaggerated the problem. By now, however, the increasing safety measures taken have greatly reduced the incidence of simultaneous death in close relatives; the solution of 'commorientes' is virtually a problem of fatal motor car and aircraft accidents with occasional cases arising from hotel fires.

The legal solutions to simultaneous death are, basically, of two types.

That operating in England and Wales states in general that, in the event of two (or more) persons dying in circumstances which make the order of death uncertain, the younger will be presumed to have survived the older.[12] In America, it is presumed that neither survived the other[13] and this rule is adopted by most central European and Scandinavian countries. France and Belgium include clauses in their codes to allow for extremes of age and for the legalistic nicety that, in similar adversity, the female is weaker than the male.[14] Since most wives are not only younger but are also less wealthy than their husbands, the clear defect of the English system is that it introduces a strong possibility that a finding of uncertainty as to which of the husband and wife survived the other may result in the male estate being diverted in ways which neither husband nor wife anticipated. This is because the test in deciding if s. 184 of the 1925 Act applies is not whether there *was* a simultaneous death but whether there was uncertainty as to which of two or more persons survived the others and the Courts appear to take the view that simultaneous death cannot be proved pathologically.[15] However, if the words 'simultaneous death' are used in a will, it is unlikely that the Courts will engage in metaphysical argument but will decide on common sense principles and on the medical evidence.[16] Scots law has recognized this imperfection and, while generally following that of England, has excluded 'spouse commorientes' from the general rule.[17] In fact, it would seem that, whenever possible, opportunity has been taken to adopt the American system – if, in England, one of the commorientes is intestate, then the estates devolve as if neither had survived the other.[18] Australia and New Zealand both followed the basic English system but New Zealand effectively reverted to the American code in 1958;[19] it is possible that legislation was precipitated when the law's manifest unfairness was demonstrated following the disastrous eruption of Mount Ruapehu the year before.

From the aspect of forensic medicine, however, it is not the differences in the systems which matter so much as that all have it in common that the presumption of simultaneous death is rebuttable by the evidence and that evidence of survival will be taken into consideration by the courts; such evidence must be provided mainly by the forensic

[12] Law of Property Act 1925, s. 184.
[13] Uniform Simultaneous Death Act, 8 Uniform Laws Annotated 608.
[14] *Code Civil*, Art. 720–722.
[15] Hickman v. Peacey [1945] A.C. 304 H.L.
[16] *Re:* Pringle, Baker v. Matheson [1946] Ch. 124, per Cohen J., at pp. 126, 129–131.
[17] Succession (Scotland) Act 1964, s. 31.
[18] Intestates Estates Act 1952, s. 1(4).
[19] Simultaneous Deaths Act 1958.

pathologist whose difficulties are compounded by the fact that no limit of time is set – survival of seconds is as significant in law as is survival for days.

Taking the commercial aircraft accident as a typical example, the useful pathological evidence may be of several types and of varying sophistication. Firstly, there is the precise cause of death. Thus, it could well be assumed that a person who had survived the crash only to die from burning would have survived longer than another who had sustained a rupture of the cardiovascular system. Such evidence should not, however, be accepted uncritically. Delayed rupture of the cardiovascular system – particularly of the atria or of the aorta – is a well-documented phenomenon (see p. 116). Moreover, the modes of death must be markedly dissimilar to be of good evidential value; thus, while the example above might well be valid, it would not be reasonable to suppose that a person with severe head injury had survived for a longer or shorter period than one with severe heart damage in the absence of other corroboration. Nor would it be right to assume that a person who had a greater overall degree of injury had necessarily predeceased someone with a single fatal injury.

The finding of carbon monoxide in the blood is objective evidence of an asphyxial death due to burning (see p. 165). A raised carboxyhaemoglobin in X compared with a negative result in Y could be taken to imply that X sustained a longer agonal period than did Y; but it would be wrong to reach the same conclusion if both showed raised values but X's level of carboxyhaemoglobin was higher than that of Y – such a difference could be related to the precise environment in which each died and to the pulmonary air intake of each, which could be affected by disease, by activity and other factors.

Further evidence of survival for a limited time may be provided in persons with fractured bones by the microscopical finding of particles of fat or of bone marrow in the lungs. Both these types of particle reach the lungs as described on p. 118; bone marrow particles provide the more unequivocal evidence because their structure indicates their origin beyond dispute. Nonetheless, bone marrow emboli are often difficult to find and a negative result might mean no more than that fragments which were present were not detected by the pathologist. Only a positive finding in indicating a definite time interval between injury and death is of true evidential value. Moreover, the *degree* of involvement of the lung in two persons cannot be used comparatively to assess the length of the survival period.

The pathological observations designed to distinguish in time between apparent simultaneous accidental deaths thus require very careful analysis. But they cannot be interpreted, unless they are sought; this implies the need for post-mortem dissection and for time-consuming and technically difficult follow-up investigations in the toxicological and microscopic fields. Quite opposing results as to the likelihood of relative survival may be obtained depending on the diligence and motivation of individual medical examiners. If justice is to be even in this sphere, the standards of autopsy must also be even – and this is unlikely to be so, particularly on an international scale. The disposal of a family estate may depend to a large extent on the precise geographical location of an aircraft crash and the routine use of 'survival' clauses in wills is therefore particularly important.

NOVUS ACTUS INTERVENIENS

It is a clear principle that a person is responsible not only for his actions but also for the logical consequences of those actions. This applies both in aggravated assault and in accidental injury. It is logical to assume that competent medical treatment will be available, if sought, for any injuries sustained. Should such treatment – or lack of treatment – be negligent and should that negligence result in a deviation from the logical sequence of events, then the responsibility for the subsequent disability or death may pass from the original incident to the later negligent action – this by virtue of *novus actus interveniens* (an unrelated action intervening). The majority of such interventions will be of a medical nature and the pathologist must provide evidence on this point in relevant cases.

The possible variations of *novus actus interveniens* are legion and no purpose would be served in listing potential causes – some may be obvious as, for example, the leaving of a surgical instrument in the abdomen following the repair of a treatable internal injury, while some may be more subtle.[20] The most vivid example in the author's experience was the accidental substitution of poisonous potassium chloride for the innocuous sodium chloride during treatment by the artificial kidney of a man injured in a road traffic accident.

Special problems associated with organ transplantation are referred to in Chapter 12. It is submitted that an element of negligence is essential to a plea of *novus actus*; an unforeseeable complication or a failure of a recognized form of treatment could not be so categorized. *Novus actus* often presents a difficult pathological problem and differences of expert opinion may be well held on such questions as the proportionate contribution to death of the original and the new events or as to whether an admitted error in treatment did, in fact, affect an inevitable outcome.

The concept of *novus actus* has an important bearing on procedure. Normally it is for the plaintiff or pursuer to prove the fact of negligence.

---

[20] *See*, for example, problems associated with the treatment of shock on p. 405.

But should the Court accept that a clear case of intervention exists, the onus shifts to the defender to show why he was not negligent. It would appear, particularly in Scottish Courts, that the proposition is rarely accepted.

Chapter 11

Head Injury

THE common head injuries which may occur either singly or in combination are bruising or laceration of the scalp; fractures of the skull – which must be divided into those involving the vault, which covers the upper and outer surfaces of the brain, or the base, on which the brain rests and through which the cranial nerves and the spinal cord pass; intracranial haemorrhage – which may be extradural, subdural or subarachnoid (*see* p. 16); laceration of the brain; and intracerebral haemorrhage. These injuries may be produced by sharp weapons or by blunt force; they may be homicidal, suicidal or accidental in origin. For practical purposes, suicidal head injuries, which will generally result from falls from a height, will be similar in nature to those of accidental origin; homicidal head injuries have only a few characteristics which distinguish them from such wounds elsewhere and will be discussed first; the bulk of this section will be concerned with accidental injuries.

The tissues of the scalp are comparatively dense and are lined internally by firm but very vascular fibrous tissue. Direct violence to the scalp which lies on the rigid vault of the skull results in a unique form of crushing between two hard objects. If the crush is of minor nature, a contusion or bruise will be produced; tracking of blood is likely to be slight in the dense connective tissue and, although bruising will usually be evident on both the outer and inner surfaces, it will commonly be more apparent on the deep aspect of the scalp. At the same time, since the scalp is held firmly over the skull, it is not unusual for the outer surface to reproduce the pattern of the weapon or object responsible for the violence. The skin will split when the compressive force is greater – the scalp is the classic place for lacerated wounds to be produced by blunt force; because the skull is convex, such lacerations may well be of linear type even when the object with which contact was made – for example, the roadway – was flat.

With the application of greater force, the underlying skull will fracture. The skull is not uniformly solid but is composed of two layers or tables of bone separated by spongy tissue. When struck, the skull will deform to some extent depending largely upon its age. A child's skull will bend before breaking; but since blood vessels will be torn in the process, head injury in children frequently shows a surprising degree of haemorrhage when compared with the relative lack of damage to the skull. Once the bounds of moulding are passed, the bone will break. In the adult, direct trauma could theoretically break only the outer table and, in these circumstances, a relatively perfect impression of the striking object would be reproduced; such a condition is very rare in practice. More usually, lines of stress fracture radiate from the point of contact while that part of the skull struck is depressed – a situation almost exactly comparable to striking the shell of a hard-boiled egg. These radiating fractures may damage blood vessels over a wide area thus explaining why death results from what seemed to be a relatively mild impact injury.

The membranes of the brain, with their accompanying blood vessels, may be crushed or torn beneath a depressed fracture; more seriously, the brain itself may be lacerated either by the actual instrument causing the external injury or by the fragments of bone which are forced inwards.

The above description illustrates the characteristics of homicidal head injuries. These may be modified by the precise type of weapon used – for instance, as between a cleaver and a baseball bat – and they may well be multiple, a factor which clearly provides evidence as to intent. Essentially, the injuries are local, are strongly related to the shape and size of the weapon and are not difficult to understand.

HEAD INJURY PREDOMINANTLY RELATED TO ACCIDENT

Fracture of the base of the skull is particularly dangerous not only because dissipation of the force needed to cause such an injury produces general effects on the brain but also because of local and indirect damage done to the blood vessels as they pass through the bone on their way to the vital centres controlling the life processes; these vessels are concentrated close to the *tentorium* and to the *foramen magnum* – the apertures through which the hindbrain and the spinal cord pass.

Fractures of the base may be continuous with those originating in and radiating from the vault of the skull. Thus, a blow to the front of the head, such as that sustained by an unrestrained front seat passenger in a car crash, may fracture the frontal bones and radiate into the anterior fossae – this is a specially dangerous injury because, in breaking into the frontal air sinuses, direct communication is established between the brain coverings and the outside air (*see below*); a blow to the side of the head, fracturing the temporal bone, is likely to radiate into the middle fossa of the base; a blow to the back of the head, as sustained in falling or being pushed over backwards, may produce a fracture which radiates into the posterior fossa and involves the foramen magnum. These fractures may be multiple and cause extensive 'comminution' or fragmentation of the bone.

Accidental force transmitted to the base of the skull is generally of two types. The commonest is that transmitted through the spine when the body falls heavily on the feet or buttocks; a fracture may be formed which surrounds the foramen magnum in a 'ring' and, in very severe cases, the spine may be driven into the skull cavity. The vault of the skull may then be burst open, giving the impression of an original massive fracture in that area. The distinction of this type of injury is of importance in forensic medicine as a similar ring fracture of the base can be caused by a severe blow to the vertex – in this case, however, the accompanying fracture of the vault will be depressed rather than of 'explosive' type. The second important transmitted fracture stems from the point of the chin – force is applied through the lower jaw to the base of the skull in the region of each ear and the middle fossae of the base shatter. Such an injury rarely results from a fist blow but is common when, say, a person falls on the chin in the roadway or when the chin is impacted on the instrument fascia of a car or light aircraft. The essential feature is the hardness of the object struck which influences the 'jolt' or rate of application of force (*Plate* 9).

CEREBRAL CONCUSSION

Head injury of more than minor severity will commonly be associated with loss of consciousness – in its simplest, short-lived, recoverable form this is known as concussion. In addition to losing consciousness, the patient enters a state of surgical shock (*see* p. 405), the severity of which greatly influences the rate of, or failure of, recovery. The precise cause of concussion is still disputed but is generally attributed to 'diffuse neuronal injury' which represents a functional abnormality of the nerve cells and of their connections rather than one with demonstrable pathological alterations in structure. The fact that no lesion can be shown is not, in itself, proof that none has been sustained; most would agree that some damage, in real terms, has been done and that this accounts for the late ill-effects of concussion from which an apparently good recovery has been made.

Concussion has several important medico-legal connotations. In the first place, it commonly produces a genuine state of retrograde amnesia for events immediately prior to injury – a concussed person is likely to be an unsatisfactory witness; secondly, the sufferer may be left with sequelae of varying severity which will be mentioned later; perhaps of greatest immediate importance, concussion is a signal of potentially severe intracranial injury – it is an indication for examining the skull by

X-ray and for retaining the patient under observation lest he develop an intracranial haemorrhage. Failure in these respects constitutes one of the more common bases of actions for negligence.[1]

INTRACRANIAL HAEMORRHAGE (*Fig.* 13)

Intracranial haemorrhage can be divided into extradural, subdural, subarachnoid and intracerebral types. The loss of blood is insignificant in comparison with the effects of the resultant raised pressure on the brain itself; this can act directly or indirectly and may result in extensive destruction of tissue. It is for this reason that the quantity and the type of bleeding – arterial or venous – are of major importance to the outcome.

Fig. 13. Four forms of intracranial haemorrhage. The dura is hatched; the arachnoid is shown as a solid black line. (The central structure is the normal ventricle of the brain).

Extradural haemorrhage refers to bleeding between the skull itself and the outer covering of the brain. It is very commonly, but not always, associated with fracture of the skull. Venous extradural haemorrhage may be due to disruption of small veins, and occasionally one of the large sinuses may give way. Tearing of a meningeal artery is, however, by far the commonest cause of this type of bleeding. Extradural haemorrhage is of particular medico-legal importance in two respects. Firstly, it is reasonably easy to treat and deaths from this cause should be rare. Secondly, there is typically an interval between injury and the onset of symptoms during which the patient, after an initial period of concussion, is per-

[1] But, overall, a fracture is present in only some 30 per cent of cases of concussion. X-ray examination, particularly in mild cases, might well be regarded as a form of insurance rather than as good medical economics. *See* Jennett B. (1976) Some medicolegal aspects of the management of acute head injury, *Br. Med. J.* **1**, 1383, for a discussion of the dilemma and the importance of a genuine medical need to justify X-ray examination.

fectly normal; there is, therefore, a tendency for patients to be discharged to home and for the onset of symptoms there to be unappreciated – it may be 12 hours before the injured person is returned to hospital by which time severe cerebral compression and brain damage may have occurred. The importance of observation of a patient who has been concussed is again stressed as is the frequent concurrence of this type of head injury with alcoholic intoxication – or the mimicry of the latter by the former; the death of such a case in a police cell is a tragedy which occurs not infrequently. If operative treatment of extra-dural haemorrhage is delayed, recovery may be complicated by emotional and intellectual disability.

Subdural haemorrhage occurs in the space between the dura and the arachnoid membrane. A large venous sinus may occasionally be lacerated but, commonly, the vessels torn are veins which are so small that no main bleeding point can be discovered either at operation or at post-mortem. This type of bleeding is not necessarily associated with fracture and results particularly from movement of the brain in relation to bone and to the relatively fixed dura mater. By its nature, subdural bleeding will take some time to produce symptoms; generally this is a matter of hours but the effect of bleeding is aggravated by concurrent respiratory embarrassment and the consequent hypoxia. This 'latent interval' may be of very great importance in the assessment of nonaccidental head injury in children; at post-mortem in such cases, it is often clear that blood has been collecting over a long period.

An interesting variation is seen in adults. Because the bleeding can be so slow, the body has time to contain the extravasation which then becomes firmly fixed to the underside of the dura by fibrous tissue. Very often, such 'chronic subdural haematomas' are symptomless – or cause a general confusion of the intellect which is attributed to 'getting on in years'. Occasionally, however, the collection of blood may continue to expand and severe symptoms may appear several months after the original injury – a cause-and-effect relationship is perfectly plausible despite the lapse of time.

Subarachnoid haemorrhage has been noted in Chapter 7 as a fairly common form of sudden natural death; it is also a frequent sequel to injury. Subarachnoid haemorrhage occurring alone must be suspected of being due to spontaneous rupture of a congenital aneurysm or of having been caused by injury to a vessel which was already weakened by aneurysmal changes. Another explanation, which has been recognized only relatively recently, is that the haemorrhage may result from damage to the vertebral artery arising as part of injury to the neck rather than to the head – the importance of this both in relation to the history of the case and the post-mortem examination is obvious; such subjects are frequently under the influence of drink. Otherwise, subarachnoid haemorrhage after injury is usually seen in combination with bleeding in other sites. In particular, there is usually some contusion of the brain, the generalized haemorrhage being due to local rupture of small vessels. Alternatively, massive subarachnoid haemorrhage may be no more than an extension of a severe intracerebral haemorrhage.

Intracerebral haemorrhage may be of two types. The first represents only contusion of the superficial areas of the brain. The distribution of such contusions as related either to bruising of the scalp or to fracture of the skull is of major importance. Injury to the brain may be local and direct – thus, if the skull is struck with a weapon and a depressed fracture is caused, the brain will be contused or lacerated at the point of impact. But brain damage as a whole – and particularly that resulting from accidents – requires a more subtle explanation which is based on the fact that, when the skull is accelerated or decelerated, the contained brain tends to continue moving; since it is attached more securely at some points than at others, it will be damaged elsewhere than at the point of application of external force. If the acceleration is rotational, sheer forces will be set up; if deceleration is linear, 'cavitation' will occur between the brain and skull as the brain tends to 'pile up' in its rigid covering. The results will be tissue damage and extravasation of blood at a distance from the point of impact and skull fracture. The cerebral contusion associated with a moving head – as, for example, one which strikes the roadway following a fall or one which impacts the windscreen in a car crash – will appear characteristically at the site precisely opposite to that of primary impact; this is known as '*contre-coup*' haemorrhage. The important diagnostic feature is that the finding of internal bruising remote from the primary external injury clearly indicates *motion* of the head at the time it was sustained.

Deep intracranial haemorrhages are also caused by indirect injury; they are also particularly associated with movement of the head and, therefore, with road traffic accidents. The lesions result from tearing of the deep arterioles – again, usually those which are the most common sites of natural haemorrhage due to disease; the distinction between haemorrhage which results from an accident and that which causes an accident may be difficult to make (*see* Chapter 10). The incompressible brain resists the extension of such haemorrhages and death may be delayed – but consciousness is not regained as so often occurs when extradural haemorrhage follows head injury. Deep haemorrhage in the absence of severe external damage is particularly common in young persons. Intracerebral haemorrhage is always serious but is almost inevitably fatal when it occurs in the brain stem, the site of the centres vital to life. Brain stem haemorrhage may be primary – that is, caused during the traumatic event; it may also be secondary to raised intracranial pressure from other causes and frequently underlies delayed death following head injury.

CEREBRAL LACERATION

Cerebral laceration may be caused directly either by an object which penetrates the skull or by fragments of bone which are driven inwards. In the event of widely radiating fractures with extensive isolation of skull fragments, there may be equivalent tears in the superficial substance of the brain.

Alternatively, severe *'contre-coup'* forces may cause actual laceration opposite the point of impact while rotational forces may drive the brain substance into the natural ridges which are found in the base of the skull. There is less restraint on the movement of the brain if the skull is fractured and, in these circumstances, the cerebrum or cerebellum may be torn from the brain stem.

The effect of cerebral laceration must vary with its location. Thus, a small laceration in the brain stem may well be fatal while comparatively major damage in the frontal area may provoke no serious sequelae in the absence of haemorrhage. In practice, laceration of the brain is commonest in the frontal and temporal lobes.

CEREBRAL OEDEMA

After trauma to the head, the patient very often falls into progressively deeper coma despite the fact that no localized haemorrhage is present; the condition of cerebral oedema, or swelling of the brain, is established.

The precise cause of this condition is uncertain. The effect is that the veins, rather than the arteries, are first compressed as the size of the brain increases while the circulation of cerebrospinal fluid is also compromised – the condition is, therefore, self-perpetuating and can cause death in its own right.

The pathological evidence of such swelling will often be referred to in the post-mortem report as 'herniation of brain substance'. The increase in pressure may force the undersurface of the temporal lobe through the tentorial opening at each side of the midbrain ('tentorial' or 'uncal' herniation) or the cerebellum may be pushed through the foramen magnum ('tonsillar' herniation). A further form of herniation which may be described in the pathologist's report results from escape of brain tissue through burr holes made in the skull in an attempt to relieve the condition.

The main significance of cerebral oedema, other than a death which is directly attributable, lies in the secondary effects of brain stem compression associated with 'tentorial herniation'. The interference with the cerebral blood flow which results may be such as to destroy the higher cortical centres while leaving those responsible for vital functions intact – the result can be a decerebrate person existing reflexly and without apparent awareness or volition.

While oedema is a common cause of the compression syndrome, similar effects can be produced by a large haemorrhage or other lesion which occupies space in the cranial cavity.

LONG-TERM EFFECTS OF HEAD INJURY

If a portion of brain is damaged by injury, there will be localized effects of varying severity and expression which depend upon the precise area involved. A detailed description of potential disabilities cannot be undertaken here – the problems are covered in textbooks of neurology.

Some mention must be made of the generalized pathological conditions or symptoms which may properly be attributed to injury. Sepsis may be introduced through an open wound of the skull – especially one involving the nose. The origin of this may be obvious if the open fracture involves the vault of the skull. Fracture of the base of the skull, which may communicate with the outside through either the nose or ear is less easy to detect and is certainly harder to repair. Generalized infection or overt abscess formation attributable to such injuries may be delayed for days or weeks. Even in the absence of infection, a distressing leak of cerebral spinal fluid may persist for some time.

Neuropsychiatric sequelae are considered in more detail in Chapter 28. Many persons suffer after head injury from chronic headache, loss of concentration and unexplained attacks of giddiness. Post-traumatic epilepsy occurs after head injury without fracture in some 3 per cent of cases and follows 16 per cent of severe head injuries.

THE PREVENTION OF HEAD INJURY

The prevention of head injury is of major concern in mining, in the construction industries in general and, of greatest general importance, in vehicular transportation.

Different forms of head protection have been developed for the various situations. Because it has to protect against impacts of very varying intensity and direction, the helmet used in transportation is the most sophisticated and merits a short consideration.

The prototype helmet on which nearly all models now in use are based was developed by the Royal Air Force, the major design feature being the separation of the skull from the hard shell by the use of a suspension harness. The importance of a good fit was apparent at an early stage of development and the need for ear flaps was emphasized by the number of head injuries which were found to originate in the temporal region. The introduction of head protection in military aviation coincided with the emergence of very high-performance aircraft; the forces involved in crashes of such aircraft generally exceed by far the protective capacity of any reasonable helmet and, currently, the main safety function of the military aviator's helmet is to protect against the buffeting associated with low-altitude high-performance flight and against the possibility of injury during the course of in-flight escape. It is disheartening to see that helmets are seldom used in the one form of flying where they would provide maximum benefit – that is, in light private aviation; there are no regulations to compel a civilian flier to protect himself in this way.

The use of helmets in motor car racing is dictated by both domestic and international controlling organizations. It would be too much to expect the ordinary driver or front-seat passenger in a family motor car to wear protective head-gear – although some lives would certainly be saved thereby – but there is undoubtedly a case for their use in open sports cars. This is because, in addition to windshield contact injuries – the prevention of which is largely a matter of shoulder harness (*see* Chapter 10) – preventable skull injury in road traffic accidents stems from secondary impact with the roadway following ejection from the vehicle.

Of all the vehicles in which this type of injury occurs, the motor cycle stands supreme and it is now compulsory by law in the United Kingdom to wear a 'crash helmet' while driving or travelling on a powered vehicle of motor cycle type;[2] such helmets must conform to designated standards.[3] It is interesting to speculate on why these regulations should have been accepted so readily while there is such opposition to the compulsory use of restraining harness in motor cars;[4] both would seem to conflict equally with the concept of individual liberty in the matter of self-protection. While it is true that helmets have an added ornamental function, their current acceptance strongly indicates that the public as a whole would agree to more stringent compulsory safety regulations.[5]

---

[2] Motor Cycles (Wearing of Helmets) Regulations 1973 (SI 1973 No. 180), made under Road Traffic Act 1972. But *see also* Motor-Cycle Crash-Helmets (Religious Exemption) Act 1976.

[3] Road Traffic Act 1972, s. 33.

[4] *See* the Parliamentary Debates on the Road Traffic (Seat Belts) Bill 1976 and its later rejection by the House of Lords (*The.Times*, 27 April, 1977, p. 10).

[5] The Courts take a similar attitude to contributory negligence in relation to safety helmets as in relation to restraining harnesses – O'Connell v. Jackson [1971] 3 W.L.R.463.C.A. This attitude to head protection applies also in industrial accidents.

Chapter 12

Transplantation of Organs and the Human Tissue Act

MECHANICAL organ substitutes are often bulky, they restrict the life style of the user, they may break down and, ultimately, some form of incompatibility arises between patient and machine – e.g. there is thrombosis of the vessels, infection and the like. The concept of transplantation of actual biological organs is, therefore, extremely attractive from both therapeutic and economic aspects.

The major difficulty in the procedure, apart from the required technical expertise, lies in the rejection by the body of foreign substances (or antigens), a principle which has been discussed in Chapter 1. The more 'foreign' the substance, the more rapid and inevitable will be the body's resistance to the graft. In the present state of knowledge, transplantation or organs, from, say, apes to man is impossible; all organs for human transplantation must be obtained from human donors. The closer the antigenic similarity between recipient and donor, the more likely is acceptance of the transplant. Antigenic similarity is, however, by no means the simple matter described under paternity testing and blood transfusion (Chapters 18 and 31); far more subtle relationships are involved and, apart from identical twins, the chances of finding two persons completely 'graft compatible' are negligible; at best, some – for example, siblings – are less incompatible than others. It follows that:

a. Transplantation must be accompanied by efforts to reduce the instinct of the recipient to reject the donated organ (immunosuppression).

b. Immunosuppression in humans cannot, as yet, be selective. The defences of the body against invasion are, therefore, reduced overall – e.g. against bacterial infection.

c. The body may still reject the graft when, ultimately, its powers to do so exceed the available immunosuppressive methods.

But any transplant must be viable in its own right if it is to be useful. A donation from a living person is more likely to succeed than is one from a dead donor and, in the latter case, success will be inversely proportional to the length of time between death and donation. Two problems of ethical and medico-legal importance arise – the lesser one of consent to make a living donation and the major issue of obtaining cadaver specimens.

The propriety of live donation of organs for transplantation depends on three main factors. Firstly, there should be a reasonable prospect of the transplant being successful; it might be legal for a man to consent but it would certainly be unethical for a physician to encourage him to do so unless the recipient were a close relation by consanguinity or a very accurate matching had been achieved.

Secondly, the benefit to the recipient must far outweigh the likely detriment to the donor. Potential donations are of three types:

   a. of tissues which are readily replaceable, blood being the most obvious example, which cause no difficulty;
   b. at the other extreme, of organs which are essential to the life of the donor. Since consent is no defence to a charge of homicide, removal of such organs in life must clearly be illegal;
   c. of one of paired organs, the remaining one of which would be capable of maintaining life so long as it were healthy; for all practical purposes, this limits consideration to a kidney. Consent to such a donation may well be properly obtained but this can be only after a very full explanation has been given. One would feel that two doctors should be required to certify that the donor has fully considered the implications, though there is certainly no requirement in law for such a practice.[1]

Finally, the donor must be capable of consent as described in Chapter 30. The major problem specific to the present discussion is whether parents or guardians can give consent for a minor to undergo a surgical procedure which can be of no benefit to him or her. Although Lord Kilbrandon appears to have given tacit approval,[2] it is doubtful if such practice would be wholly desirable because it is unlikely that a child would fully understand a complex subject and because the possibility of a child subsequently needing his own donated organ may be greater than is so in an adult.

A major advantage of living donation is that it allows time for full appraisal of all aspects of the case. No such latitude is available in

---

[1] The South African Union Anatomical Donations and Post Mortem Examinations Act 1970 does require certification by two doctors in the case of donation of 'naturally irreplaceable tissue'.

[2] As quoted by Meyers D. W. (1970) *The Human Body and the Law*, Edinburgh, University Press, p. 123.

cadaver transplants – kidneys must be removed from the dead body within 30–60 minutes of circulatory failure and, in general, can be stored no longer than 12 hours. The moment of death has been described by Simpson as 'the starting pistol for a race to save life'.

Organs for transplantation must be healthy and it follows that, apart from some occasional cases of fatal natural cerebral disease, violent deaths will provide the major source of donations. Apart from those professionally concerned with the transplant procedure there are, thus, two groups of persons with a practical interest in the provision of cadaver organs. The medico-legal authorities, represented by the Procurator Fiscal or the Coroner, and those 'lawfully in possession' of the dead body. The position of both of these must be considered.

The main problem related to those 'in lawful possession of the body' lies in the definition of 'lawful possession' as now applied. The discussion involves three parties – the deceased, the authorities in charge of the place where the body died and the next of kin.

Under English, Scots and American common law, the deceased has very limited rights as to the disposal of his body and, in the event of conflict, the wishes of the next of kin would normally be supported rather than those of the dead person irrespective of how the latter had expressed his intentions. The common law position appeared to be supported by the Secretary of State for Health and Social Security in 1973.[3] Statute law is, however, tending to replace common law. In America, the Uniform Anatomical Gift Act has done much to regularize and standardize the situation; the Human Tissue Act 1961 now serves the same purpose in the United Kingdom.

Section 1 of the British Act deals, firstly, with the situation when the deceased has asked during his life that his body should be used for transplant donorship. Then, the 'person lawfully in possession of the body' after his death may authorize the removal of any part of his body for use as requested. In the absence of a specific request, subsection (2) empowers the 'person lawfully in possession' of the body to authorize removal of organs 'if, having made such reasonable enquiry as may be practicable, he has no reason to believe (*a*) that the deceased had expressed an objection to his body being so dealt with after his death and had not withdrawn it; or (*b*) that the surviving spouse or any surviving relative of the deceased objects to the body being so dealt with'.

The Act thus poses three uncertainties of importance to those engaged in transplant surgery.

Firstly, what constitutes 'reasonable enquiry'? A recent authoritative opinion believes this must be interpreted in relation to the time available;[3] it would appear to be *unreasonable* to carry enquiries beyond the

[3] *Br. Med. J.* (1973) **3**, 360.

point in time when a viable transplant would be unlikely.

Secondly, it must be decided whether the Act is speaking of those 'in possession' of the body – who are clearly the hospital authorities – or of those 'with a right to possession' – who are the next-of-kin; obviously, there may be a saving of time and, possibly, an increase in available treatments, if the former interpretation is correct. There is some doubt on this at the time of writing. The English Medical Defence Union expressed firmly the opinion that it was the executors or relatives of the dead person who had to authorize the removal of any organ. On the other hand, Lord Kilbrandon in Scotland and Lord Edmund Davies in England clearly believe that, for the purposes of the Act, the Hospital Board are lawfully in possession of the body. In this, they have the support of the British Medical Association.[3] The Act itself infers the correctness of this view – in Section 1 (6), undertakers are specifically excluded as being in possession of the body for the purpose of authorizing organ donation while, in Section 1 (7), allowance is made for the delegation of authority within the hospital. If there is no authority, how can this be delegated?

The third question – that of the legal significance of a living person's declared desire to dispose of his body after death – has already been raised; the effect on such 'authorizations' as 'kidney donor cards' is obviously a matter of concern. If the relatives are 'in lawful possession' of the body, they may well be legally entitled to refuse to authorize organ donation even under Section 1 (1) of the Human Tissue Act.[4] One cannot help feeling that, if put to the test, modern opinion would approve the principle that, so long as the instructions given are reasonable and not contrary to public health or decency, a person has a right to dispose of his body in the same way as of anything else he controls in life.

All these considerations are, of course, subject to the authority of the Fiscal or the Coroner. Nearly always they will be 'the appropriate authority' for disposal of the body and it is axiomatic that there must be no interference with a body so constrained unless specific permission is granted – unauthorized removal of tissue is expressly prohibited under

---

[3] *Br. Med. J.* (1973) **3**, 360.

[4] Although accompanied by the proviso that the matter can be finally determined only by the Courts, NHS Circular 1975 (Gen) 34, issued in May 1975, leaves no doubt that the person lawfully in possession of the body is the Health Board or Area Health Authority responsible for the hospital. Only if and when the deceased's executors or relatives ask for the body to be handed over to them do they take over lawful possession of the body from the Board. It is further stated that, if the relatives or executors ask that the body be handed over to them after an authorization under Section 1 (1) has been given, this action does not revoke the authorization which continues to be legally effective. The Circular states that, if the deceased during his lifetime had recorded an appropriate request, then it would, in these circumstances, be reasonable for the authorization to be acted upon.

the Human Tissue Act s.1 (5). But since speed is essential and no authority wishes to obstruct unreasonably a potentially life-saving measure, most Fiscals and Coroners agree to prior discussion of cases – which, incidentally, allows time for inquiry – and the consequent immediate granting of permission in the event of death.[5] Previous inquiry will dispose of the possibility that the removed organ may have been of importance to the medico-legal investigation – in practice, this will only be of major concern in heart transplantation. The possibility, although remote, of the entry of a plea of *novus actus interveniens* does suggest that patients whose death is likely to be the subject of criminal proceedings should not be used as transplant donors; the decision rests, however, with the appropriate authority.[6]

It is everywhere appreciated that persons dying in hospital as a result of previous violence may well be maintained in a state of animation by machine and, before any third parties become involved, these cases present a frightening dilemma on two counts – 'what is death?' and 'who is responsible for death if "life" is dependent on a machine?'.

Many attempts have been made to relate death to scientific tests, particularly to a negative tracing on the electroencephalogram, but none is entirely satisfactory. The United Kingdom legislature has refused to provide any such definition, preferring to leave each case to the judgement of the physician in charge. The following quotation from a statement by the World Medical Association in 1968 sums up the position:

This determination [of death] will be based on clinical judgement supplemented if necessary by a number of diagnostic aids (of which the electroencephalograph is currently the most helpful). However, no single technological criterion is entirely satisfactory in the present state of medicine, nor can any one technological procedure be substituted for the overall judgement of the physician.[7]

The definition of 'physician' is important. Most authorities would certainly agree with the recommendation of the Advisory Group on Transplantation Problems (1969) that two doctors should collaborate in making such an important and debatable decision. Furthermore, it must be regarded as mandatory that the physicians pronouncing life extinct should have no professional association with the transplant team.[8]

The question as to who causes death when the machine is turned off

---

[5] Such 'permission' is still confined by the interpretation of s. 1(1) and 1(2) of the 1961 Act.

[6] R. v. Potter (*Med. Leg. J.* (1963) **31,** 195). In this unusual case, a man was committed for trial by the Coroner on a charge of manslaughter. His victim was used as a 'beating heart' donor (*see below*). At the subsequent trial he was convicted only of common assault.

[7] British Medical Association *Handbook for Members* (1970) p. 73.

[8] Positively enacted in the Uniform Anatomical Gift Act of the USA.

does not arise if this procedure is adopted – the patient is already adjudged dead and is certified as such. It is worth reiterating that death is an absolute concept and its recognition is a technical, not an ethical, exercise; the 'switch operator' has clearly no part in the process. This is, however, not to say that temporary removal of support may not be used as a test of death; it may be, and is, very properly so used particularly in respect of defining 'brain death'.

The terms 'brain death' and 'beating heart donor' are now widely used and require some explanation. It will be clear from what has been said before that the functional success of a transplanted organ is related inversely to the length of time it has been anoxic – that is, deprived of an efficient circulation. It would, therefore, be of immense value to recipients if the function of the heart and lungs of a dead person could be mechanically maintained until the kidneys were removed for immediate transplantation. Such conditions can be achieved relatively easily in some instances, particularly those involving death from head injury; the 'beating heart' donor is a feasible entity.[9] The traditional importance of the heart beat as a parameter in the definition of death must then be superseded by the failure of the primitive brain's ability to stimulate the vital cardiorespiratory functions; if it can be shown to be permanently incapable of doing so unaided, then 'brain death' has occurred and the death of the organism can be certified although individual parts may be kept alive in a 'support only' situation. Very stringent criteria are laid down for justifying this clinical diagnosis. These include the exclusion of hypothermia or drug overdosage as causes of coma; there should be no spontaneous respiration over a period of 3 minutes' observation and no spontaneous movement; no brain stem reflexes should be present; the pupils must be dilated and corneal and gag reflexes must be absent; there must be no response to pressure above the eyes and eye lag on moving the head must not occur. If all these tests are unequivocal on two occasions 12 hours apart, then the brain stem can be said to be dead.[10] Very obvious possibilities for transplanting organs of greatly improved quality are then opened up. It is, however, often inadequately appreciated that concepts such as 'brain death' are not intended to increase the authority of the transplant surgeon but rather to improve the methods of establishing the fact of death so that maximum benefit can accrue to the recipient. Moreover, the acceptance of 'brain death' is urged by neurosurgeons, many of whom regard the artificial maintenance of a subject with irrecoverable failure of the brain as inhumane.

---

[9] There is, indeed, a medico-legal possibility – and perhaps reality in the United States – that to transplant anything other than the 'best possible' organ could be construed as medical negligence.

[10] Brain death. *Br. Med. J.* (1975) **1**, 356.

While the vast majority of the medical profession would accept these principles, unqualified public approval is, presently, less certain; perhaps one of the most unsatisfactory aspects of the current position is the general failure to establish acceptable international criteria.[11]

The beating heart donor introduces a further minor administrative medico-legal problem in that a certificate must be supplied in respect of a death which is clearly to be the subject of a Fiscal's or Coroner's postmortem examination. In practice, this presents little difficulty as both authorities have the power to override the terms of a certificate should the need be indicated by their inquiries. In addition, it is common practice for the pathologist who is to perform the autopsy to be present when the organs are removed from the cadaver.

There is little doubt that the subject of organ transplantation is now dominated by public opinion and it is probable that a major advance in statute law will only be achieved when kidney donation, which is now recognized as an established method of saving valuable lives, is separated from the more experimental and flamboyant procedures, of which heart transplantation generates the most emotion. This probably stems from the fact that, in a cardiac transplant, one is removing an organ which is still supporting life no matter how imperfectly and is replacing it by something which must, in the present state of knowledge, fail sooner rather than later – at which point the situation is irretrievable. No such absolute limitations affect kidney transplants which are usually performed only as a substitute for mechanical supports to which return can reasonably be made in the event of biological rejection. The failure of the Renal Transplantation Bill to reach the Statute Book in 1968 on technical considerations seems to have been most unfortunate.

The British Transplantation Society has put forward, as a matter for discussion, the suggestion that the Human Tissue Act 1961 should be amended so as to allow the person lawfully in possession of the body to authorize removal of organs without having to take positive steps to ascertain whether there were objections on the part of the next of kin[12] – put another way, the onus would be on individuals to 'contract out' of a cadaver donor system in the event of objection. The author's limited experience with public opinion on the matter suggests that the modification would be unacceptable; in practice, the very great majority of cases likely to provide organ donations are accompanied to hospital by relatives whose opinions must be sought and respected.

---

[11] The interested reader is referred to a most useful review by van Till A. (1975) How dead can you be?, *Med. Sci. Law* **15**, 133.

[12] British Transplantation Society (1975) The shortage of organs for clinical transplantation: Document for discussion. *Br. Med. J.* **1**, 251.

Chapter 13

Asphyxia

ASPHYXIA is here defined as the result of interference with the oxygenation of the red blood cells. Tissue hypoxia due to anaemia, which is a deficiency of the red blood cells themselves, is therefore excluded from discussion.

Asphyxia is of five main types (*see Fig.* 3, p. 13):

   a. Mechanical – in which the airways are blocked in an unnatural fashion.
   b. Pathological – where the transfer of oxygen to the lungs is prevented by disease of the upper air passages or of the lungs themselves.
   c. Toxic – whereby poisonous substances prevent the uptake of oxygen.
   d. Environmental – or an insufficiency of oxygen in the inspired air.
   e. Iatrogenic – or caused by the medical profession and mainly associated with anaesthesia.

All of these have some medico-legal significance which is probably greatest in the case of mechanical asphyxia.

MECHANICAL ASPHYXIA

Atmospheric oxygen may be excluded from the lungs at various levels.

Firstly, the nose and mouth may be obstructed – the process of *suffocation*.[1] Secondly, the glottis – or upper entry to the air passages – may be blocked as in *choking* due to impaction of food or of a gag. The most important level of occlusion in the context of forensic medicine is at the larynx, where the process is generally described as *strangulation* – if this is accomplished by hand alone it is manual strangulation or *throttling*; strangulation by ligature or cord may also be performed manually, the most specific example being *garrotting*, or it may result from

---

[1] Total occlusion of the nose and mouth by liquid – that is, drowning – is described separately in Chapter 14. Although suffocation also results from burial in trenches following land falls etc., the results are then very comparable to those described later under 'traumatic asphyxia'.

suspension, i.e. *hanging*. Still lower in the air passages, the whole trachea or a main bronchus may be blocked following *inhalation* of foreign bodies or of stomach contents. Finally, the muscles of respiration may themselves be immobilized, for example, by crushing; the condition known as *traumatic asphyxia* results.

Suffocation

Unnatural suffocation in infancy presents one of the most difficult problems in forensic pathology. It is a simple matter to place a pillow over a baby's face leaving, as likely as not, no evidence of external pressure. The only signs demonstrable at autopsy will then be those of anoxia in general, which can be summarized as:

a. Cyanosis. In the absence of oxygen, most of the oxyhaemoglobin will be converted to and remain in its reduced form; the colour of this is of dark plums which will be seen in the skin. This sign is of little medico-legal value for two main reasons. In the first place, death itself is a matter of permanent tissue anoxia; some degree of cyanosis is therefore found in most natural deaths and may be very marked in those due to cardiac failure. Secondly, an asphyxial death must be of relatively prolonged type if there is to be sufficient conversion of the blood pigment as to be readily identifiable as to cause.

b. Venous congestion. Failure of the right side of the heart, with stagnation of blood in the veins, is an accompaniment of all asphyxial deaths save those which terminate suddenly. Congestion of the lungs is most common but, as this is a frequent finding in natural heart failure, its significance is but slight; major diagnostic importance is confined to systemic congestion – that is, congestion of the skin and of the organs other than the lungs. A main result of venous congestion is capillary rupture and consequent formation of *petechial haemorrhages* which are almost always found in asphyxial deaths.[2] The distribution of these haemorrhages is of diagnostic importance and is greatly influenced by:

i. Impairment of the venous exit from the capillaries. Thus, pressure on the veins of the neck while the heart continues to beat, as in strangulation, will cause local pressure in the capillaries of the head – petechiae will, therefore, be pronounced in the eyes and on the face.

ii. The nature of the tissue. The capillaries will give way more readily where they are least supported – thus petechiae will appear to be more concentrated in fatty fibrous tissue such as the eyelids.

iii. General visibility. Other than on the skin, petechiae will be

[2] This evidence of asphyxia was first described in infant suffocation by a French police surgeon; as a result, the haemorrhages are frequently referred to as 'Tardieu spots'.

most readily visible when confined by a transparent membrane. Internally, therefore, they are seen most frequently on the lungs beneath the pleura or on the heart beneath the pericardium. In infancy, they are often obvious beneath the covering of the thymus gland and, in severe asphyxia, they will be seen underneath the inner covering (mucosa) of the pharynx, larynx and other hollow organs.

iv. Intensity of congestion. The intensity of congestion may be such as to cause the petechiae to coalesce into larger haemorrhage; if the pressure builds up still further, the covering material may rupture and frank bleeding will occur.

Although back pressure is a major factor causing the petechiae, a deficiency of oxygen alone will damage the capillaries; since such a deficiency must occur during any process of dying, the question arises as to whether petechiae can be found following natural death. There is certainly no shortage of written authority to the effect that they *can* be.[3] In these circumstances, the 'spots' are usually confined to the pleural surface of the lungs, most often between the lobes. The distinction between 'natural' petechiae found in this situation and those resulting from asphyxia is essentially a matter of quantitation; the former are generally few in number and must be sought with determination.

c. Oedema. Hypoxic damage to the capillaries will result in increased permeability of their walls which will allow the passage of fluid plasma rather than of particulate red blood cells; oedema (or 'water in the tissues') will accompany asphyxia provided the hypoxic stimulus is relatively long lasting. The process is generally best demonstrated in the lungs. Again, the distribution of oedema may be important as its production will be exaggerated by intravascular pressure – thus, oedema of the face, tongue and pharynx is a feature of strangulation.

The suffocated infant, therefore, may well show no more than generalized congestion with the formation of petechial haemorrhage on the surface of the lungs, heart and thymus; the changes are nonspecific and their interpretation must depend to a large extent on the circumstantial evidence. Suffocation by the hand may leave identifiable evidence because the generalized congestion of asphyxia will not develop at the points of pressure; there may be similar findings on the back of the head if the baby's face has been forced into a pillow. Such appearances must be distinguished from the normal effects of hypostasis which are present in 'cot deaths' (*see* p. 248); in these cases, the baby has often been

[3] *See*, for example, Polson C. J. and Gee D. J. (1973) *Essentials of Forensic Medicine*, 3rd ed., Oxford, Pergamon, p. 367; Gordon I. and Shapiro H. A. (1975) *Forensic Medicine*, Edinburgh, Churchill Livingstone, p. 68.

dead for some time before discovery and pressure areas of pallor will have formed – since the child is invariably moved by distraught parents, the consequent anomalous position of these areas may give rise to some confusion.

Can suffocation of accidental type occur in infancy? Most authorities would agree that it is an improbable occurrence because a baby suffocating with its face into a pillow will move reflexly so as to breathe; but there may be cases when, because of entanglement in a harness or bedclothes, movement is impossible and true accidental suffocation can result. Suffocation by overlaying, essentially a matter of overcrowding, is now rare; occasional instances are associated with drugs and drunkenness (Chapter 20).

Accidental asphyxia in older children focuses attention on the specific hazards of 'plastic bags'. Numerous tragedies have occurred due to such activities as 'playing spacemen' when a 'helmet' of polythene, attracted to the nose and mouth by respiration, becomes moulded firmly to the shape of the face; if the airway occlusion is sudden, rapid death may result with the classic signs of asphyxia. The great majority of plastic bags are now marked as 'dangerous' and others are perforated when their intended use permits.[4]

The Sexual Asphyxias

Plastic bags also play a part in the interesting group of conditions known as sexual asphyxias; these may also include features of strangulation.

These deaths are characterized by an almost exclusively male distribution and by an equally common association with transvestism together with the use of some asphyxial mechanism, such as a plastic or other bag; a masochistic tendency is often shown by tying the hands or binding the torso and by the superimposition of some form of suspension by a neck ligature. The sexual nature of the condition may be emphasized by a display of pornographic literature.

These features taken together virtually eliminate the involvement of another party, particularly when, as is usual, the victim has taken precautions to preserve his solitude. Occasionally, however, the possibility that the dead man was the victim of a sadomasochistic partnership needs to be excluded – death may be very rapid in any high emotional state, particularly when the neck is involved and, should it occur, any others involved are likely to leave the scene. The common problem in the classic sexual asphyxial death is, however, to distinguish between accident and suicide; unless there is specific evidence to the contrary, such deaths should generally be regarded as accidental, being due either to an

---

[4] See Toy (Safety) Regulations (S.I. 1974 No. 1367) arising from the Consumer Protection Act 1961.

unexpectedly rapid loss of consciousness or to failure to escape from the manufactured conditions.

Obstruction at the Laryngeal Opening

Gagging is seldom intentionally homicidal. More commonly, death occurs accidentally when the mouth has been stuffed with material to stifle calls for help – this may have been premeditated as when immobilizing a night watchman or done on impulse, say, during the course of a sexual assault. Suicidal gagging must be very rare. The author has personal experience of one case in which a depressed hospital patient forced his handkerchief down his throat. Death may be of an asphyxial type but sudden death due to reflex vagal inhibition of the heart is a strong possibility.

Accidental gagging – or choking – can also follow impaction of a bolus of food in the larynx. This may be associated with drunkenness but is most commonly seen in elderly persons who bolt their food as a symptom of senile dementia – the process of mental ageing – or who cannot masticate efficiently without teeth. Death is almost always sudden and is due to stimulation of the vagus nerve. An asphyxial type of death may follow if the food passes the larynx and lodges in the trachea; impaction of something smaller – for example, a nut – in a main bronchus may result in death of almost any degree of suddenness ranging from vagal stimulation to death far removed in time due to bronchopneumonia or lung abscess. This type of death needs to be distinguished from that due to aspiration of regurgitated stomach contents – discussed later in the chapter – which is far less satisfactorily defined.

Obstruction at the Neck

Strangulation is that aspect of asphyxia which most often results in serious criminal charges. It is, therefore, considered here in some detail.

1. Manual Strangulation

Except in unusual circumstances – for example, in retributive gang warfare – it is doubtful if throttling is often the result of deep premeditation; far more frequently, exasperation or fear provokes a murderous impulse which, in the absence of any weapon, is satisfied by 'wringing his or her neck'. The circumstances surrounding the crime and the precise type of a strangling are, therefore, of great importance in assessing the mind of the assailant at the time. Much may be reflected in the mode of death and the pathological evidence may be of particular significance in the final evaluation.

Throttling can be accomplished single-handedly, in which case the thumb of a right-handed assailant is pressed into the right-hand side of the victim's neck close to the angle of the jaw, or bimanually, when each thumb is used to exert pressure; in the event of attack from behind, it is the fingers of each hand which act as the main constricting agent.

The local signs of throttling may consist, therefore, of bruising or superficial abrasion of the neck corresponding to a number of thumb or finger pads. Both structures involved – the neck and the fingers – are relatively soft and bruises, although often obvious, may have indefinite edges; the appearances may well be clearer some hours after death when the process of blood stasis has produced a general pallor of the area. The edges of the bruises may show elliptical abrasions caused by the finger nails of the assailant.

The signs of death from throttling depend upon the precise mode of death; this also applies in other types of violence to the neck. There are, essentially, four mechanisms:

a. The windpipe is occluded. In this case, the changes will be those of generalized oxygen deficiency and, because of the associated struggling, petechial haemorrhages are likely to be prominent. Pulmonary oedema will have been provoked if the anoxia has been prolonged and may show itself as froth at the nose and mouth if the pressure has been intermittent. This finding is not specific and occurs in prolonged hypoxia of many other types.

b. The venous return is obstructed. Anoxia in the brain results from stagnation of the blood and, because this is a gradual process, the cumulative effects of local oxygen lack will be prominent – thus, suffusion of the face with many petechial haemorrhages will be found; but generalized signs of asphyxia will be slight because the rest of the body is adequately oxygenated. There is some division of opinion amongst authorities as to how long is the agonal period in such cases. Some believe that, in throttling with the hands, the pressure must be applied for two minutes or more to cause death.[5] Such estimates cannot be based on experiment and there is no doubt that two minutes is a lengthy period for sustained activity. Others[6] hold that most stranglings are over within half a minute – irrespective of the intervention of factors discussed below at (*c*) and (*d*). This latter estimate has been borne out in studies of accidental strangling and would seem to be the more reasonable.

c. The blood supply to the brain is cut off by pressure on the carotid vessels. Except in strangulation by suspension (*see below*) this can be little more than a theoretical possibility as, firstly, it is mechan-

<hr>

[5] *See*, for example, Camps F. E., Robinson A. E and Lucas B. G. B. (eds.) (1976) *Gradwohl's Legal Medicine*, 3rd ed., Bristol, Wright, p. 333.

[6] The author is indebted to Professor C. K. Simpson for a personal communication on this point.

ically difficult to achieve the necessary compression through the tissues and, secondly, an alternative blood supply to the brain is available through the arteries of the vertebral column. Pressure on the carotid arteries is far more likely to cause:

    d. Death from vagal inhibition of the heart. As described in Chapter 1, a sudden unexpected and, particularly, abnormal sensory stimulation may result in an equally sudden and abnormal reflex through the motor component of the vagus nerve; the heart is arrested and death occurs with great suddenness. The carotid plexus in the neck is particularly sensitive and pressure at this point may well be the predominant cause of this type of sudden death; alternatively, fracture of the laryngeal cartilages may provide the main reflex stimulus.

As discussed in deaths associated with anaesthesia (Chapter 31), autonomic reflexes are likely to be less inhibited when the higher control centres are functionally depressed and it is certainly the author's impression that vagal activity is more common in death due to strangulation when the victim is moderately to severely affected by alcohol — often of the order of 200 mg per 100 ml blood; there is support for this observation in the literature.[7]

    Injuries to the tissues of the throat and larynx provide the most important findings in the post-mortem dissection following manual strangulation. Bruising is the most constant of these and is found at all depths corresponding, in the main, to the pressure marks under the fingers; posterior bruising of the larynx may be caused by pressure against the spine and the base of the tongue may be affected by traction as much as by direct pressure. The thyroid gland may, itself, show bruising.

    Fracture of the laryngeal cartilages is another diagnostic finding. The most frequent fracture involves the superior cornu of the thyroid cartilage, the natural position of the thumb in manual strangulation being to rest on the ligament which joins the thyroid cartilage to the hyoid bone. The hyoid is, therefore, also often involved due either to upward displacement by the thumb or to downward traction as the point of attachment to the thyroid is broken. Associated haemorrhage is a most important post-mortem observation; this is the acid test of injury in life. It is, however, well established that bruising can occur as a result of the dissection itself — particularly around the neck structures. For this

---

    [7] *See* for example, Simpson K. (ed.) *Taylor's Principles and Practice of Medical Jurisprudence,* 12th ed., London, Churchill (p.359) 'States of narcosis and drunkenness may considerably shorten the period (of time taken to die from asphyxation)'.

    Gonzales T. A. *et al.* (1954) *Legal Medicine,* 2nd ed. New York, Appleton-Century-Crofts (p.472): 'Alcoholic individuals may be asphyxiated easily by manual compression of the neck and succumb without revealing any demonstrable signs of violence at autopsy'.

reason, it has been suggested that the cranial cavity should be dissected first in any case of suspected throttling; the potential for artefact is thus reduced by releasing the pressure in the engorged veins. The laryngeal cartilages can be broken during removal of the neck organs but this should not occur other than in unskilled hands. Finally, the possibility that an injury discovered derived from a previous episode far removed in time, cannot always be entirely discounted; such a fracture will, of course, be bloodless.

The pathologist is almost always asked for his opinion as to the force required to cause a fracture of the larynx. Such an assessment is bound to be to some extent subjective. However, damage to the larynx beyond fracture of the cornua of the thyroid and hyoid – for example, fracture of the main wings of the thyroid – will imply 'considerable force'; this type of fracture may result from the karate-blow type of assault rather than from simple throttling. Cartilages which are calcified are certainly easier to fracture than are those which are young and supple – but this is a comparative estimate only which still fails to answer the question of how much force was applied in the individual case. In order to improve the objectivity of the assessment, it is advised that the larynx be X-rayed in every case in which fracture is discovered (*Plate* 10). But it must be remembered that the muscles and ligaments will tend to realign any broken ossicles; a fracture may well be present but may not be visible in the X-ray because of this tendency to a normal position and because of variable calcification in the area.

2. Strangulation by Ligature

Strangulation by ligature without suspension is not uncommon as a form of homicide. Apart from the classic premeditated crime of garrotting – in which the assailants used their own prepared form of ligature – the material used to strangle is usually that which happens to be near at hand; because of the close association with sexual assaults and of the rarity of an original intention to strangle, nylon stockings or pantihose are most frequently found in adult cases; the victim's own scarf is also often used.

The ligature may or may not be knotted in homicidal strangling; although the former is more common, the assailant sometimes depends upon his own strength to maintain the pressure on the neck. This is usually sufficient to cause actual obstruction of the windpipe and must involve pressure on the veins. The usual post-mortem appearances are those of generalized anoxia with exaggerated appearances in the head; rapid death from vagal inhibition of the heart can, however, occur. The ligature causes a mark which is characteristically horizontal and of regular depth; it nearly always passes in front of the neck across the membrane connecting the hyoid and thyroid cartilages which are fractured far less commonly than in the case of manual strangulation. Very little external evidence of the presence of a ligature may remain if it is composed of soft material and is removed immediately after death. Cord or rope may, however, leave a distinctive pattern while irregular finger-nail scratches, inflicted by the victim in an attempt to loosen the constriction, are highly suggestive of homicidal strangling.

Suicidal strangulation by ligature is uncommon but certainly occurs. It is generally associated either with an intricate system of tourniquet application or with the use of elastic material which will spring back to give powerful constriction after having been knotted – nylon stockings behave effectively in this way. At the same time, this effect may be accidental rather than suicidal – self-strangulation is used as a form of exhibitionism. Accidental strangulation either by self or by another in horseplay may occur in the absence of a tied knot when death is of a reflex type (*Plate* 11).

The umbilical cord is occasionally used to strangle a newborn infant – the question then arises as to whether the cord can encircle the neck so as to cause fatal accidental strangulation either *in utero* or during the act of birth. Few would dogmatize that either cannot happen and, in cases of precipitate labour, the cord may be markedly tightened. Such cases must arouse suspicion but, no matter how great this may be, the onus is still with the prosecution to prove the *fact* of a separate existence before a charge can be upheld. A separate existence will scarcely ever be possible in accidental strangulation by the cord but proof *may* be forthcoming in cases of child murder or infanticide; the problem is discussed in Chapter 19.

3. Strangulation by Suspension

Death from hanging may be judicial or quasi-judicial. Judicial hanging in the United Kingdom[8] gave rise not to an asphyxial death but to disruption of the cervical spinal cord due to a separation fracture of the neck induced by the massive jolt following a drop of some 7 ft; the common fracture site was at the level C2–3. Asphyxial hangings of the 'Western' film type were resurrected in the quasi-judicial circumstances of partisan warfare but, nowadays, death by hanging is almost entirely suicidal with a small accidental element.

The suicidal nature of the case is nearly always apparent from the circumstances – although an attempt to disguise a homicide as a suicidal hanging is not unknown.[9] Arrangements involving some elaboration are often made and steps are usually taken to offset the possibility of

---

[8] Abolished under the Murder (Abolition of Death Penalty) Act 1965 apart from potential use in the event of treason.

[9] R. v. Emmett-Dunne, General Court Martial, Dusseldorf, 1954.

detection before death; as a consequence, it is not unusual for suicidal hangings to have been dead for some days before discovery.

The main post-mortem findings are those of facial congestion coupled with severe hypostatic changes in the legs and forearms; the former may, however, be absent if the carotid arteries have been compressed. The ligature mark in the neck is deep and is maximal opposite the point of suspension; it often passes between hyoid and thyroid cartilages in front, rising to the point of an inverted V, corresponding to the knot of the noose, either in the midline posteriorly or behind one ear. The internal appearances will be those of generalized anoxia but, even if death has resulted rapidly from vagal stimulation, the effects of blood pooling will still result in severe changes which are visible externally; anomalies of lividity may indicate the possibility of simulation. Fractures of the laryngeal cartilages may occur in hanging but are by no means invariable; much depends upon the age of the subject. The ligature may be so firm and applied so rapidly that vital reaction is absent; a false impression of a post-mortem origin may be gained.

Accidental hanging is generally sexually orientated and is associated with the sexual asphyxias previously discussed; simple exhibitionism may, however, end disastrously. Death can be due to vagal inhibition of the heart even though steps have been taken to prevent a fatal outcome – for example, by having the point of suspension so low that the feet touch the ground. It is, in fact, surprising how many 'successful' suicides occur thus – the combination of motivation, nervous tension and mechanical cerebral hypoxia, which may be of great suddenness, combine to produce death in a situation which appears readily recoverable. Such deaths are well documented in conditions which eliminate the possibility of homicide.

Other forms of accidental hangings scarcely need special mention though many need careful differentiation from homicide – the baby strangled in its restraining harness is one example. Industrial accidents of many types can be imagined. A somewhat bizarre form of accidental hanging may occur in sport or military parachuting when the neck becomes entangled with the shroud lines; the severe jolt often imparted gives rise to intimal laceration of the carotid arteries – a minor sign at post-mortem dissection which strongly indicates a sudden stretching of the neck in hanging incidents of all types.

Obstruction in the Lower Air Passages
Drowning, discussed in Chapter 14, is an obvious form of obstruction involving the lower respiratory tract. But it is also possible effectively to 'drown' in one's own body fluids – the accumulation of fluid in the lungs is known as pulmonary oedema, which forms part of the syndrome of hypoxia described above.

The condition is not specific to mechanical asphyxia. It occurs in all forms of hypoxic death including those of central origin such as barbiturate poisoning. It is also a natural result of heart failure – an ineffective left ventricle is unable to clear the blood returning from the lungs; very severe oedema is commonly present in death due to coronary insufficiency. A similar manifestation of 'heart failure' is seen when the volume of the circulating blood is increased beyond the capacity of the left ventricle; this occurs when fluids are transfused over liberally into the body and is a form of iatrogenic asphyxia which is discussed in Chapter 31.

Pulmonary oedema commences within the alveoli but it may be so intense that the bronchioles and bronchi are filled with fluid. Irritant gases produce extremes of the condition – the early war gases chlorine and phosgene are examples of such direct acting substances but even tear gas may produce severe pulmonary reaction in high concentration.

The interpretation of obstruction of the lower airways by inhaled stomach contents presents a practical problem in forensic pathology. This is certainly a common post-mortem finding which is particularly frequent in hypoxic deaths. Although it is easy to presume a cause-and-effect relationship, a diagnosis of asphyxia due to inhalation of stomach contents may well be a misconception; it is widely held that vomitus in the air passages is usually there because of, rather than as the cause of, tissue anoxia[10] and this may be especially pertinent to 'cot deaths' (p. 248). To complicate matters further, the act of vomiting itself may cause the appearance of petechiae by suddenly raising the venous pressure. In practical terms, the presence of inhaled material from the stomach should not be accepted as the precise cause of death unless products of digestion can be demonstrated microscopically in the small air passages; a valid diagnosis is often associated with conditions which depress the reflex ability to expel foreign material from the lungs – head injury and intoxication due to drugs or alcohol are frequent causes.

Restriction of Chest Movement
Pressure on the chest sufficient to inhibit respiratory movement will cause asphyxia – the condition must be unnatural and is known as traumatic asphyxia. Circumstances likely to produce this effect are self-evident – crushing under rock falls, pinning in a vehicular accident, crushing in a crowd – particularly if the crowd collapses – are all common accidental causes of traumatic asphyxia. The pathological findings are characteristic – there is intense congestion with widespread formation of petechiae in the tissues, especially in those of the upper thorax and neck; occasionally, there is little or nothing to be seen externally. It

---

[10] See Knight B. (1976) *Legal Aspects of Medical Practice*, 2nd ed., Edinburgh, Churchill Livingstone, p. 149.

is just possible that the mechanism of traumatic asphyxia could be used homicidally by the assailant sitting on the victim's chest – some such method, coupled with manual suffocation, was admitted by Burke and Hare, hence the descriptive title of 'burking'.

PATHOLOGICAL CONDITIONS

Any pathological condition of the lungs which interferes with the free interchange of gases across the alveolar capillary membrane will cause some degree of tissue hypoxia. Bronchitis, emphysema and pulmonary fibrosis are the main conditions but, although they are a major cause of mortality in the general population, they have only limited medico-legal significance.

Many pathological pulmonary conditions are intimately associated with work and are likely to be the subject of compensation for industrial injury. They are discussed in some detail in Chapter 15.

The presence of lung disease may result in severe strain on the right side of the heart – that side which is responsible for pumping blood into and through the lungs; a failing heart in this situation is known as *cor pulmonale*. While most sufferers exist in a state of chronic ill health, an acute exacerbation may be a cause of sudden death resulting in a Coroner's or Fiscal's Inquiry.

The presence of a condition predisposing to tissue anoxia will compound the effects of any other asphyxial mechanism; the pre-existing condition of the victim's lungs may, therefore, have considerable bearing on the evaluation of a case of, say manual strangulation. This concept of synergism holds for all the main categories of asphyxia discussed.

TOXIC ASPHYXIA

Toxic asphyxia is of two main types. Either the capacity of the haemoglobin to bind oxygen is impaired, or the enzymatic processes whereby the oxygen in the blood is utilized by the tissues are blocked.

Conversion of haemoglobin to the compound methaemoglobin is effected by many industrial poisons (*see* Chapter 22). This change produces more frightening signs than genuine pathological effects and the only haemoglobin derivative which is of major practical medico-legal importance is carboxyhaemoglobin – formed by the combination of haemoglobin with inspired carbon monoxide. Cyanides are outstanding examples of enzymatic poisons. These two substances will, therefore, be treated individually.

Carbon monoxide poisoning

Until a few years ago, the most readily available source of this asphyxiant was the domestic gas supply which contained some 5–15 per cent of carbon monoxide (CO); this supply is now widely provided by natural gas which, although asphyxiant in that it is irrespirable, has no positive toxic qualities. Most carbon monoxide with which the public comes in contact nowadays derives from the combustion of carbon containing material; carbon dioxide (CO_2) is the end product of ideal combustion but, since very few flames are totally efficient, all gas produced by fire contains some carbon monoxide. Carbon dioxide is relatively unimportant as its physiological effects can be compensated save in an enclosed environment (*see* p. 161); the affinity of haemoglobin for CO is, however, some 300 times that of its affinity for oxygen. There are two dangerous outcomes – the formation of carboxyhaemoglobin (COHb) is cumulative and, consequently, a potentially fatal proportion of respirably inert COHb in the blood can be derived from only a small concentration of CO in the inspired air.

In practice, therefore, two factors are needed to endanger life through carbon monoxide poisoning – firstly, there must be combustion and, secondly, the removal of the products of combustion must be inefficient.

The most common sources of poisoning include:

   a. Solid-fuel, gas or oil fires fitted with inadequate flues or used in rooms without sufficient ventilation. Oil heaters in bedrooms (including caravans) or geysers in bathrooms present as obvious examples.
   b. Internal combustion engines having defective exhaust systems – or operating within closed garages.
   c. Mines – where the perpetual minor fires leave pockets of contamination.

With the exception of the last circumstance, death from carbon monoxide poisoning may be homicidal, suicidal or accidental.

Homicidal poisoning must be extremely rare because of its uncertainty of success although one could conceive of a town gas supply being deliberately opened in the presence of a sleeping or otherwise unconscious victim; infanticide attempts combined with suicide are probably less uncommon. The use of carbon monoxide in the course of murder, presumably as a sexual stimulant, has been recorded but would not constitute the prime weapon in such an instance.[11]

Suicidal poisoning was most often associated with the gas oven in the past; the motor car exhaust is now the most frequent source of the poison for this purpose. The true nature of a suicidal CO poisoning is

---

[11] *See* Camps F. E. (1953) *Medical and Scientific Investigations in the Christie Case*, London, Medical Publications Ltd.

likely to be shown by the intricate arrangements made – not only to ensure a concentrated delivery of the gas but, often, for the comfort of the subject. Additional suicidal agents – such as drugs – may well have been used. Death ensues in some 5 minutes in an oven; car exhaust gas, which contains about 6 per cent carbon monoxide, can also kill in a matter of minutes but this time will be greatly influenced by variations in the efficiency of delivery and ventilation.

Several other factors affect the individual's susceptibility to CO. As with all poisons, the elderly are likely to be killed more easily than the young and the presence of disease which, of itself, contributes to or kills through tissue hypoxia must be taken into account – coronary insufficiency is an obvious example. Similarly, an anaemic person will succumb more quickly than will the normal as it is the sum of hypoxic factors which matters. It follows that the symptoms of carbon monoxide poisoning will also depend on the physical state of the individual. Thus, it is generally stated that conversion of 30 per cent of the haemoglobin to carboxyhaemoglobin results in dizziness and headache, incoordination appears at 50 per cent saturation, unconsciousness at 60 per cent and death at 70–80 per cent; but these are proportions relative to the total oxyhaemoglobin available and it is this total which conditions symptoms. Moreover, the more rapid and deep is the respiration, the more contaminated air will be inspired and the faster will be the accumulation of COHb. From the purely legal aspect all these factors will be relevant when problems of survival arise as they may well do if members of a family are found dead in a room or caravan; they also greatly influence the medical assessment of accidental CO poisoning.

Accidental intoxication by carbon monoxide is of interest on two counts – firstly, it may of itself be the cause of death and, secondly, it may be the cause of a vehicular accident and, indirectly, of death from trauma.

All sources of carbon monoxide are associated with accidental poisoning. These include space heating appliances, water heaters of the geyser type and the exhausts of stationary cars left with engines running. Fumes from the latter contaminate the compartment either through a faulty exhaust or heater system or as a result of escape into the air of a closed garage. Leaking pipes or loose taps conducting town gas must also be considered; mining accidents can occur but, thanks to safety measures taken, are now rare. Death is almost invariably associated with a degree of unawareness – senility, sleep, alcoholism or preoccupation with other matters are obvious examples. Accidents connected with senility are those of forgetfulness in turning off taps, failure to remember open taps when recharging coin-operated meters and the like. Accidents in sleep are usually associated with open-flame heating apparatus. It must be remembered that individuals may react differently, that carbon monoxide tends to layer and that concentrations in a room will vary greatly according to the positions of draughty windows and doors. The maximum concentration of CO in the air of a room will not be very great and the effects are spread over a relatively long period; alterations in the environment will exaggerate differences in clinical response and, when there are several persons in a room, it may well be that some will wake up or be roused when others are already dead – such a result by no means rules out accident. Alcoholism may be a particular feature predisposing to death amongst down-and-outs who are huddled around inefficient braziers or boilers especially if these have inadequate flues (*Plate* 12). Preoccupation may be a feature of deaths in garages while making car repairs; the combination of preoccupation and exercise leads to sudden deaths during sexual activity – often in cars in which the heater is left running. Perhaps the bathroom geyser is the only apparatus likely to be lethal to a person normally aware and occupied; the usual small size of the room exaggerates the danger of failing to turn off the flame before entering the bath.

Carbon monoxide is a potential – and actual – cause of death due to traumatic injury in motor cars and in aircraft; the problem is discussed in Chapter 10. For the present, it is necessary merely to emphasize that only low levels of COHb – sufficient to cause no more than distraction or disorientation – are needed to cause a vehicular accident and, further, that there will be a marked synergistic relationship with other adverse physiological factors such as fatigue. The forensic pathologist and toxicologist will, therefore, be dealing with concentrations of COHb which are only slightly raised and which must be interpreted with care and in relationship to the accident as a whole.

Poisoning by cyanide is uncommon but has historical interest; it is also the most significant example of histotoxic asphyxia – tissue enzymes are blocked by the process known as molecular substitution and are unable to transfer the oxygen in the blood. Death is essentially due to poisoning of the respiratory centre which is especially sensitive to hypoxia. If death is not sudden, the high proportion of oxyhaemoglobin in the venous blood may show itself through the bright-pink colour of the skin and internal organs; the colour must be distinguished from that of carboxyhaemoglobin and from the effects of cold, including post-mortem refrigeration. Delayed death only occurs in cases of ingestion of cyanide salts; hydrocyanic acid is one of the most rapidly fatal poisons known.

Hydrocyanic acid is used as a gaseous fungicide or, more commonly, rodenticide; its use is specifically controlled.[12] Cyanide salts are used in the steel industry and in other industrial processes; they are common laboratory chemicals; the most open route to the public depends upon

[12] Hydrogen Cyanide (Fumigation) Act 1937.

their use in photography. Natural sources of cyanide include bitter almonds, the kernels of many fruit-stones and the leaves and fruit of some plants.

Despite this wide distribution of very toxic substances, death from cyanide poisoning is now rare. Homicidal poisoning seems to be a matter of history only – although cyanides were used for the genocidal killings of the 1940s; accidental poisoning occurs mainly in industry and in laboratories; the greatest number of cases now reported are suicidal with a strong preponderance of subjects who are in daily contact with the poison – e.g. chemists and photographers.

Poisoning from natural sources of cyanide is very rare. A number of very old cases involving bitter almonds themselves, or the essential oil, have been reported. The significant quantities of cyanide contained in fruit-stones are only available after laborious extraction and cyanide poisoning from plants is extremely unlikely. There are, however, general dangers for children eating berries with which they are unfamiliar and these are emphasized in Chapter 22.

ENVIRONMENTAL ASPHYXIA

Reduction in the available oxygen to a level inconsistent with life arises as a medico-legal problem most commonly in relation to enclosed spaces – too many people may be closetted in too small a space or the space may be too small to support a single human life. The former may be murderous in intent – the 'Black Hole of Calcutta' is history's most vivid example – or a matter of reckless indifference; occasionally, overcrowding in small, cold rooms may cause the accidental death of whole families living in ghetto conditions. The second category is commoner and is typified by a child being trapped inside a disused refrigerator or trunk; it is generally clear that such instances are accidental – although the precise nature of the accident, particularly of the part played by other children, may be in doubt – but the pathologist has to be aware of the possibility of the disposal of a child dead from other causes. Adults can also be locked in containers accidentally though such circumstances would almost always be highly suspicious; at the time of writing, a particularly horrifying homicidal variant has been reported in which several victims of gang warfare were deliberately locked in a safe. Accidents of industrial type may also result in anoxic deaths – mining and submarine disasters are obvious examples.

There is often some difficulty in deciding whether to attribute a death of this type to oxygen deficiency or to poisoning by excess carbon dioxide; the author believes that the former is correct unless carbon dioxide is introduced into the environment in some way other than as a product of normal respiration. Both physiological mechanisms are, however, operative and the process of asphyxiation in an enclosed environment is self-accelerating. As oxygen is utilized, the concentration of carbon dioxide builds up; an increase in CO_2 reflexly increases the respiration activity which, in turn, accelerates the depletion of oxygen; a rapidly fatal vicious circle is established, gross biochemical changes being super-added to lack of oxygen.

Environmental asphyxia due to altitude must be mentioned although, being virtually confined to aviation, it has but slight medicolegal implications. Death truly due to high-altitude hypoxia is rare. Mountaineers and those living at heights are able to adapt to the conditions; balloonists were early historic casualties but are scarcely a large group now; emergency oxygen is available to airline passengers and, so far as is known, has never failed when required.

Hypoxia at altitude is of greater importance in two other respects. In the first place, a person who is particularly susceptible to oxygen lack is at increased risk as ascent is made. An altitude of the order of 5000–6000 ft (1500–1800 m), which is quite safe for normal fit persons, may precipitate fatal myocardial ischaemia in the presence of an already inadequate coronary circulation; similar altitudes could precipitate a crisis in a person with sickle cell disease. The ability of hypoxia to cause an aircraft accident is of even more significance. Precision performance falls off rapidly with decreasing oxygen pressure and it is generally accepted that 10 000 ft (3000 m) is the effective upper limit at which a man can operate an intricate machine without supplemental oxygen; above 30 000 ft (9000 m) this supplement must be supplied under positive pressure. The effects of hypobaric hypoxia are quite insidious, the victim being wholly unaware of his decreasing efficiency; it follows that failure of the oxygen supply to a military aviator or undiscovered loss of pressure in cabin-type aircraft[13] are potential causes of accidents. Sudden loss of pressure ('explosive decompression') in a large aircraft – such as might be caused by the detonation of a bomb or by major structural failure – is a complex pathological problem; death and injury may result from turbulence in the cabin, anoxia, the effects of low pressure and of cold and, of course, from the likely crash.

IATROGENIC ASPHYXIA

Some degree of hypoxia may occur whenever a general inhalation anaesthetic is administered, the relative avoidance of this being a measure of the anaesthetist's vigilance and skill. Since oxygen lack in these circumstances is often imposed upon patients who are particularly susceptible by reason of disease, there is a real possibility of death due to hypoxia under anaesthesia. The medico-legal importance of the subject is great and it is treated separately in Chapter 31.

[13] This is, of course, an impossibility in major commercial aircraft which have multiple detection means available.

Chapter 14

Fire, Water, Heat, Cold and Neglect

THIS chapter deals with a number of conditions which, while being mainly related to asphyxia, have a wider interest than the simple production of tissue anoxia. Those which are not so associated are logically related through at least one line of interest.

INJURY AND DEATH FROM BURNING

Legally, burns include the destruction of tissue through the application of any form of heat or of any chemical substance. There is no distinction in law as to the degree of burning – to burn someone in any way is a serious assault and the use of corrosive substances is a specific aggravation in Scots Law.

Burns may be natural – as in exposure to non-ionizing solar radiation or due to lightning; they may be due to dry heat – generally from open fires but also from such articles as hot plates, hot-water bottles etc.; burns due to moist heat are commonly known as scalds; corrosive substances have their own individual pathologies; and burns due to electricity and X-rays should be included in this classification.

The distribution of these types of burn varies with age. Under the age of three, a high proportion are due to scalding; scalding also occurs in later childhood but accidental setting light to clothes is more important in this age group and is the most significant source of burning in old age; in normal adult life, accidental burns associated with vehicular transport are common but the great majority of cases stem from industry which provide examples of dry, wet and corrosive burning. However, with the exception of those due to lightning and man-made electricity (*see below*), the local medical effects of all burns are similar; this section will deal with burns due to fire as being the most typical, the most common and, medico-legally, the most important form of thermal injuries.

Burning in the human varies from simple reddening and blistering of the skin to severe charring and destruction of deeper parts of the body; the author was involved in the investigation of one aircraft disaster in

163

which no less than 23 bodies remained unaccounted for – it could only be assumed that they had been effectively cremated. It was at one time customary to classify burns according to their appearance; it is more rational to speak in terms of depth. If there is loss of only partial thickness of the skin, it should be self-healing, whereas full thicknes loss will require skin grafting; very deep burning will inevitably cause some loss of function or lead even to amputation. This classification, essentially related to treatment, is also helpful in assessing the hurt and inconvenience sustained. The immediate prognosis of a burn depends to a great extent on susceptibility to pain – which is mainly a matter of conditioning and of age. Once over the initial impact, the outcome of a burn involving loss of skin is largely dictated by the escape of body fluids the severity of which correlates, within limits, with the area rather than the depth of burning. There is a massive loss of water, protein and electrolytes from the raw areas and severe surgical shock arises if treatment is inadequate. Subsequently, the results of a burn are related to the risk of overwhelming infection. Children and the elderly are more susceptible to secondary infection and septicaemia than are young adults. The general rule is that burning which destroys more than 70 per cent of the skin is likely to be fatal irrespective of the treatment; the elderly may not survive a 20 per cent burn.[1]

Severe burns due to fire may be accidental, suicidal or homicidal. The first is by far the commonest and is a particular hazard of childhood and of old age; catching the clothes in an open or an electric fire is very liable to occur in both age groups.[2] Statutory protection is given to children both in England and Wales and in Scotland[3] where it is declared an offence for a person over the age of 16 unreasonably to expose a child under the age of 12 (age 7 in Scotland) in his or her care to the dangers of contact with an open fire grate or any heating appliance in such a way as to cause injury. Children are also prone to scalding by boiling fat and similar things to which they are drawn by inquisitiveness. There is a clear association between infirmity and burning in the aged; frank illness may lead to a sequence of collapse, concussion and burning while in the unconscious state. Acute alcoholism also plays an important part in accidental burning; the combination of intoxication and smoking in bed is extremely dangerous and the latter practice is illegal in hotels in the United States of America.

---

[1] The calculation of the area is based on the 'Rule of Nine'. The head and neck represent 9 per cent of the body area; each arm 9 per cent; the front and back of the trunk each 18 per cent; and each leg 18 per cent.

[2] Current Regulations require that a guard be fitted to all domestic heating appliances whether they be coal, gas, electric or oil fires. The spaces can still be sufficiently large for clothing, etc., to penetrate.

[3] Children and Young Persons Act 1952, s. 11 as amended; Children and Young Persons (Scotland) Act 1937, s. 22.

Mass accidental burnings are a risk whenever large numbers of persons are congregated in an enclosed area. The likely situations are obvious and need no detailed discussion; tenements, hotels, dance halls, theatres, etc., provide the common examples. Prevention of disaster is a matter of rigid application of building regulations and of provision of adequate escape facilities; major loss of life in conflagrations stems, in perhaps the majority of cases, from the difficulty of applying such regulations retrospectively.[4]

Burning in transport accidents must be mentioned. It is far less common than might be anticipated in automobile accidents but it is by no means rare in aircraft accidents; although the latter do not constitute a numerically important cause of unnatural death, it is noteworthy that the more 'survivable' an aircraft accident is in terms of crash forces, the more likely is death when it occurs to be due to burning – there is clearly room for improvement in the design of seats, passenger restraints and emergency escape procedures.

Suicidal burning is very rare but may be adopted when maximum publicity is sought – igniting one's own kerosene-drenched body has become something of an extreme form of political protest. Otherwise this form of suicide must generally be associated with severe mental derangement; the author has experience of only one case where the subject also drank over a pint of paraffin, presumably in the hope of dying by explosion. The practice of suttee – or ritual suicide by a widow on her husband's death – has ceased even in the most rigid Hindu communities.

Homicide by burning must also be very exceptional owing to the uncertainty of success. But murder by fire after having immobilized the subject – say by injury or by drugs – or, more probably, attempted concealment of a murder through post-mortem incineration are not at all unlikely; many of the classic examples of inspired forensic pathology have derived from such attempts.[5] The distinction of antemortem from post-mortem burning is, therefore, essential. The demonstration of 'vital reaction' (see Chapter 4) around a burn is of minimal value in this context as the body will almost always be severely charred. Major importance attaches to the demonstration of products of combustion either in the form of soot in the air passages or upper gastro-intestinal tract or as carboxyhaemoglobin in the blood – values of 20–50 per cent are common. For reasons which are sometimes unclear, the two parameters do not always follow one another logically,[6] but it is virtually

---

[4] Fire Precautions Act 1971.

[5] For example, R. v. Rouse, 1931, Northampton Assizes; R. v. Dobkin, 1943, C.C.C.

[6] This problem is discussed in detail by Blackmore D. J. (1973) in: Mason J. K. and Reals W. J. (ed.) *Aerospace Pathology*, Chicago, College of American Pathologists Foundation, p. 196.

impossible to force soot deeply into the tissues of a cadaver while no more than traces of carboxyhaemoglobin would be likely to result from post-mortem diffusion of gas from the atmosphere. In the event of fractures having been found, the discovery of bone marrow or fat emboli in the lungs (*see* Chapter 10) would strongly suggest that the bony injuries were sustained in life; it has been claimed that burning by itself will cause fat embolism but the author has not been able to substantiate this observation. The most certain evidence of a cause of death other than burning would be a finding positively indicating that cause – such as the discovery of a bullet or of evidence of manual strangulation.

Burning of itself causes artefacts which are to be distinguished from antemortem injury; the lawyer should have some knowledge of them as they may appear as unqualified factual statements in post-mortem reports. The most common of these artefacts are muscle contractures which often result in the so called 'pugilistic attitude'; this is simply due to heat coagulation of protein and is not evidence of a defence reaction. Contraction of the skin may lead to splits which are very like incised wounds. Boiling of body fluids in enclosed spaces may lead to apparent intravital haemorrhage; the most common type presents as a false extra-dural haemorrhage. Burning may of itself cause bony fractures; these are common in the bones of the arms and legs but are also seen in the skull where they may result in severe loss of bone. The combination of artefactual haemorrhage and fracture can pose a most difficult patho-logical problem.

Death from burning may be immediate – the intense pain may cause reflex inhibition of the heart or the thermal injury may simply be so severe as to be incompatible with life. Alternatively, death may be asphyxial in type; fire victims do not die from carbon monoxide poison-ing *per se* – the discovery of COHb is rather a measure of survival in a fire environment. Early stupefaction can occur but this is probably due to the inhalation of other poisonous substances – e.g. cyanides – which are combustion products of many man-made materials. The distinction of the mode of death is of more than academic interest; it may be im-portant evidence in the application of the laws of succession (*see* Chap-ter 10). Delayed death from burning is nearly always due to traumatic shock which is often complicated by infection spreading from the damaged areas; even should the problems of fluid loss and toxaemia be overcome, acute renal failure may have occurred and the response to dialysis is universally bad when this condition follows burning. Death more remote in time may result from pneumonia due to enforced and prolonged immobilization and it is possible – though not everywhere agreed – that the effects of prolonged stress may be such as to exhaust the capacity of the adrenal glands to sustain life.

It scarcely needs emphasis that the long-term results of survival from severe burning may be disfiguring and disabling and that such features must be considered in assessing damages. Some effects may not be immediately apparent – blindness, for example, may be threatened not only by the immediate fire but by an increasing inability to close the eyes or blink as the injured tissues contract. Overall, accidental burning results in a substantial reduction in the efficiency of the young and active population.

DEATH FROM ELECTRICITY

Electricity is used on a vast scale even by persons with negligible understanding of its behaviour. The fact that it causes so few deaths is a tribute to the safety engineering which has accompanied the development of the electrical industry.

The outcome of an electric shock depends upon physical factors in the discharge and on the physiological state of the subject.

The determinants in the discharge are the current (measured in amperes), the voltage (or electromotive force of the current, measured in volts), the time over which the discharge is passed (amperes × seconds = coulombs) and the type of current – whether direct or alternating. The major factors in the subject include his resistance to an electrical discharge, his body weight – children are more susceptible than are adults – his earthing and his degree of preparedness.

The relative importance of the discharge factors depends significantly upon the period of application. Ultra-short exposures are unpredictable in their effects which depend upon the precise state of excitability of the heart when the shock is received. If the electric current is passed for less than three seconds, the danger is related both to the magnitude of the current and to the duration of the shock. Applications of longer than three seconds depend almost entirely on the amperage for their lethal effect; the latter to some extent dictates the former as a high current initiates muscle spasm – the subject is unable to release the conductor and long exposure results. Direct current is less hazardous to life than is alternating. The danger of the latter increases with the frequency and probably reaches its peak at the frequency of the public supply – 50 hertz (cycles per second) in Britain and Europe and 60 Hz in the USA. Alternating current becomes less dangerous once the power frequency range of 1 kHz is passed, ultra-high frequencies being only a source of intense heat.

The voltage of the discharge is important when related to the resistance of the subject. The latter is almost entirely a matter of skin moisture; a completely dry person would have an exceptionally high resistance and might well tolerate voltages of the order of those used in supply systems. The skin is generally of such conductivity that voltages above 200 are likely to be fatal due to the limb-to-limb passage of a current of over 50 mA. Efficient movement of current depends, in ordinary circumstances, on the efficiency of earthing – a subject standing on wet ground is at far greater risk than is one on a dry surface. In the worst conditions, an alternating current at 25 V and 50 Hz has been fatal. Short duration impulse shocks are used in agricultural electric fences; pulses of the order one tenth of a second in each second are usually considered nonlethal but children of small body weight have been killed in exceptional circuit conditions. All workers with electricity will testify to the protective effect of preparedness for a shock; this is scarcely surprising since death from electric shock involves a considerable element of reflex nervous activity.

As to the relationship between electricity and accident, suicide and homicide, the last can be virtually dismissed save, perhaps, in the context of the 'battered baby' (see Chapter 20). Even judicial electrocution – which involved the passage of a double current of very high voltage followed by one of great intensity – is now of extreme rarity. Suicidal electrocution has been reported but is now very uncommon despite the ready availability of the methods; the diagnosis can seldom be in doubt owing to the complexity of the arrangements made – a factor which also serves to eliminate homicide (Plate 13a).

Accidents are overwhelmingly responsible for death due to electricity and are of several types:

Industrial accidents are kept to a minimum by stringent safety precautions but nevertheless continue to occur as a result of genuine mishap or flouting of the regulations due to overconfidence. Direct contact may not be necessary if very high tension cables are involved as arcing may occur at a distance of a few millimetres. Domiciliary accidents are more common and are of three main types: the apparatus may be defective, due often to fraying of insulation; attempts may be made to repair equipment without disconnecting it from the mains supply while using makeshift tools, a particular hazard of housewives; or apparatus may be dangerously used – the most common example involves the use of electric equipment in the bathroom where conditions for electrical conduction are optimal. Neutral fusing which, in the event of dissolution, can give a false indication that the apparatus is 'dead', is a hazard peculiar to older apparatus of British manufacture. Iatrogenic accidents are of much medico-legal importance as they will almost invariably lead to actions for negligence. Electroconvulsive therapy, in which convulsions are deliberately precipitated by electrical stimulation of the brain, is occasionally used in the treatment of mental disorder and is the greatest source of such injury and death; traumatic injury may be sustained during the actual convulsion and deaths have been reported due to the electric shock itself. Polson and Gee[7] have drawn attention to the hazards of electricity used in association with 'invasive' diagnostic or therapeutic techniques – i.e. those which involve penetration of the skin or of a mucous membrane; since the resistance of the skin is eliminated and blood is an excellent conductor, death may be caused by misapplication of very low intensity currents. The same authors (at p. 317) have also reported on the use of electricity as an *auto-erotic stimulant*. The present writer has seen one case in which a penile vibrator was connected to a mains plug; when the dead body was discovered, the plug was not actually in the socket and no marks were found on the penis – the cause of death could not, therefore, be attributed to electricity with certainty.

The diagnosis of death due to electric shock may, in fact, be difficult – electric marking is not always present. Characteristically, however, there is a mark which may correspond to the shape of the electrode and shows a central area of necrosis surrounded by a white zone which is, in turn, encircled by a blush of dilated vessels. A true burn of parchmented or charred type may result if the current has been prolonged. An 'exit' mark may also be present and may take on the shape of the exit contact.

Death is predominantly physiological when due to the electric shock itself; the post-mortem findings are, accordingly, often slight and generally nonspecific. Three modes of death are described. In the least common, the respiratory centre of the brain is directly affected if the current passes through the head; a variant hypothesis is that vagal stimulation causes cardiac arrest. Alternatively, the entire musculature may be involved in the spasmodic contracture described above; death is then akin to that in traumatic asphyxia (*see* p. 156) and accounts for those cases of electrocution which show the post-mortem changes usually associated with mechanical hypoxia. The most common cause of death is said to be ventricular fibrillation – that state in which the ventricles of the heart beat so rapidly as to be ineffective pumps. It is of interest that the current passing must be of fairly critical intensity to produce this effect – the deliberate application of a high-intensity current is used medically as a *treatment* of ventricular fibrillation and this may account for some remarkable survivals which are reported following the passage of very high intensity electric shocks (any counter-shock, including painful injury, can act as a defibrillator). There are two major points of medicolegal interest associated with death from fibrillation. Firstly, it has been reported that death may not be immediate and can be preceded by volitional movement. Secondly, and of far greater importance, cardiac function may be restored; prompt resuscitative measures are therefore essential and artificial respiration can be successful even after having

[7] In *Essentials of Forensic Medicine* (1973), 3rd ed., Oxford, Pergamon, p. 316.

been applied for very long periods.

Finally, it should be mentioned that death may be caused by, but not be due to, electrocution. Thus, the fatal outcome may be due to burning if the clothes are set alight; alternatively, death may result from traumatic injury if a high-intensity shock precipitates the subject from, say, a high ladder.

Lightning as a Source of Electrocution

A lightning flash incorporates several physical features. These include the application of an electric current of extremely high intensity, the effects of primary 'flash' and secondary thermal burning and the pressure effects of a high intensity blast wave (*see* p. 111). The subject struck may, therefore, sustain injuries of traumatic type – including fractures – which must be distinguished from those due to homicide. Superficial skin burns of a leafy or arborescent type are characteristic, when present, of lightning strike. Beyond this aspect of differential diagnosis, lightning strikes are of no medico-legal importance being always occurrences of unpredictable, accidental type. Despite the apparent ferocity of a lightning strike, it is noteworthy that death occurs in less than half the subjects who are treated promptly.

DEATH FROM HYPERTHERMIA

Although it has little medico-legal significance, a note on hyperthermic death is added for the sake of completeness. The human body is fairly well adapted to hot climates; sweating is the main protective mechanism and severe effects may follow abnormalities of this function.

Direct effects of heat on the brain may lead to heat stroke. The thermoregulating mechanism of the body is affected and the body temperature rises precipitously in association with a failure to sweat. The condition is essentially due to exposure of the head to direct heat usually in an arid climate. This type of death could be criminally associated with deliberate exposure of soldiers or prisoners; some cases were the subject of war crimes.

Heat exhaustion is, medically, a different condition and arises in two forms. Anhidrotic heat exhaustion – that is, heat exhaustion due to failure of sweating – is secondary to a form of skin disease which occurs in hot, damp climates and is of no concern in the present context. Hyperhidrotic heat exhaustion, due to excessive sweating, could well form the subject of a medico-legal inquiry. In this condition, sweat flows so freely that enough sodium chloride is lost as to provoke severe physiological effects unless it is purposefully replaced. This is the characteristic exhaustion of the long-distance runner or of the soldier on forced march but the pure condition is not often seen in outdoor activity – the really dangerous situation arises when heat stroke is superimposed. Heat exhaustion has considerable importance in industry and is a hazard to stokers in ships, etc., where the effects have been declared industrial accidents.[8]

DEATH DUE TO DROWNING

Although closely related to asphyxia, death from drowning is not a simple matter of oxygen lack. This certainly occurs but an additional, and perhaps main, effect of water inhaled in the lungs is to alter the biochemical balance of the blood; how this occurs depends upon the medium of immersion.

Drowning in salt water is closest to a true asphyxial death and, generally, there is ample evidence of a struggle to breathe; petechiae, however, rarely form in the lungs due, possibly, to the mechanical pressure of the inhaled water upon the capillaries. During the death throes, water not only passes into the lungs but is gulped into the stomach and is forced into the middle ear. Death may result from total immersion for some 2–3 minutes.

The mechanism differs in fresh water which is removed from the lungs and transferred to the blood stream far more quickly than is sea water. During this process, which, by raising the blood volume, is dangerous in itself, the protective covering of the alveoli – so called 'surfactant' – is removed and this, amongst other results, causes the classical frothing at the mouth. Such frothing is not specific to drowning – it occurs in burning and in virtually any condition associated with pulmonary oedema – but it is very good evidence of death having been due to drowning when found in a body removed from the water. The fresh water passing into the pulmonary capillaries dilutes the plasma and an osmotic differential is built up between the plasma and the interior of the red blood cells. Water then passes into the cells which burst, liberating large quantities of intracellular potassium; a state of *hyperkalaemia* results which poisons the heart. Death from drowning in fresh water is, therefore, predominantly cardiac rather than asphyxial in nature and, consequently, is more rapid. It is fair to add that not all authorities are convinced this sequence occurs in the human.

The naso-pharynx and larynx are particularly sensitive to unusual stimuli; the sudden impact of cold fresh or salt water on the back of the throat is a classic potential cause of vagal inhibition of the heart. Those who have fallen out of boats, slipped into canals and the like may, therefore, show none of the standard signs of drowning and often present a

[8] For example, Maskery v. Lancashire Shipping Co. Ltd. (1914) 7 B.W.C.C.428; Ismay, Imrie & Co. v. Williamson [1908] A.C. 437; but *see* Pyper v. Manchester Liners Ltd [1916] 2 K.B. 691 when death due to heat stroke was not considered the result of injury by accident.

difficult pathological problem. Persons who slip in the bath, particularly children, may die in this way; indeed, a *normal* type of drowning in the bath would, in itself, be a suspicious circumstance.[9]

Death from drowning may, again, be accidental, suicidal or homicidal. Accidental drowning is commonly associated with steep-sided, unnatural water courses or containers. Thus, children tend to drown in water tanks, brewery workers may actually drown in the vats and adults falling into canals are less able to extricate themselves than are those who fall into rivers. Alcohol is a very important factor in the latter situation and ill health may also contribute to accidental drowning; epileptics may drown face down in only inches of water. Unconsciousness from any cause will produce the same effect and a person falling into a dock may sustain concussive head injury in the process; the importance – and difficulty – of distinguishing such an injury from one due to an assault needs no emphasis.

Suicidal drowning is surprisingly common – even by walking out to sea, a method which must give ample scope for reconsideration. The placing of weights in the pockets or the tying of legs may be indications of suicide but such methods will also be adopted in criminal activity. The distinction of suicide from either homicide or accident must depend, to a large extent, on the circumstantial evidence. In this connection, Simpson[10] stresses the importance of the location of the hat; the handbag in the case of a woman is, perhaps, an even better distinguishing feature.

There are many variations in homicidal drowning. The possibility of immersion in the bath has already been discussed. Pushing a non-swimmer into inshore water would scarcely be an elective method of murder due to the likelihood of rescue; such cases are more likely to be in the nature of culpable homicide – the actual drowning being the result of a brawl on land. On the other hand, even the best of swimmers will die if thrown from a boat in the open sea; a conclusive distinction between murder and accident might well be impossible on pathological grounds and, indeed, a charge of murder may be brought in the absence of a cadaver. However, the most likely association between criminality and 'drowning' is the disposal in the water of a body already dead; as in incineration, the pathological problem is to distinguish between ante-mortem and post-mortem immersion.

This is often complicated by severe putrefaction following failure to recover bodies from the water for relatively long periods. Not only do the pathological findings change – fluid, for example, passes from the

---

[9] George Smith, who drowned his 'brides in the bath' is, nevertheless, thought to have done so through the medium of vagal stimulation – the method being suddenly to immerse the woman's head by lifting her feet.

[10] In *Forensic Medicine* (1974) 7th ed., London, Edward Arnold, p. 95.

lungs into the pleural spaces – but, during the period of immersion, there is opportunity for destruction of tissue by fish and crustaceans. Additionally, artefacts simulating antemortem injury can be produced by contact with rocks, ships' propellors and the like. The rare condition of cadaveric spasm is probably most often found in drowning; it is almost certain that the casualty was alive on entering the water if weeds or flotsam are discovered firmly clenched in the hand. On the other hand, the finding of mud or weeds in the upper air passages has been criticized as good evidence of respiratory movements while under water – it has been stated that such foreign bodies can enter a dead body; it is difficult to generalize on this – the interpretation depends on the amount of foreign material involved and the depth of its penetration. Two further approaches to the diagnosis of inhalation of water are theoretically available. Firstly, there is the biochemical concept that a high concentration of electrolytes entering the lungs from sea water will be reflected in a higher chloride content in the blood of the left side of the heart than in that of the right; the converse should hold if the pulmonary blood is diluted by fresh water. The test is, however, relatively insensitive – a difference of at least 25 mg chloride/100 ml blood must be demonstrated – and becomes nonspecific with the onset of putrefaction. It generally gives a good result when the diagnosis of death from drowning is obvious; it fails in just those instances where help is needed. The demonstration of other sea water constituents – for example, magnesium – may be of more value while others have drawn attention to the low specific gravity of the blood in the left side of the heart which is found in deaths from drowning irrespective of the type of water concerned. The second test of inhalation depends on the demonstration of diatoms within the body. These are silica-covered organisms of minute size which are found to a varying extent in both salt and fresh water – the precise type of diatoms discovered in the cadaver has been used as an indication of the exact place of death. Most diatoms will be found in the lungs but it is generally held that organisms must be discovered in the systemic circulation – for example, in the bone marrow – to give proof of inhalation *intra vitam*. This is to guard against the possibility of passive entry of water into the lungs after death; the test has also been criticized on the grounds that airborne diatoms are widespread in some districts. The problem seems to be simply one of quantification – the finding of many diatoms is good evidence of drowning but, if only a few are discovered, the result must be considered equivocal. The extreme resistance of the organisms to all forms of digestion makes the test especially valuable in the fact of severe putrefaction.

Drowning is associated with one specific form of delayed death – post-immersion pneumonitis. This inflammatory condition is the result of the structural damage inflicted on the lungs by inhaled water. It may come on only hours after an apparently successful rescue and has a high mortality.

DEATH FROM HYPOTHERMIA

Hypothermic deaths of medico-legal importance fall into two major groups – firstly, those associated with fit persons exposed to the cold, as an example of which immersion in water forms a logical link with the preceding section; secondly, there are the cases involving elderly, unfit persons who die in conditions associated with subnutrition.

In contrast to its relatively good defences against a hot environment, the human body adapts very poorly to cold; the protective mechanism of shivering operates only when the body temperature has actually fallen. The warmest clothing compatible with function, and not artificially heated, will fail to protect a man at rest from a fall in body temperature when that of the ambient temperature is −20° C; it will not keep him in comfort at an ambient temperature of 0° C or less. The subject is at grave risk when the body temperature falls to 30° C, evidence of life is difficult to detect at 27° C and recovery from a fall in temperature to 24° C is unlikely. Shivering ceases when the body temperature has fallen to 33° C and, after that, the only defence open to the body is one involving shifts of blood from the periphery to the deep core. This causes profound physiological changes to which the body may be unable to adapt. Concurrent alcoholism accelerates death probably by interfering with these protective vascular responses.

The body temperature falls with surprising speed. It is doubtful if many persons could survive for more than 15 minutes in the North Sea in winter. Clothing may postpone the end and fat persons will survive longer than thin. The author has seen one case in which three partially clothed children equipped with life jackets were precipitated into the Bristol Channel in very cold weather; there was no evidence of drowning and death was estimated to have occurred in about 10 minutes. A moribund condition of persons removed from the water may be due either to drowning or to hypothermia but the treatment of the one condition is likely to be lethal in the other. The diagnostic dilemma confronting the attending physician may be one of great complexity.

As metabolism approaches zero, so do the body's requirements for oxygen; sufficient quantities of the gas may, in fact, be dissolved in the plasma. States of 'suspended animation' can, therefore, occur. The most outstanding example reported is that of a young boy who travelled for 9 hours in the unpressurized nosewheel compartment of an aircraft at 29 000 ft (8800 m). Death in these circumstances would be expected either from hypoxia or from hypothermia; occurring together, they resulted in unconsciousness which was rapidly reversed in hospital. Any condition greatly reducing the body's need for oxygen – for example, narcotic poisoning – coupled, perhaps, with a low atmospheric temperature as in extreme poverty, might simulate death so closely as to deceive the examining physician; it is conceivable that conditions in the mortuary refrigerator might perpetuate the simulation and cases have occurred when life has been discovered on the autopsy table. Hypothermic deaths do, therefore, require very careful certification and this applies particularly to the classic case of the elderly person living alone in poor conditions.

The post-mortem diagnosis of death due to hypothermia is largely circumstantial and a matter of exclusion. The circulation of blood is affected and leads to the development of a type of surgical shock; characteristically, the inefficient circulation results in the presence of microthrombi – or widespread clotting of the blood in the small vessels. Haemorrhage into the bowel and acute inflammation without bacterial invasion of the pancreas also occur in a high proportion of cases, the underlying mechanism being the same. Very likely, however, nothing specific will be found. Deaths of this type are unlikely to be anything more than a sociological problem although, occasionally, the management of an old people's home might be called into question.

DEATH DUE TO NEGLECT

Neglect is, in practice, divisible into two categories – self-neglect and the neglect of children; occasional cases of deliberate neglect of old persons occur but these must be rare.[11] While skin ulcers, parasitic infestation and the like are an integral part of neglect, it is the accompanying starvation which is the most important factor contributing to death. 'Starvation' consists of subnutrition – which is the intake of an insufficient quantity of food – and malnutrition – which is feeding of inadequate quality. Malnutrition can and does occur as a separate entity; subnutrition must always include some degree of malnutrition.

The usual case of neglect, therefore, presents as an emaciated body which shows multiple trophic ulcers, is verminous and shows evidence of severe vitamin deficiency. The inevitable weakening of the body may open the way to wide dissemination of natural disease but disease may, of course, be the primary cause of the marasmic state; this distinction between cause and effect is of great importance in the event of criminal charges being pressed. The typical case of neglect must have been taking or been provided with *some* sustenance to have survived a sufficient time for the other changes to develop; total starvation is fatal in some two weeks, but life may be prolonged for up to ten weeks so long as fluid

---

[11] There is an interesting discussion of manslaughter by neglect in *Br. Med. J.* (1977) 1, 722.

is available.

Self-neglect commonly represents a failure of society itself, often abetted by the individual's ignorance or fault – alcoholism being a frequent precipitating factor. Other cases of self-neglect have a psychiatric background; certainly not all elderly persons suffering from malnutrition are impoverished although the fear of impending poverty may motivate the condition. Neglect in the well-to-do may be not so much true self-neglect as the result of an incapacity to get about; the possibility that the condition derives, effectively, from neglect by family or society must be considered. If criminal charges are to be brought, there has to be more than simple neglect – there must be evidence of deliberate intent to cause harm or of a reckless indifference to the well-being of a person in the charge of the accused. Nevertheless, all cases of apparent self-neglect deserve intensive forensic study because, irrespective of the elimination of criminality, this is an area of community preventive medicine in which the medico-legal services can be properly involved.

The hunger strike is one aspect of self-neglect – virtually suicidal in nature – which has recently returned to public interest. This situation raises fascinating problems in criminological and medical ethics: the point at which a doctor should actively engage in saving life against the wishes of the subject, thereby committing an assault and often apparently associating himself with a political bias, is one which needs careful assessment – it is fortunate that the great majority of cases are resolved by the politicians themselves and, thus far, no case brought against the doctor by a prisoner so treated has succeeded.[12]

Child neglect is by far the most important aspect of the subject. There in no doubt that some parents are so ignorant as to be incapable of adequately caring for their children but, in many cases, child neglect must have criminal undertones. The obligation placed upon a parent, or other person legally liable to maintain a child, to provide adequate food and clothing, to obtain medical care and to provide housing – or, in the event of these being impossible, to take steps to procure such advantages – is statutory throughout the United Kingdom.[13] The pathologist has often a difficult task in the interpretation of a death due apparently to child neglect. The mere discovery of subnutrition or malnutrition is not evidence of criminal neglect while the role of intercurrent disease may be very difficult to assess; much will depend upon the ancillary evidence – often this will be in the form of unusually severe skin disease. Death due to neglect should be a rarity as efficient social services are widely available to arrange for adequate care and protection while

---

[12] The subject is well discussed in: The law and forced feeding. (1974) *Br. Med. J.* **2,** 737.

[13] Children and Young Persons Act 1933, s. 1(2); Children and Young Persons (Scotland) Act 1937, s. 12(2).

recovery is still possible. Neglect is a fault of omission; the faults of commission associated with child maltreatment are discussed in Chapter 20.

Child neglect includes abandonment or exposure which, in the event of death, could amount to infanticide, child murder, culpable homicide or even murder. The pathological contribution will be likely, in these cases, to be equivocal as the findings will not be those of neglect but rather those of simple hypothermia. Infants are more susceptible to the cold than are adults but the post-mortem diagnosis can seldom be made other than on the basis of exclusion.

Chapter 15

Industrial Injury and Disease

IT IS axiomatic in a developed society that persons should be compensated for disability attributable to their working conditions. Ideally, such compensation should be payable irrespective of contributory fault and, while not excluding the possibility, should be free from the uncertainties of litigation on the bases of negligence or of contributory negligence. Such a system has been in operation in the United Kingdom since 1948 when the original National Insurance (Industrial Injuries) Act became operative. The relevant legislation is now consolidated in the Social Security Act 1975.[1]

All persons employed in an insurable occupation are automatically insured – through contributions from employees, employers and the Exchequer – against disablement, incapacity or death resulting from an injury by accident arising out of and in the course of employment. The definition of injury is wide, including any physiological injury or change for the worse, and that of accident is equally embracing, being 'an unlooked-for-mishap or an untoward event which is not expected or designed'. The course of work need not be the proper course – for example, failure to take such safety measures as have been ordered has no effect on the payment of benefits (s. 52). Accidents due to skylarking or misconduct by another also attract benefit (s. 55).

There are, however, limits to which an insurance fund can stretch and disputes as to definition[2] are bound to occur; nor is industrial disease an entirely straightforward subject.

Injuries which are self-evident – that is, those which involve external mutilation – will not be discussed here; not only are these beyond dispute but they are so various that a detailed description would be impossible. But the term 'accident' also includes injuries sustained in circumstances which are accidental merely by virtue of being unexpected. These circumstances need not be exceptional; an unexpected

---

[1] Previous legislation is repealed in Social Security (Consequential Provisions) Act 1975. Northern Ireland has its own Act (Social Security (Northern Ireland) Act 1975).

[2] Examples being the definition of 'place of work' in relation to transport and physical boundaries. A person is generally held to be at his place of work if he is in transport provided by his employers (positively enacted, s. 53) but not when in his own; an accident occurring in the grounds of a factory would also probably qualify for compensation.

178

event may be brought about by the routine engagement in work and it is immaterial that the work did no more than exacerbate known pre-existing disease.[3] A person more prone to accident than normal is still covered by the Act; thus, a known epileptic who has a fit at work and, as a result, suffers injury still sustains an industrial injury.[4]

Disease contracted at work is dealt with in two main categories. There is first a disease which results from a single occurrence at work – and this is clearly an accident. The precise moment of injury need not be defined in all circumstances; a nurse contracting tuberculosis was clearly infected at a certain time although the precise exposure which was responsible for infection cannot be ascertained. In certain circumstances, however, there is continuing exposure to a work hazard and a disease contracted as a result is a matter of process rather than of accident. To qualify for insurance benefits, the second category of disease must be prescribed by regulations. These diseases are loosely defined as those which can be attributed with reasonable certainty to the occupation and which do not constitute a risk to the whole population; sufferers from such diseases are treated for insurance purposes exactly as if they had sustained an accidental injury. A list of prescribed diseases is given in Appendix I.

Benefits for industrial injuries are available as:

a. Injury Benefit payable as an allowance during the period in which the insured is unable to work through injury. It is not payable in respect of pneumoconiosis when it is replaced by special benefit. Injury Benefit is given for 156 days disregarding Sundays and is then replaced by

b. Disablement Benefit which is payable according to the disability (including disfigurement) sustained expressed as a percentage of total disablement. Less than 20 per cent disability is paid in gratuity form; otherwise it is distributed weekly. The disablement pension can be increased by an unemployability supplement and, *inter alia*, in respect of special hardship or exceptionaly severe disablement.

c. Death Benefit is payable as a pension to a widow until remarriage – at which time a gratuity is paid. The amount payable is naturally modified by the number of dependants of the dead person.

Problems as to whether an injury is to be regarded as industrial are decided by an Insurance Officer; referral or appeal is to a local tribunal consisting of a chairman and a representative each of employers and employees. There is a further right of appeal to a National Insurance

---

[3] Clover, Clayton & Co. Ltd. v. Hughes [1910] A.C. 242; Oates v. Earl Fitzwilliam's Collieries Co. [1939] 2 All E.R. 498.

[4] Tankard v. Stone-Platt Engineering Co. Ltd. (1946) 174 L.T. 277.

Commissioner. Cases of special difficulty may be heard by a tribunal of three Commissioners. The degree of disablement is, however, decided by Medical Boards consisting of two or more medical practitioners. Appeals from their decisions are made to Medical Appeal Tribunals consisting of a chairman and two consultant medical practitioners; both the board and the tribunal may reverse their assessments if there are reasonable grounds. Final appeal against the decision of a Medical Tribunal is to a Commissioner, such appeal being permissible only on a point of law.

Specific regulations are made as to prescribed diseases – in particular, the establishment of special medical boards and the appointment of special medical officers – and provisions are made in regard to the pneumoconioses[5] which cover initial and periodic medical examinations and also allow for suspension or nonemployment of persons found to be suffering from pneumoconiosis. Attendance at, and provision of facilities for, such examinations are compulsory. Byssinosis, or dust disease following inhalation of cotton dust, was, at one time, considered separately but is now benefited in the same way as any other occupational dust disease. A list of prescribed occupations is given at Appendix J.

The Role of the Lawyer in Industrial Compensation

A worker seeking industrial benefit may be represented – and, indeed, need not be present – at hearings of the local tribunal and before the National Insurance Commissioner. The main function of these appeal bodies is to decide whether or not the ruling of the Insurance Officer as to the definition of an industrial accident is valid.[6]

Decisions, unless setting a precedent, will largely depend upon previous rulings which can be studied under the heading of 'Commissioners' Decisions'; these are published individually or bound under categories of benefit in the continuing 'Index and Digest of Decisions'. The list of conditions which have been held to be industrial accidents is steadily lengthening – some of the more extreme examples including a nervous shock resulting from watching a fatal accident which involved a workmate, a 'drop foot' sustained as a result of continual kneeling (this being something of an extension of accident as opposed to process) and coronary thrombosis arising during the act of tightening a nut.

It follows that not only must the lawyer be aware of these decisions but that, in the case of death, these should have been founded on good medical evidence. Ideally, all deaths occurring at the place of work

---

[5] Pneumoconiosis is defined as fibrosis of the lung due to silica dust, asbestos dust or other dust and includes the condition of the lungs known as 'dust-reticulation'.

[6] It is the Secretary of State who is charged with the duty of deciding whether the *occupation* was insurable under the Act (s. 93).

should be reported to the Fiscal or the Coroner irrespective of the certifying doctor's opinion as to the causative association with the deceased's occupation[7] and the cause of death should be certified as a result of post-mortem dissection; such a procedure would at least narrow the fields of dispute as to fact. It has been noted that appeal from the decisions of the Medical Appeal Tribunal can be made only on points of law; the role of the lawyer is then self-evident.

Both the solicitor and the advocate may be further involved in industrial litigation in so far as there is an ultimate appeal from a decision of the Commissioner to the High Court on a point of law. Much civil litigation is initiated by employed persons against their employers based on negligence resulting in loss, injury and damage; in a proportion of these, the provisions of the Law Reform (Contributory Negligence) Act 1945 are invoked when the damages fall to be reduced on account of the contributory negligence of the injured party himself. There have recently been a significant number of successful actions for negligence against employers by workers who have contracted prescribed diseases. All such cases appear to have been settled out of court and are therefore unreported, but damages of £7500 have been awarded to a man with coal miners' pneumoconiosis.[8]

The medical nature of conventional 'accidents' at work is generally readily understandable and the logical sequence implied in disease contracted as a result of an accident is also normally clear. The nature – and rationale – of the prescribed diseases may not, however, be common knowledge in legal circles and a brief description is apposite.

THE PNEUMOCONIOSES
As stated above, the pneumoconioses are defined as fibrosis of the lung resulting from exposure to dust; they are listed in Appendix J.

Fibrogenic dust may be mineral or vegetable in nature. The former is by far the more important and, while all occupations associated with mineral dust carry some risk, three conditions are outstanding – coal miner's pneumoconiosis because of its frequency in the United Kingdom, silicosis because it is, perhaps, the underlying basis for the clinical manifestations of the majority of mineral dust diseases and asbestosis because of its severe effects and because it is a particularly good example of how workers other than miners – perhaps even the general population – may be affected by dust.

Coal Miners' Pneumoconiosis
Some 35 000 certified cases of coal workers' pneumoconiosis are on

---

[7] See the Brodrick Report, para. 6.33 (*Report of the Committee on Death Certification and Coroners.* 1971, Cmnd. 4810. London. HMSO).

[8] *Sunday Times*, 1 February, 1970.

record in the United Kingdom. About 500 new cases are certified each year.[9]

Pulmonary changes are often originally symptomless and are gauged radiologically; but this may not necessarily be so and the interrelationship of pneumoconiosis with other lung disease poses a considerable clinical problem which may result in differences of expert opinion when litigation or problems of compensation arise. The disease is divided into simple and complicated forms and, in view of the difficulties of clinical assessment, the former is empirically quantified on the radiological appearances. The lesions seen in the X-ray are known as nodules and these are classified according to size (Group p nodules are up to 1·5 mm in diameter, Group m from 1·5 to 3·0 mm and Group n between 3·0 and 10·0 mm). The severity of the disease is further classified by its distribution, Category 1 diseases being limited to defined portions of the lungs while Category 3 denotes affection of the whole of both lungs; Category 2 is intermediate (*Plate* 13b).

Complicated pneumoconiosis is alternatively known as progressive massive fibrosis (PMF). Nodules larger than 10 mm in diameter appear and coalesce to produce extensive destruction of the lung with severe symptoms of respiratory distress. The incidence of PMF rises with the extent of the simple disease but, while the two must be in some way connected, the relationship is by no means a simple one. Coincidental tuberculosis probably plays a major part in the extension of the primary disease; the effects of coincident tuberculosis are treated as though they were the effects of pneumoconiosis.

It is officially stated[10] that simple pneumoconiosis is not itself a cause of disability and does not reduce the expectation of life. Certainly other respiratory diseases are often present as no more than coincidentals but the total validity of this pragmatic view is, at least, open to challenge.[11] The main conditions which are agreed as complicating simple pneumoconiosis are chronic bronchitis and emphysema; provided the primary disability is not less than 50 per cent, any disability due to these is added to the assessment of the dust disease for the purposes of benefit.

Because of the clinical difficulties involved, compensation is largely based on 'rule of thumb' observations. The suspected case is examined by two members of the Pneumoconiosis Panel and is certified as suffering from pneumoconiosis if they agree that Category 2 disease is present – Category 1 disease is sometimes accepted if the subject is young. The

[9] The approximate comparable figures for pneumoconiosis as a whole are 40 000 and 800.

[10] Ministry of Social Security (1967) *Pneumoconiosis and Allied Occupational Chest Diseases.* London, HMSO.

[11] *See*, for example, Davies D. (1974) Disability and coal workers' pneumoconiosis, *Br. Med. J.* **2**, 652.

degree of disability is assessed on the basis of the vital capacity of the lungs – which is a measure of the amount of oxygen the lungs can make available to the body – and on the forced expiratory volume of the breath – which is a measure of the effectiveness or impairment of the elasticity and, hence, efficient function of the lungs. No appeal is normally available against the decision of the Pneumoconiosis Medical Panel save, in special circumstances, to the central Pneumoconiosis Medical Board; rejection of a claim does not prohibit repeated applications.

This valiant attempt to ensure a uniform procedure, the rationale of which is readily demonstrable, causes some problems which are particularly related to the difficulties of correlating clinical symptoms, which may have several different origins, with the radiological appearances, which are related to a single causative factor. It is often difficult for a legal adviser to understand how one man with apparently appreciable respiratory distress can be denied benefit while a much fitter colleague is a certified pneumoconiotic; yet it can and does occur.

Further causes of confusion may attend the result of post-mortem dissection. The Registrar of Deaths is obliged to report to the Procurator Fiscal or to the Coroner any deaths due to or arising from industrial disease or poisoning (*see* Chapter 2).[12] The Coroner must also notify the Pneumoconiosis Panel of the date and place of the postmortem examination and the Panel may be represented there; no such obligation rests on either the Procurator Fiscal or the Registrar in Scotland. While the Rules prevent a Coroner asking a member of the Pneumoconiosis Medical Panel to carry out the dissection,[13] there is an informal arrangement whereby the thoracic organs are later made available to the Panel.[14] Thus the Coroner's certificate of death – whether it be by virtue of his own Form B or of a Certificate after Inquest – may include pneumoconiosis as relevant to death whereas the Pneumoconiosis Medical Panel may decide that there is no entitlement to Industrial Death Benefit; the converse may also hold. The important fact is that the report of the Coroner's pathologist is only indirectly associated with death benefit in so far as the Pneumoconiosis Medical Panel will usually take into account the results of the Coroner's inquiries and these may also be used as evidence on appeal against the decision of the Insurance Officer; in the final analysis, however, it is the opinion of the Pneumoconiosis Panel which exerts the main influence on the Insurance Officer.

---

[12] In neither case is there a requirement for a doctor, who is willing to provide a certificate as to the cause of death, to draw attention to any occupational condition which, in his opinion, has no association with that cause.

[13] Coroners' Rules 1953, Rule 3(d).

[14] Home Office Circular 79/69.

The importance of post-mortem dissection and of the availability of the evidence to the equitable settling of cases is obvious.

Silicosis

Silica in its large particulate form causes no more than a harmless reaction to a foreign body. But when the size of particles is small, a fibrotic reaction is set up which has profound effects on the lungs. Silica is, in essence, the primary source of the pneumoconioses and is likely to be dispersed whenever rock is drilled or sand is particularized as in the cleaning of blast furnaces, building in sandstone, grinding and the like. Coal dust as such is relatively innocuous in the absence of silica; true silicosis in coal miners generally occurs only in those confronted with the harder seams – that is in anthracite miners and in the 'hard headers' who drive the tunnels to reach the face. Gold mining is particularly dangerous as a source of the disease.

The lesion in silicosis is that of formation of fibrotic nodules due to the locally poisonous properties of silica when dissolved – possibly in the form of salicic acid. The process is self-perpetuating, the amount of fibrosis is disproportionate to the quantity of dust and the end result is massive destruction of lung tissue with death from a combination of cardiac and respiratory failure. In the process, the original isolated nodules coalesce to form what is known as massive conglomerate nodular silicosis; alternatively, a form of progressive massive fibrosis, not unlike that seen in coal miners' pneumoconiosis, may arise.

Silicosis is clearly associated with tuberculosis and potentiates the virulence of the organism causing the latter disease. There is, however, no fully acceptable evidence that silica stimulates the formation of cancer.[15] Thus, silicosis differs markedly from the third of the most important dust diseases – asbestosis.

Asbestosis

Asbestos occurs in two main types – chrysotile and amphiboles of which there are three varieties, crocidolite, amosite and anthophyllite. The fibres of the former are long and are used mainly for the preparation of asbestos clothing; those of the latter are shaped like needles and are used to make roofing, tiles and insulating material.

As with all dust disease, asbestosis consists of fibrosis of the lung tissue which can be finely nodular or dense and massive. Since asbestos is virtually indestructible, its effects on the lung are progressive even after removal from the dusty environment. Fibrosis of the lung does

---

[15] Two haematite mines in Cumbria, separated by only 30 miles, showed a marked difference in the incidence of lung cancer. In the mine associated with soft clay substrate, cancer was not an occupational hazard; the incidence of cancer among workers in the hard rock mines was some 70 per cent above the general level. The difference, however, might well have been due to radioactivity – cf. the iron ore miners in Czechoslovakia.

occur in asbestos mines but, because the main offending condition is the 'asbestos cloud', those who are exposed to asbestos in its purified – or purifying – form are at greatest risk. Asbestos is used in very many industrial processes but maximum exposure outside the factories concerned with preparation occurs in the building trade, in shipbuilding, where it is used mainly as a thermal insulator, and in the manufacture of brakes, clutches and the like. The danger is particularly great during the destruction of asbestos products when masses of very dry dust are dispersed in relatively uncontrolled conditions. There is, therefore, a potential hazard to the public in the vicinity of large reconstruction projects.[16]

Although simple asbestosis may cause lethal dysfunction of the lungs, and may be associated with tuberculosis, the danger which distinguishes asbestosis from almost all other forms of pneumoconiosis is its incontrovertible association with malignant tumours of the lung. Asbestos workers have a death rate from the common form of lung cancer – bronchogenic carcinoma – which is some ten times that of the general population. This increase is almost entirely taken up by an association with smoking. Asbestos workers who do not smoke are scarcely at an increased risk unless exposed to exceptional concentrations. Bronchogenic carcinoma is probably associated with all types of asbestos and with a relatively long exposure but one particular form of cancer – mesothelioma – appears to be particularly associated with exposure to crocidolite or 'blue asbestos'.[17] It is very rarely associated with chrysotile and never with anthophyllite. There is some evidence that mesothelioma occurring in miners results from exposure to an asbestos/manganese complex but it is workers in an atmosphere laden with the dust from prepared asbestos products who are at greatest risk; the exposure to blue asbestos need only be short and, of major medico-legal significance, there is always a long incubation period – the condition may not manifest itself for some 20–40 years after exposure. A cause-and-effect association may be difficult to prove – or defend – at such a distance in time; the provisions of the Limitation Acts 1963 and 1975, which extend the period in which an action for personal damages can be brought in the event of there being no symptoms for some time after an untoward event, must be invoked in any suit for negligence.

Other Prescribed Diseases

The pneumoconioses are so distinct and of such importance that they have been given particular prominence. Other prescribed diseases are less common and are of such diversity as to preclude a full description

---

[16] Very rigid precautions are laid down in the Asbestos Regulations 1969.

[17] Mesothelioma may be greatly reduced in future due to the virtual banning of crocidolite under a Code of Practice in the asbestos industry.

outside a work confined to industrial medicine. The reader will be able to understand the great majority from a simple view of Appendix I; some specific aspects of poisoning are, however, considered in Chapter 22.

SAFETY AT WORK

Safety at work has been regulated by two main statutes – the Mines and Quarries Act 1954 and the Factories Act 1961.[18]

The Factories Act laid down provisions,for health, safety and welfare in factories – which include premises designed for the making, adapting, cleaning or demolition of an article, slaughterhouses and a host of other designated places where work is carried out – and established an Inspectorate of Factories. The Inspectors have wide powers of entry to relevant premises and to examine documents. From the medico-legal point of view, the most important sections are those which deal with the notification of accidents, which must be so notified in the event of death or disablement for more than three days of an employee; particularly dangerous occurrences must be notified even if there is no major personal injury.

Certain industrial diseases must also be notified by a doctor to the Chief Inspector of Factories – these include poisoning by lead, phosphorus, arsenic and mercury or infection by anthrax when contracted in a factory. Subsequent to the original Act, poisoning by beryllium and cadmium have been added to the list together with a number of other diseases which are listed in Appendix K.

The Employment Medical Advisory Service Act 1972 amends the 1961 Act in relation to the medical arrangements in places of work. Factory doctors have been replaced by Employment Medical Advisers who form the medical wing of the Health and Safety Executive (see below); the medical advisers are granted the full powers of an Inspector as defined in the Factories Act and they will investigate the cause of death, injury, disease or poisoning resulting from employment.

In England and Wales and in Scotland, the Minister may direct that a full investigation be held into the causes and circumstances of any accident occurring or of any disease acquired in a factory – it is not uncommon for a legal man to be appointed as the Assessor and lawyers will be involved on behalf of the parties concerned.

Deaths resulting from a notifiable disease or accident must be reported to the Coroner or to the Procurator Fiscal. The former is obliged

---

[18] Somewhat similar provisions appropriate to the work areas implied in the titles are contained in the Agriculture (Safety, Health and Welfare Provisions) Act 1956, the Offices, Shops and Railway Premises Act 1963, and the Mineral Workings (Offshore Installations) Act 1971.

to hold an Inquest with a jury at which any interested party may be legally represented. In Scotland, the same situation is covered by the inquiry which is held under the Fatal Accidents and Sudden Deaths Inquiry (Scotland) Act 1976 but such an Inquiry will not normally be held if a Ministerial Public Inquiry has been ordered.

Mines and quarries are defined basically as places where persons are employed in the getting of minerals. The massive Mines and Quarries Act 1954 contains provisions as to health and safety which are similar to, but more extensive than, those detailed in the Factories Act. Notification of death or serious injury must be made not only to the Inspector of Mines but also to the nominee of the trade union concerned; this, of course, applies also to specified disease. Coroners' Inquests must also be held before a jury and the Inspector of Mines must be informed and given reasonable opportunity to be present at the inquest. The Minister may direct an Inspector's investigation or a Public Inquiry, the latter again rendering a Fatal Accident Inquiry unnecessary in Scotland. The 1954 Act stipulates that the Inspector has the power to direct that the site of an accident or dangerous occurrence be left undisturbed so long as is reasonably necessary for the purposes of an examination; it also provides for some control of safety factors by the workers themselves.[19]

The Health and Safety at Work, etc. Act 1974 makes an attempt to provide a comprehensive system of law designed to integrate the safety and health of work people and the public. It establishes a Health and Safety Commission and an Executive who may direct that a public inquiry be held into the circumstances of a mishap.[20] None of the more directly medico-legally important provisions of the earlier Acts discussed above are, however, altered.[21]

---

[19] Section 120; s. 123.

[20] With the usual dispensation for a Fatal Accident Inquiry in Scotland.

[21] A minor amendment (incorporated at p. 36) to the Coroner's Amendment Act 1926, s. 13(2)(c) is required.

Chapter 16

Medico-legal Aspects of Sport

GENERALLY speaking, medico-legal aspects of sport are governed by the doctrine of *volenti non fit injuria*. However, this cannot always hold. There are several interests involved in organized sport – including those of the participants, the promoters and the public – and while the Roman crowds no doubt felt themselves well entertained, it is unlikely that the early Christians were happy with their representation. So much is now materially at stake in what once were games that the law must become involved; injury and death at sport are now integral parts of forensic medicine.

It is not intended to consider all potential injuries which can arise in risk sports; most are relatively obvious and few – other than accidental gunshot wounds which are discussed in Chapter 9 – have particular medico-legal significance other than in relation to standards of professional medical care – negligence in treatment of a knee injury occurring in a man who made his living from football would be likely to attract greater damages than would be the case in similar circumstances involving an elderly bank clerk. But those sports which are, in effect, legalized assaults require separate consideration, and there are other more general aspects of forensic medicine which can conveniently be discussed under this chapter heading.

BOXING AND WRESTLING

Springing from its roots in illegal prize-fighting and being most obviously associated with 'intent to inflict bodily injury', boxing has inevitably attracted the greatest forensic attention among sports.

Attitudes to boxing have altered dramatically in a lifetime. In the amateur sphere, the annual school boxing tournament has fallen so far from its position as the event of the year that the Royal College of Physicians has concluded 'it must be generally questioned whether there is any justification for including boxing as a school sport'.[1] It is fair to point out that, against this view, there are many who regard organized boxing as a controlled method of unleashing normal violence and, as a

---

[1] Royal College of Physicians (1969) *Report on the Medical Aspects of Boxing.* London, Royal College of Physicians.

result, a positive contribution to the reduction of violent crime. On the professional side, there is no doubt that stricter controls introduced since the Second World War have transformed the image of boxing. Perhaps the administrative changes have been accelerated by the campaign against the sport which has been based to some extent on its mortality and, more importantly, on the associated long-term morbidity.

There are, in fact, surprisingly few acute fatalities in boxing. Between 1955 and 1958, only one death was attributed to boxing in the United Kingdom out of 50 deaths occurring during sport – astonishingly, during the same period, 14 persons were killed playing cricket.[2] It is claimed that there have been less than 20 deaths from boxing since 1945. When it occurs, death is most commonly due to intracranial haemorrhage; intracerebral bleeding into the midbrain is the injury said to be most specific to boxing, but subdural bleeding, with its attendant latent period, is, in practice, less uncommon; abnormal stimulation of the autonomic nervous system, as by blows to the neck or to the solar plexus, are occasional causes of sudden death.

Far greater interest centres on the long-term effects of boxing – traumatic encephalopathy or 'punch drunkenness'. There is no doubt as to the reality of this syndrome although its frequency may have been exaggerated. The precise mechanism is unknown but it probably results from a succession of attacks of 'diffuse neuronal injury' described in Chapter 11 as the cause of concussion. The condition, which is characterized by defects of memory, slurring of speech, unsteadiness of gait and clumsy movements, appears related to persistent repetition of severe injury to the head – it is, therefore, one which occurs in poor-quality boxers forced by economic necessity into frequent bouts beyond their capability and who consequently receive more than average punishment; there is also some evidence that punch-drunkenness is associated with the length of each bout – while the brain can recover from five contests of three rounds each, it has no interval in which to do so during fifteen consecutive rounds. The *Report on the Medical Aspects of Boxing* concluded that, while the likelihood of severe disablement due to brain damage was rare in boxers, there was evidence of a lesser degree of damage in a high proportion of persons who had boxed professionally for over ten years.

This being so, the effects of boxing should be preventable by regulation and, certainly, much effort is put into this aspect of the spectacle. A strict medical code has been enforced in British professional boxing since 1953 and includes general annual examinations of licensed boxers as well as immediate pre-fight medical check-ups. The number of bouts is controlled by the Medical Commission of the British Board of Boxing

[2] Parliamentary Debates, House of Lords, 1962, vol. 240, col. 366.

Control who also have the power to withdraw a man's licence on the grounds of ill health. Appointed doctors are present at the ringside to advise on fitness to continue the fight and to assess the injury in the event of a knockout; an injured boxer must be suspended until he is declared fit for another bout. Moreover, an investigation is mounted if a boxer loses four fights in succession.

In view of all these precautions, a death in the ring can scarcely be regarded as anything other than accidental; this, however, depends upon the regulations being observed. Death resulting from a deliberate mismatch could certainly attract a charge of culpable homicide as would one which could be attributed to premeditated failure to stop a fight which was clearly leading to severe injury. Disability sustained because of inadequate pre-fight medical examination could be, and has been, construed as being attributable to medical negligence.[3]

It may seem inequitable that the *voluntary* provision of medical care can lead to litigation when such care is seen to fall short of acceptable standards; there are, for example, no comparable controls in professional wrestling, yet this causes no adverse comment. There would, however, be a popular demand for medical supervision of wrestling should the need become apparent; the fact that death or severe injury is virtually unknown in professional 'all-in' wrestling in the United Kingdom can probably be left to speak for itself – interestingly enough, there is a considerable morbidity in Eastern Europe. It is doubtful if boxing would have survived the political attacks of the early 1960s had it not set its own house in order; public opinion, having forced a standard, requires that standard to be maintained.

SUDDEN DEATH IN NON-CONTACT SPORTS

Occasional deaths occur in apparently healthy young adults engaged in strenuous exercise such as long-distance running, protracted swimming or severe marching. Sometimes the environmental conditions are obviously extreme and can be held responsible for the death – e.g. in severe heat death may be due to heat stroke or heat exhaustion (see Chapter 14) or, at the other end of the spectrum, an enforced stop may lead to death from exposure; many deaths of this type result from ignoring authoritative advice or from inadequate planning.

Very often, however, the cause of death is obscure and may only be assumed after a diligent search has revealed some unusual abnormality; equally, no cause may be demonstrable and the death is, in effect, physiological. The abnormal conditions discovered are generally those

---

[3] Polson C. J. and Gee D. J. in *The Essentials of Forensic Medicine*, p.184, quote a case of retinal detachment in which a claim against the Medical Officer of the boxing club was settled for £4600. There was an element of contributory negligence in this case.

which might be expected to leave the heart dangerously short of oxygen in the event of excessive demand – in particular, anatomical abnormalities of the coronary circulation or an unusual degree of atheroma. The importance of these conditions in a medico-legal context is twofold – firstly, they would not have been recognizable by routine medical tests for fitness and, as a corollary, no blame for the death can reasonably be attached to the organizers of the activity. A number of such deaths have been attributed to blood disorders which are sensitive to hypoxia; sickle cell disease has been cited and other unusual conditions[4] may cause collapse and dangerous sequelae if not sudden death. Selection both for employment and for recreation on the basis of sickle cell trait is seldom practicable in the absence of symptoms; nevertheless, persons known to have the trait should be warned of the possible dangers and doctors responsible for certifying fitness should obtain written acknowledgment that appropriate advice has been given. Some form of abnormal reflex nervous stimulation – or, equally nebulously, an acute failure of an essential endocrine gland such as the adrenal – must be supposed in those cases in which no cause of death can be discovered; the author has been impressed by the number of these deaths which appear to be associated with very full stomachs – this suggests the former possibility, but such diagnoses are rarely satisfying.

SPORTS AND STEROIDS

Competition in any walk of life leads to the search for advantages of doubtful morality. International sport is no exception and, in the last decade, much attention has focused on the use of a group of hormones known as *anabolic steroids* as intended aids to the improvement of physical performance.

There is no doubt that the total muscle mass is increased by their use but it may well be that this is achieved through water retention rather than by an increase in the size and number of fibres;[5] much of the physical result attributed to steroids has been ascribed to psychological effects, including a euphoric attitude to hard training. The balance of evidence would seem, however, to be that, provided the subjects are already highly trained, steroids can significantly improve performance – and this applies particularly in power events. It has been pointed out that standards in women's field sports improved very rapidly from 1968 and it could well be that this coincided with the general introduction of

---

[4] For examples the condition known as 'march haemoglobinuria' in which the red blood cells break down in the particular circumstances of strenuous exercise. The main danger lies in associated acute renal failure.

[5] A distinction which is of no consequence in 'body building' competitions; steroid adjuvants are permitted by the organizers of these events.

steroids – there is little doubt that the habit of steroid medication is now fairly widespread among high-grade athletes.

Against their probable benefits must be balanced the ill effects of steroids, particularly as there is a strong probability that some self-medicators will inevitably over prescribe, especially if there has been a good response to small doses. The side effects involve hirsutism, spotty skin (acne), prostatic enlargement and, of greater importance, some degree of liver damage. There is loss of libido and, perhaps, loss of fertility. Many of these effects are due to the associated androgen (or 'maleness producing') effects of the steroids. More serious effects on growth, etc., may, therefore, result from the use of these hormones in high dosage in prepubertal subjects. As with any substance used essentially to alter the physiology of the body, withdrawal should be gradual lest a sudden imbalance be precipitated.

Laboratory tests for anabolic steroids are available, but are expensive and require considerable expertise; control of their abuse in sport is, therefore, difficult – prohibition without detection is an unsatisfactory state of affairs. The Technical Commission of the International Federation of Sports Medicine has condemned the use of steroids by healthy sportsmen but the onus of discovery and elimination rests on the governing bodies of the sports concerned.[6]

Other forms of 'doping' have been – and may well still be – used in competitive sports; the amphetamines, for example, had a vogue as stimulants. The amphetamines, in particular, are unlikely to pose any problem in British athletics, being now Class B controlled drugs[7] – they are also readily demonstrable in body fluids. The difficulties in screening for known drugs which are excreted in the urine or saliva are not, in fact, so much technical as emotional and political; very adequate control can be exercised over race-horses.

SEX AND SPORT

Problems in the differentiation of sex are discussed in relation to marriage in Chapter 17. In recent years, comparable problems have arisen in competitive international sport where intimate medical examinations of competitors as a routine would be unacceptable. This is, therefore, an appropriate place to draw attention to some of the unexceptional methods available for the determination of the genetic sex on a screening basis; such methods depend upon the positive demonstration of either the Y chromosome or of what may be the XX agglomerate.

The latter process is that most commonly used and depends upon the fact that a high proportion of female cell nuclei show one or two dots of

[6] Br. J. Sports Med. (1975) 9, 111.
[7] Misuse of Drugs Act 1971 (see Chapter 23).

chromatin, easily visible under the microscope, beneath the nuclear membrane – the so-called 'Barr bodies'. These bodies are well seen in the skin or smooth muscle when a surgical biopsy is taken but this is, of course, impossible for routine use. Screening on a large scale is facilitated by the fact that the surface cells of the mucosa of the mouth are a good source of diagnostic Barr bodies. It is quite practicable to rub the inside of the cheek with a blunt edge, to transfer the cells removed to a slide and to stain them. The proportion of cells showing Barr bodies is not high. One must find them in at least 2 nuclei out of every 100 cells examined to make a firm diagnosis of femininity.

A variation on this theme is the demonstration of sex chromatin or 'Davidson' bodies in the polymorphonuclear white cells of the blood. These appear as drumstick appendages to the multilobular nuclei. They are not easy to distinguish with certainty from other nuclear excrescences which occur independently of XX chromosomes and they are, again, by no means universal in the cells. The classic test for femininity involves discovery of six drumsticks. If these are found in less than 300 consecutive polymorph cells then the subject is regarded as 'chromatin positive' – this being a properly purist way of expressing 'femininity' through the finding of chromatin bodies.

The only advantage to be gained in sport from a sex transfer is for a chromosomal male to masquerade as a female – the deception need not be deliberate and may be due to genuine error. The tests described above therefore suffer from being of a negative nature. It is the *failure* to demonstrate chromatin bodies which indicates a deception. It would be preferable to demonstrate the Y chromosome positively and this can be done using, again, either desquamated cells from the inside of the mouth or white blood corpuscles; a positive result depends on the ability of the Y chromosome to fluoresce when treated with the dye quinacrine. The technique is considerably more complex than is that involved in searching for female chromatin masses. The portion of cells which are clearly 'Y positive' varies from 15 per cent to 80 per cent with different observers; a very occasional cell which is apparently male may be found in normal females. Most people would regard the technique as currently in the development stage (*Plate* 14).

Problems of false sex are of decreasing importance in sport largely due to their increasing ease of discovery. Sexing by cells is, however, widely used in population studies and in the investigation of infants of doubtful genital sex – the chromatin bodies are developed *in utero* and much psychological difficulty can be avoided by an early diagnosis.

DEATH AND INJURY IN THE CROWD

The extent of violence in a crowd depends on two main characteristics –

the quality of the crowd and its quantity as related to available space.

As to quality, it is a matter of common observation that the corporate nature of crowds at sporting events has changed dramatically in the last 20 years, so much so that a proportion of spectators at some events appear to attend with the express intention of being violent and others must take steps to defend themselves. Despite intensive police action, offensive weapons find their way into stadiums and injuries ranging from those due to kicking, through bottle injuries, to those involving the use of razors and knives are sustained each week. Violence may, of course, be continued after the event itself. Apart from the unusual environment in which they are inflicted, the injuries do not differ materially from those which are described elsewhere and they need no further consideration here. Some forms of traumatic injury and death which are related to the number and density of persons are, however, typified by sports crowds and can conveniently be discussed in this section.

A human being can tolerate considerable crowding in normal circumstances and in a normal atmosphere. Minor physiological disturbances such as fainting or collapse due to heat exhaustion occur frequently but, provided the subject can be removed from the crowd, no lasting injury results. Danger is associated with loss of 'herd' control which may be accidental or impulsive. The former is exemplified by the collapse of a stand or of crowd control barriers and the latter by a crowd's reaction when attempting to move in difficulty or under threat of danger.

In the event of crowd collapse, death may result from traumatic asphyxia. This has already been mentioned in Chapter 13. The sheer weight of bodies – the condition is very rare except on inclined terraces or when the subjects are supine – prevents the use of the thoracic and abdominal muscles of respiration. An element of suffocation by occlusion of the nose and mouth may be added. A feature of this type of death is that the blood vessels are also compressed; the classic appearances of asphyxia – congestion and petechial haemorrhage – are characteristically exaggerated in traumatic asphyxia.

Similar deaths will occur if the crowd piles up at an exit, particularly when the route funnels downwards. The conditions are self-generating as those who find themselves obstructed by others in front attempt to escape the crush of those behind. Panic ensues and injuries due to trampling may well predominate; the extreme of such a situation is seen when a pressing danger such as fire is propelling the crowd forward. A remarkable example of a human 'stampede' occurred in the London underground in 1942 when 173 persons died while taking shelter from an air raid. The disaster was precipitated by one or a few persons stumbling and obstructing the free flow of people.

In either type of event, death may be delayed for some days and be ultimately due to the 'crush syndrome'. This condition, which is certainly not confined to crowds,[8] results essentially from the crushing of the muscle masses and release of degeneration products. Death is due to acute renal failure, but, in practice, recovery is the rule in those who survive the initial trauma. A major medico-legal issue arising from crowd deaths centres on the responsibility of the owners of the stadium for the safety of spectators. A simple disclaimer written on a ticket would certainly not absolve the promoters from blame and the heavy damages awarded to the estates of those killed at Ibrox Park, Glasgow, indicate that negligence is proved unless all reasonable safety precautions have been taken on behalf of the crowd. The definition of reasonable precautions in these circumstances would seem to be difficult – this was one of the twilight areas of liability referred to by the Pearson Committee as meriting consideration.[9] The subject is one on which there has been recent legislation.[10]

A NOTE ON HAZARDS OF DIVING

An appreciable number of recreational divers die each year and the exploitation of North Sea oil has recently focused attention on the hazards of professional diving. The diver is essentially at risk on three counts – the effects of pressure, the need for an artificial respiratory environment and the dangers from marine predators.

The pressure increases by 101 kPa (1 atmosphere) with every 33 ft (10 metres) of depth. A great excess of air is therefore needed to fill the lungs and this expands during ascent; the same principles apply to gases dissolved in the body fluids.

While breathing air at depth, the diver may suffer from both nitrogen narcosis – a condition which has been likened to acute alcoholism – or from acute oxygen poisoning which can occur when this essential gas is inhaled under pressure (over 300 kPa) and causes convulsions of central cerebral origin. In either case, the diver may die from the direct effects, he may become incoordinated and mismanage his task or his apparatus, he may drown or he may ascend precipitously.

Rapid ascent leads to massive expansion of the lungs and to release of bubbles of gas – nitrogen being especially significant – from the body fluids. Pulmonary distention is of no consequence provided the airways are opened; rupture of the alveoli and blood vessels may occur if the glottis is closed and, in severe cases, death may result from air embolism

---

[8] It is mainly seen in persons buried under falling rocks or masonry and is common in garage accidents when the subject is impacted between two vehicles. Train accidents provide a number of cases due to the often lengthy process of extricating survivors (cf. the accident at Moorgate underground station in 1975).

[9] Royal Commission on Civil Liability and Compensation for Personal Injury, second circular, 1974.

[10] Safety of Sports Grounds Act 1975.

– or blocking of the circulation by bubbles of gas (*see also* p. 232). Release of gas into the tissues causes severe pain in the joints ('the bends'), difficulty in breathing ('the chokes'), pain in the air-containing ear or skull sinuses (barotrauma) or death due to widespread air embolism. Repeated compression and rapid decompression leads to cavitation of, and permanent damage to, the central nervous system and the bones. Known as caisson disease, it is a hazard of all work undertaken at pressure and is prescribed (Appendix I, disease No. 27). Caisson disease is a problem for the professional diver rather than for the sportsman.

The hazards of diving may be compounded by anxiety (overbreathing) or by hypothermia (*see* p. 174), either of which may be fatal in their own right. The prevention of diving fatalities rests on good training, maintenance of apparatus, adjustment of the artificial atmosphere – for example, by the substitution of nitrogen by helium, the correlation of depth of dive with the apparatus available[11] and on the rigid application of decompression schedules – the deeper the dive, the longer time must be allowed for ascent.[12]

Somewhat similar, though generally far less severe, exposures to the hazards of decompression result from ascent in unpressurized high-altitude machines. Serious effects, which include some unique and baffling deaths due to postdescent shock, are limited to professional aviators and astronauts; prevention rests on pressurization either of the cabin environment or of the man by a pressure suit. The effects of high and low pressure may, however, be summative; occasional holidays have ended tragically through taking a 'last quick scuba dive' before the aircraft, the cabin pressure of which is equivalent to a height of some 5500 ft (1800 metres), leaves for home – diving should not be practised within 24 hours of an intended flight.

The sea has its share of dangerous animals. Many have poison apparatus in tentacles, gills or fins and are most dangerous at spawning time. Marine venoms are generally toxic to the central nervous system and, while most 'stings' cause little more than local pain, others may be rapidly fatal. As with all poisons, the effect is to some extent dependent upon body weight and children are, therefore, more susceptible; highly poisonous fish are virtually limited to tropical waters.

Fish are carnivores and some may attack man; of these, the shark is pre-eminent – but, even so, is probably unfairly maligned. The size and aggressiveness of sharks, of which there are many varieties, is very roughly proportional to water temperature. The teeth of the shark cause extensive laceration and death from shark-bite can result rapidly from

---

[11] Simple skin diving must be limited to depths of less than 45 ft (15 metres).

[12] The formula commonly used in the United Kingdom is based on Royal Naval Diving Tables.

haemorrhage; occasionally, drowning may be precipitated by panic. The moods of sharks are unpredictable; adults have died from shark-bite sustained while paddling. Shark netting or shark patrols are essential where bathing occurs in infested tropical or subtropical waters.

Chapter 17

Medico-legal Aspects of Marriage and Pregnancy

A NUMBER of legal problems which are of immediate concern to the medical profession, or which can be resolved only on the basis of medical opinion, surround the state of matrimony. The subject is fundamental to forensic medicine though cases for decision are relatively rare.

DISPUTED SEX

Marriage is defined as the union of a man and a woman and, on occasion, the definition of sex may be difficult. A declaration of nullity could properly follow if it were shown that the sex of one spouse was not that supposed.[1]

The sex of a person can be judged on various criteria. Firstly, there is the chromosomal or genetic make up. As has been discussed elsewhere (p. 4), the possession of a Y chromosome in the cell nucleus determines maleness. If a Y chromosome is discovered on testing, it is reasonable to assume that the person is a male, save in very rare circumstances when, as a result of abnormal division of the sex chromosomes, there is, in effect, a preponderance of X chromosomes and the subject is bisexual to a varied extent. Mosaicism, or the presence in one body of both male and female cell populations, may produce even more bizarre anatomic anomalies. Such cases usually become apparent at puberty and are of no concern in relation to marriage.

Secondly, the sex may be indicated by the gonads – basically, whether there are testes or ovaries. Again, there are instances in which the testes fail to develop normally and, as a result, the Y chromosome does not exert its influence on the general sex characteristics. In the extreme of the condition, the subject may have clearly female appearances yet have XY chromosomes.

Thirdly, there is the appearance of the external genitalia and here there may be very great difficulties. The commonest abnormalities are failures of the development of the normal male genitalia when a gross

---

[1] Matrimonial Causes Act 1973 (S.11(c)); but this Act does not apply in Scotland where the same situation would be covered by common law.

condition of *hypospadias* may leave the genitalia closely resembling those of a female. Alternatively, there may be excessive secretion on the part of the adrenal gland which leads to great hypertrophy of the female genitalia and to a spurious appearance of maleness. Cases of either type may easily be mistaken at birth[2] but are usually discovered during childhood and at puberty; again, these cases are of little significance in the context of marriage but they may be of considerable psychiatric importance as the subject may have been reared incorrectly for some years.

Fourthly, there is the person's own psychological assessment of his or her sex which may be contrary to all the other evidence; in its most advanced form, this state is known as transsexualism.[3] The importance of this abnormal state is that it may lead to surgical intervention – generally to remove the male genitalia and to fashion others simulating those of the female; femaleness is maintained by treatment with female sex hormone (oestrogen).[4] In very unusual circumstances, a person who had been so treated might 'marry' another of the same genetic and gonadal sex. Such a marriage has been declared null in England on the twin grounds that both persons were male and that normal intercourse – which means intercourse *per vaginam* and not through an artificial vaginal passage – could not occur.[5]

OTHER REASONS FOR NULLITY OF MARRIAGE

Sexual intercourse is a most important factor in a functioning marriage and, as discussed above, must be of normal type and must involve penetration of the vulva to be acceptable in law as true intercourse. Inability on the part of either spouse to consummate the marriage in this way enables the Court, on the appropriate proceedings being taken, to declare a marriage null provided that the failure is due to an irremediable defect or deformity which the other party was either ignorant of at the time of marriage or did not believe to be incurable. Consummation of marriage depends on successful coitus; sterility is immaterial.[6] The pro-

---

[2] There is provision in both the relevant English and Scottish Acts for the correction of registration as to sex; the name may also be changed. In Scotland, a Register of Corrections is maintained. This does not, however, apply in cases of 'sex change' – whether surgically assisted or accomplished by natural anatomic changes (X Petitioner 1957 S.L.T. (Sh. Ct.) 61).

[3] Not to be confused with transvestism which is the wearing of clothes of the opposite sex; transvestism may, of course, be a prominent sign of transsexualism.

[4] Myers D. W. (1970) *The Human Body and the Law*, Edinburgh University Press, p. 52, argues that such surgery is of doubtful legality in England, consent to a severe and unlawful physical invasion not being possible. The wide discretion given to doctors in Scotland might, however, lead to a more lenient view there.

[5] Corbett v. Corbett [1971] P.83.

[6] R. v. R. [1952] 1 All E.R. 1194.

creation of children is not, in law, a principal intention of marriage and, therefore, neither the use of contraceptives nor the practice of coitus interruptus constitute grounds for a declaration of nullity.[7]

The Court must, in practice, base its decision on medical evidence and, in England, appoints its own medical examiners to whom both parties must submit for examination. In Scotland, however, it is for the pursuer to lead what evidence he or she can; the courts will not normally order a defender to undergo an examination. Obvious defects may be apparent externally, the extreme being sufficient to induce a genuine error as to sex although, as described above, such cases are unlikely to persist until marriage. Even so, a true penis may be of such small size as to be incapable of penetration and a vagina may be so rudimentary as to inhibit entry of a normal male organ.

Most often, however, the allegation will be based on impotence in the male. Statutory impotence exists in England in boys under the age of 14 but, since marriage below the age of 16 is unlawful, this has no present relevance. In neither English nor Scots law is there an upper age limit beyond which there is a presumption of impotence.

Impotence may be physical in origin – it is a frequent, though not invariable, accompaniment of paraplegia – or it may have apparently no more than a psychological basis. Demonstration of the former may be easy for the doctor but, in the presence of normal genitalia, the latter may be hard to prove in the face of a resolute defence.

Impotence in the female in the sense of failure to have orgasm is clearly not grounds for annulment but frigidity – or hatred of intercourse – to the extent that the vagina was thereby stimulated to a state of persistent spasm would be competent grounds were it possible to prove its existence. Occasional women reach the same condition by reason of the pain experienced in sexual intercourse. Physical disease other than malformation in women is a relatively uncommon cause of impotence.

Impotence arising from any cause after the marriage has been consummated cannot be grounds for a declaration of nullity. There is, however, a famous case in which a declaration was made despite the fact that there was a child who was the undisputed offspring of the couple concerned.[8] It was held that entry of the sperm and fertilization of the ovum could occur without legal penetration; medically speaking this is so, though it must be a fortunately rare occurrence.

There are other bases for nullity which are, in the main, statutory but as to which medical evidence may occasionally be called. A bigamous marriage is one obvious example but, medico-legally, perhaps the most important are that a marriage is null if one of the parties was aged less

---

[7] Baxter v. Baxter [1948] A.C. 274; White v. White [1948] P.330.
[8] Clarke v. Clarke [1943] 2 All E.R. 540.

than 16;[9] certain degrees of consanguinity and affinity are a lawful impediment and, in general, the relationships exist whether in the legitimate or illegitimate state;[10] a marriage can be annulled if one party was of unsound mind or mentally defective as defined in the Mental Health Act 1959 or, in Scotland, if there was insufficient understanding at the time of the ceremony; there are grounds for annullment in England and Wales when one partner was suffering from venereal disease at the time of marriage – provided that the petitioner was unaware of the situation when the marriage took place; pregnancy by another man at the time of marriage unsuspected by the petitioner is grounds for annullment in England and Wales but not in Scotland – contrariwise, a false threat of pregnancy as a spur to wedlock does not constitute grounds for nullity.

PREGNANCY

Aside from these considerations, and the criminal connotations which are discussed in Chapter 19, pregnancy is of obvious medico-legal importance in civil litigation involving problems such as divorce and succession. The question of paternity will loom large in these issues and Chapter 18 is devoted to the scientific basis of its settlement. For present purposes, it is intended only to recapitulate the circumstantial evidence which bears on the probability of conception being as averred by one or other party.

Certain presumptions as to age and pregnancy are made – at least in relation to perpetuity law. These include, firstly, that a young woman is capable of conceiving a child in her 13th year and, secondly, that an old woman is past childbearing in her 56th year.[11] As to the lower age limit, it has been pointed out that many very youthful pregnancies result from incest and such an instance has been recorded in a girl aged $12\frac{1}{4}$ years. The most extreme cases reported are those of a Peruvian girl who is said to have given birth at the age of $5\frac{3}{4}$ and of another pregnancy which occurred in a child $6\frac{1}{4}$ years old. These, however, must be regarded as freak occurrences and it would be reasonable to accept the 13th year as the

---

[9] Matrimonial Causes Act 1973 (s. 11), but see p. 256 as to sexual offences in such a circumstance.

[10] The list in Scotland is a formidable one. A man cannot marry (and the reverse applies for women) his mother, stepmother, grandmother, daughter, stepdaughter, granddaughter, sister, half-sister, aunt, great-aunt, niece, great-niece, former wife's mother, former wife's daughter, adoptive mother, adopted daughter. A very similar list is provided by the Marriage Act 1949 in England and Wales. Under both jurisdictions, marriage between cousins is permissible as is marriage to a former wife's sister, aunt or niece (Marriage (Enabling) Act 1960).

[11] Perpetuities and Accumulations Act 1964. Quoted by Coode C. A. (1968) *The Law of the Individual*, London, Sweet & Maxwell, p. xv. There are no general presumptions in Scots law.

practical lower limit for young birth with, perhaps, the 12th year as the earliest at which conception is possible. At the upper end, it is generally agreed that impregnation is unusual after the age of 45 but that exceptions here are more numerous and more acceptable; each case must be considered individually as to probability. It has certainly been held that inability to bear children after the age of 53 was a rebuttable presumption.[12]

The duration of pregnancy is of greater medico-legal significance. The normal average gestation period is regarded as 280 days but this depends on numerous factors including the length of the menstrual cycle which may vary quite markedly from the norm of 28 days. Additionally, allowance must be made for the possibility that fertilization of the ovum does not occur immediately following coitus; although spermatazoa lose their viability rapidly in the vagina (see Chapter 21), they can survive for some 48 hours in the receptive environment of the uterus and, exceptionally, have been demonstrated as fecund 5 days after injection.

Such physiological variations will account for divergences from the normal of at most 10 days; there is no doubt, however, that less explicable cases do occur and the courts are prepared to accept wider limits in reaching decisions as to paternity when the length of a pregnancy is the main or only evidence. What is, perhaps, the extreme decision held that a husband was not entitled to a divorce on the grounds of adultery simply because a child was born 349 days after the last intramarital coitus.[13] A similar claim involving a gestation of 360 days was, however, upheld.[14] Medical investigations have also indicated that a period of 354 days from coitus to live birth is not impossible,[15] while a recent newspaper report described the birth of a normal child to a woman who believed herself to have been pregnant for 13 months.[16] This case is currently unreported in the medical press and may have been an example of superfetation. This condition arises from the fertilization of ova liberated from the ovaries at different monthly ovulations. It is generally believed that, even if it be accepted that a second ovulation can occur in the presence of a normal fetus, it must be incredibly rare; it is possible, however, that a fetus could die in utero and a second impregnation occur before the onset of a menstrual period – the appearances would therefore be of a grossly prolonged gestation period. Superfecundation is a different and well-accepted concept whereby two ova released at the

---

[12] These cases are reported in Glaister's Medical Jurisprudence and Toxicology, 13th ed. (1973), Edinburgh, Churchill Livingstone, pp. 360, 371.

[13] Hadlum v. Hadlum [1948] 2 All E.R. 412.

[14] Preston-Jones v. Preston-Jones [1951] 1 All E.R. 124.

[15] McKeown T. and Gibson J. R. (1952) The period of gestation. Br. Med. J. 1, 938.

[16] The Scotsman, June 9, 1975.

same ovulation are fertilized by two different acts of coitus; such an event would be distinguishable from the bearing of binovular twins only in exceptional circumstances.

Problems as to the minimum length of a pregnancy are complicated by the fact that short pregnancies may terminate either as abortions, stillbirths or premature births – medical viability in the latter depending to a large extent on the efficiency of the obstetric services available. Legal viability (*see* Chapter 19) is, however, a different matter and refers only to a fetus of 28 weeks' gestation. It has been held that the fact that a premature child lived when the notional history of marital intercourse indicated that it could only have been of less than 28 weeks' gestation was not proof of illegitimacy.[17] The precise age of a newborn infant, whether alive or dead, may, therefore, be of very considerable medico-legal importance and the process whereby it is assessed is discussed in Chapter 19.

ARTIFICIAL INSEMINATION

Artificial insemination of a woman who is unable to conceive a child through coitus with her husband may be chosen as an alternative to adoption. It is practised in two forms – insemination by the husband (AIH) or by an unrelated donor (AID). In each case, the seed is introduced into the cervical canal by means of a syringe.

Artificial insemination with the semen of the husband poses no problems other than its possible effect on a plea of nullity on the grounds of impotence in either spouse. The Departmental Committee on Human Artificial Insemination[18] recommended that the birth of a live child through the medium of AIH should be a bar to subsequent proceedings for nullity by either party; the question has not, however, been decided in the courts.

Artificial insemination by donor is, on the other hand, loaded with forensic problems for all concerned – including the medical practitioner who may be called to advise on or to complete the procedure.

From the doctor's point of view, the most important feature is the consent of both husband and wife to the process. It is possible that a doctor who became involved without the consent of the husband might be guilty of serious professional misconduct (*see* Chapter 30); when obtained, such consent can only be valid after the most complete explanation of the procedure and of the associated complexities. The presence of a single donor in a district could lead to problems of consanguineous marriage in future generations. It has, therefore, been

---

[17] Clark v. Clark [1939] P.228.

[18] *Report of the Departmental Committee on Human Artificial Insemination* (1960), Cmnd. 1105, London, HMSO, para. 108.

suggested that a doctor who is aware of the semen donor's identity in a case in which he is involved should keep careful notes of the process lest these should be of importance in the future. The ethics of professional confidence might then be seriously at risk and it would seem that any such notes should properly be destroyed on the death of the practitioner.[19]

Donation of the semen is not without its problems. Speller[20] has suggested that the donor's own spouse might have grounds for divorce if it were known that he was the father of another woman's child. It is advised that the name of any donor of semen should be kept secret, that the donor should not know to whom his semen is being given and that any married donor should obtain valid consent to his role from his wife.

As to husband and wife, the Departmental Committee already cited has urged that the birth of a child as the result of AID with mutual consent from the spouses should be a bar to proceedings for nullity.[21] On the other hand, it was recommended in para. 117 that the acceptance of AID by a woman without her husband's consent should be grounds for divorce. This, however, is one of the few aspects of AID which have been decided in the courts; it has been held in Scotland that, in so far as there is no mutual coitus, AID cannot be construed as adultery on the part of the woman concerned.[22] The situation might be different in England under the Matrimonial Causes Act 1973. Coode[23] looks at the same problem from a rather different angle and points to the absurdity of supposing that a husband who consented to his wife accepting a semen donation would be guilty of condoning the matrimonial offence of adultery.

The position of the child resulting from insemination is, at least in the author's mind, doubtful. There is certainly a presumption in both English and Scots law that a child born in wedlock is legitimate but this presumption is rebuttable; the current literature clearly implies that proven AID, in showing that the husband is not the father of the child, is a *prima facie* rebuttal. Speller advises the family doctor that: 'the husband and wife should be told plainly that in law any child born (as a result of AID) will be illegitimate and that it should be registered as such'.

---

[19] It has been recommended that the criteria for a choice of donor additional to those described in the text should include that he is not a relative of either spouse, he should be potent, should be of age, his age should not exceed 40, he should have children of his own and his race and charateristics should resemble as closely as possible those of the husband of the woman to be inseminated (quoted in *Glaister's Medical Jurisprudence and Toxicology* (1973), 13th ed., p. 367).

[20] In *Law of Doctor and Patient*, (1973) London, H. K. Lewis, p. 42.

[21] Para. 156. Nevertheless, Knight, at p. 195 of *Legal Aspects of Medical Practice*, 2nd ed., states that a decree has been granted in just such circumstances.

[22] MacLennan v. MacLennan 1958 S.C. 105.

[23] In *The Law of the Individual*, (1968) London, Sweet & Maxwell, p. 2.

The Departmental Committee on Human Artificial Insemination (at para. 187) recommended that there be no amendment of the law relating to legitimacy or registration of birth and there can be no doubt that to register a child parented by AID as that of the mother's husband would constitute a false registration. It has been suggested that the *MacLennan* case throws doubt on this interpretation on the grounds that, if there is no adultery, the child cannot be illegitimate; this, however, is to confuse the two quite separate items of adultery and biological parentage. It seems fairly clear that an AID child is treated as an ordinary child of the union if the fact of artificial insemination is not manifest in the registration; if it were at any time established that the child was not a true offspring of the spouses, the birth entry would have to be altered. If the true paternity is revealed in the register, the child is considered as is any other illegitimate child.

In practice, many of these problems have been dissipated by recent legislation and regulations. The possible disadvantages to a child born as a result of AID have, in common with all illegitimate children, been very largely removed by the provisions of the Family Law Reform Act 1969 (ss. 14 to 19) and of the Law Reform (Miscellaneous Provisions) (Scotland) Act 1968; so long as there has been no false registration, the child may, in any event, be legally adopted within the terms of the Adoption Act 1958; and the shortened form of birth certificate does not state the father's name. Despite these conditions, there are sufficient difficulties associated with the practice of AID to recommend the view of the Departmental Committee that, while it should not be held to be a criminal offence, the practice of AID is to be discouraged strongly.

STERILIZATION

A woman may be surgically sterilized – that is rendered incapable of bearing children – by removal of the ovaries, by section, ligation or diathermy of the fallopian tubes or by removal of the uterus. Similarly, a man may be made unable to procreate by removal of the testes or by section of the vas deferens on each side. Removal of the ovaries or testes, which is castration, may cause considerable hormonal upset and is undertaken only in exceptional circumstances.

Sterilization may be the primary object of, or merely incidental to, the operation. A man may have both testes removed because they contain tumours; but by far the most common form of unavoidable sterilization is associated with the removal of the female uterus – either for the eradication of a tumour or as a relief of problems in menstruation.

There is no serious medico-legal difficulty associated with sterilization which is imposed as a price for treatment of a medical condition. A woman – one can, for practical purposes, exclude a man in this context –

is entitled to consent to or dissent from medical treatment for herself whether she is married or not; it seems perfectly clear that a husband has no right of veto nor has he any redress against the surgeon who operates on his wife without his consent so long as the decision was reached in non-negligent fashion. This implies fully-informed consent by the wife; ideally this should include consent by the husband after the patient has given permission for him to be brought into discussion. But Speller[24] has also pointed out that a doctor who refrained from necessary gynaecological treatment *because* of lack of consent on the part of the husband might find himself in a difficult professional position.

Primary sterilization is a different matter. It poses a basic problem of ethics as to whether a surgical procedure not designed for treatment of a medical condition is sufficiently 'against the public interest' as to constitute criminal assault and, therefore, to be beyond the protection of consent. Sterilization may be performed, among other reasons, as a punitive measure, on eugenic grounds or as a form of birth control. The first, although permissible in some states of the USA, is so foreign to British thought as to need no consideration. The second is rather different. There can be no question but that eugenic sterilization without consent must be an assault. But, with consent, sterilization has at least been advocated by the Departmental Committee on Sterilization[25] in certain cases of mental defect and of hereditary disease; the risks are, however, formidable and no legislation to this end has been passed. The nature of consent in such cases poses an inherent problem – if a person is suffering from disease of the mind to the extent that he ought to be sterilized, can he give a valid consent? It would also seem that parents ought not to be able to consent to a nontherapeutic operation on behalf of a minor; there can rarely be any compelling reason why sterilization should not be postponed until the subject is aged 16.[26]

The ethical issues relating to sterilization as a form of birth control appear to have been settled. Public interest is dictated by public opinion and this has changed dramatically. Both the English and Scottish Medical Defence Unions have advised their members to the effect that sterilization carried out as a method of birth control is a legitimate undertaking.[27] It is doubtful if it would ever have been criminal in Scotland owing to a lack of evil intent. Vasectomy has now been specifically

---

[24] In *Law of Doctor and Patient*, p. 37.

[25] *Sterilization. Report of Departmental Committee* (1934). Cmnd. 4485, London, HMSO.

[26] The relevant ages in Scotland would probably be those of puberty – 12 years in the case of a girl and 14 for a boy. The sterilization of an English minor on eugenic grounds was banned on a judicial opinion in 1975. The whole subject is well discussed in: Sterilisation of minors, *Br. Med. J.* (1975) 3, 775.

[27] *Br. Med. J.* (1960) Legality of sterilisation: a new outlook. 2, 1516.

authorized under the National Health Service (Family Planning) Amendment Act 1972. Abortions performed under the Abortion Act 1967 are combined with sterilization in some 16 per cent of cases and there may also be good psychiatric indications for the operation in many sterilizations which are apparently of 'convenience' type. Myers,[28] however, draws a distinction between sterilization (e.g. by tying the tubes) and castration; although limiting his argument to the operation in the male, he believes that the latter is an offence which consent cannot legalize.

The secondary problem of the *nature* of the consent is far more important. There seems no doubt that, in the absence of medical grounds, sterilization of a married person must be validated by consent of both the subject and the spouse. An aggrieved spouse might well have grounds for an action for tort or delict against the doctors concerned and one-sided consent might possibly afford grounds for divorce to the other party; on the other hand, sterilization before marriage is not grounds for a Declarator of Nullity.

There remains the problem of civil liability in the event of failure of sterilization; this is probably the main medico-legal hazard associated with sterilization as a method of contraception.

It is often insufficiently understood that sterilizing operations cannot always guarantee infertility. Some techniques are more efficient than others but, in general, the certainty of success is related proportionately to the extent of mutilation. The ethical problem thus resolves itself into balancing the immediate effect against the possibility of a later wish to reverse the procedure – say, on remarriage or on the death of an existing child.

This poses a real dilemma. The success rate for reversal of sterilization by vasectomy in the male is unlikely to be better than 25 per cent and many surgeons would decline to perform an operation which was specifically limited by the patient to one which could be undone. Reversal in the female is likely to be more successful – up to about 70 per cent – but the original operation must have been of limited extent and the risks of an ectopic pregnancy (*see* p. 88) are definitely increased following a reparative operation; sterilization techniques which virtually eliminate the possibility of failure must be regarded as irreversible.

Using a good technique with competent hands, the risk of pregnancy following female sterilization is very small indeed – but it would be a brave man who averred that it was nonexistent without removal of the uterus. Sterilization in the male is by no means so straightforward. When the subjects are tested for the presence of sperm in the ejaculate, it is found that a small number of motile organisms are still present 6

---

[28] In *The Human Body and the Law*, p. 18.

months after the operation in some 40 per cent of the men treated. Very occasionally, sperm are found later in those who were apparently sterile 3 months after operation but, in these instances, the organisms are generally immobile and probably dead. The most serious complication is spontaneous recanalization of the ducts which may occur in up to 1 per cent of cases; instances have been reported even following surgery of moderately severe type.

All these considerations must be explained to the patient and to the spouse before consent can be valid.[29] Having done so, the usual rules covering medical negligence apply – if the patient fully understood the risks, if the operation was properly performed and if the procedure was one which was accepted by competent colleagues in the profession, then the mere fact of pregnancy would not be proof of negligence. The proper procedure must, however, include adequate follow-up; this consists of routine examination of the ejaculate[30] and, of major importance, pathological proof by microscopy that the correct tissue was removed. It scarcely needs pointing out that if a husband who had been sterilized brought an action on account of an unexpected pregnancy in his wife, it would be quite reasonable for the surgeon to question the paternity of the child.

DIVORCE

Divorce in England and Wales can only be granted on the basis of an irretrievable breakdown of marriage.[31] There are a number of specific conditions which are taken either together or individually to indicate that this situation exists. These include adultery and that the petitioner finds it intolerable to live with the respondent,[32] intolerable behaviour and desertion; in addition there is an 'agreed' ground in that the couple have lived apart for at least 2 years and there is no objection by the respondent to the decree being granted – if there has been a separation for at least 5 years, a decree can be granted even in the face of opposition.

The position is now very similar in Scotland. The common law ground of adultery and the several other possible bases for divorce detailed in the Divorce (Scotland) Act 1938 are now consolidated under the general heading of irretrievable breakdown of marriage in the Divorce

---

[29] In the case of a woman, it would be wise to obtain consent for more extensive surgery than is generally undertaken to cover the possible need for emergency treatment of a haemorrhage, etc.

[30] An acceptable regimen would be to require 2 negative specimens 2 weeks apart taken 2 months after the operation followed by a third negative specimen 1 month later before pronouncing the subject sterile.

[31] Matrimonial Causes Act 1973 (s. 1).

[32] But the two phrases are independent – Cleary v. Cleary [1974] 1 All E.R. 498.

(Scotland) Act 1976. Behaviour on the part of the defender can be regarded as intolerable irrespective of his or her mental state. The Divorce (Scotland) Act 1964 is also repealed but the 1976 Act continues to encourage reconciliation; cohabitation for a period of up to three months for the purpose of reconciliation is not regarded as condonation of adultery.

There is, therefore, surprisingly little forensic medicine associated with divorce. The greater part will involve proof or disproof of adultery and this, in turn, is mainly a matter of paternity. Occasionally, however, the length of pregnancy will be decisive as may be evidence of venereal disease which could not have been contracted from the spouse. Forensic departments are often presented with bed linen, cushions and the like to establish the presence or absence of seminal stains; while these are usually presented in the hopes of proving adultery, it seems that, even if the stains are positively seminal and proven to be of a different secretor group (see p. 219) from the husband, such evidence can rarely be more than indicative of unseemly conduct on the part of the wife.

There remains cruelty, for proof of which there need be no evidence of physical injury; nevertheless, such evidence, if present, would carry much weight and the medical practitioner may have an important part to play here if a woman seeks his advice and assistance; this must include an assessment of injury to health other than by physical means.

But what if the doctor notices evidence of physical illtreatment in a female patient when she has consulted him for other reasons? There is strong evidence that nonaccidental injury in married women is a problem comparable in extent to that in children (see Chapter 20).

There is currently very little medical literature on the subject probably because there are essential differences in the aetiology and management of these two types of household violence.[33] The wife who is being illtreated is adult and capable of taking her complaint to the appropriate authorities. There is no need for the doctor to protect a helpless patient, as applies to babies, and, if there is no need, there may be no justification for disclosure of confidential information; indeed, there is evidence that many women, whether because of genuine choice or of fear, would themselves resent such an intrusion.[34] The role of the doctor is perhaps limited to counselling not only as to his woman patient's course of action but also as to the advisability of the husband being induced to seek medical help; in contrast to fathers who injure their children, many of those who seriously assault their wives are older and

---

[33] The most useful reference is the *Report* from the Select Committee on Violence in Marriage (1975), Vol. 1, H-C.553–i, London, HMSO.

[34] But a number of wives do seek help, especially from voluntary organizations. *See* Gayford J. J. (1975) Wife battering: a preliminary survey of 100 cases, *Br. Med. J.* **1**, 194.

suffer from psychiatric disease – in the event of trial, a higher proportion of hospital orders are made than in cases of child abuse. The keeping of accurate records by the doctor, particularly including an assessment of the mental state of the woman and of injuries noted in examination but of which no complaint is made, is of equal importance; such evidence might be invaluable in subsequent criminal[35] or civil proceedings.

[35] Gordon holds that, in Scots law, an assault may be aggravated by being committed by a husband on his wife. (Gordon G. H. (1967) *The Criminal Law of Scotland*. Edinburgh. W. Green & Sons. p. 765.) Nevertheless, police involvement in domestic affrays is relatively infrequent.

Chapter 18

Elementary Genetics and Testing for Parentage

THE normal human nucleus, which defines the 'personality' of the cell, contains 46 chromosomes arranged in two sets of 23 pairs, one set being derived from each parent. The sex cells, ova or spermatozoa, are therefore unique in containing only a single series of 23 chromosomes, but this series is formed from a random choice between one of two paired chromosomes present in each parent. Certain severe abnormalities are the direct result of an abnormal number of chromosomes being present – mongolism is, perhaps, the classic example.

Chromosomes consist of large numbers of genes. These are formed from deoxyribonucleic acid (DNA) and function as templates from which further identical genes can be formed at will through the medium of ribonucleic acid (RNA) which acts as a 'messenger' or carrier of a carbon copy. The original genetic pattern of the fertilized ovum is thereby maintained as the fetus and free living body are developed.

Save in abnormal circumstances, each paired chromosome will contain one of a pair of genes which refer to the same genetic characteristic; each gene is derived from either the father or the mother but both cannot come from a single parent. These paired genes are known as *alleles*. The allelic genes may be the same, in which case the individual is said to be *homozygous* for that particular factor or they may be different, resulting in the *heterozygous* state.

In the simplest heterozygous state, one of the pair of genes will express itself – or demonstrate its presence – and is therefore said to be *dominant*; the other member of the pair is known as *recessive* – it is still present and available for transmission to the offspring but is overshadowed or obscured by its dominant partner. This can be illustrated in simple fashion by hair colour for which characteristic the 'black hair' gene is dominant over the 'red hair' gene. Reference to *Fig. 14* shows that, if a man (or woman) homozygous for black hair mates with a woman (or man) homozygous for red hair, all the offspring will be heterozygotes but all will be black-haired because the gene for red is recessive. But if two such heterozygotes mate, one of four offspring will be red-haired and three will be black-haired; two of the latter will, however, be 'carriers' of a recessive gene for red hair. It is pointed out in passing that this is a theoretical reason for prohibiting certain degrees of consanguineous marriage. Many harmful genes are recessive – it is scarcely possible for a truly disadvantageous gene to be dominant and for the strain to survive – and normal random mating leads to their natural suppression; 'in-breeding' must, however, increase the possibility of such recessive genes meeting as alleles – the harmful gene is then free to express itself with increasing frequency.

Fig. 14. Homozygous and heterozygous matings. Either of the genes present in one parent may be paired with either of the genes present in the other. *See* text for explanation.

Reverting to the example of hair colour, ordinary observation will show that the position has been oversimplified since only a few people in whom it is not a racial characteristic have jet-black hair. In other words, dominance, save in some well-defined all-or-nothing situations, is relative; the capacity of a dominant gene to express itself is described as its degree of *penetration* – a gene of weak penetration may express itself only rarely when all the circumstances are in its favour. This is the justification for genetic counselling and for some legal abortions (*see* Chapters 19 and 20); if a very weakly-penetrating harmful gene expresses itself once in a family, the conditions which encouraged that expression are likely to recur though, of course, they may not necessarily do so.

Some genetic variations are *sex-linked*. The sex chromosomes are designated X and Y; a normal female possesses the homozygous alleles XX while the male is XY. The combination YY is biologically impossible since Y is available only in a spermatozoon. Sex linkage is illustrated in *Fig.* 15 on the simple premise that a recessive gene is positioned in that area of the X chromosome which is absent in the male. A dominant 'unaffected' X arm suppresses the abnormal gene in the female; expression of the abnormality can only occur in the male while the female remains a 'carrier' – the only way for a female to express a sex-linked gene is for her to possess two abnormal X chromosomes, a possibility which is unlikely in the absence of 'in-breeding'.

If genetic studies are to be useful, the genes must be demonstrable. Some genes express themselves as *antigens* and can, therefore, form *antibodies*; either may be used to demonstrate the other in the laboratory. Antibodies which are stimulated in a person who does not possess the corresponding antigens are described as immune – they arise in response to the presence of a foreign antigen and repeated exposures

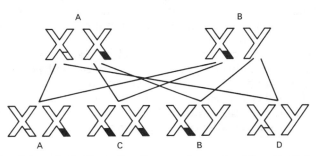

Fig. 15. Sex linkage. In the illustration, the normal gene absent from the Y chromosome is designated in black, while the abnormal variant is white. A is a female carrier of the abnormal gene which is suppressed by the normal; B is a normal male. Their possible progeny are as follows: A, A "carrier" female similar to her mother. C, A normal female—the disease has been eliminated from that strain. B, A normal male. D, A diseased male—there is no normal sex-linked gene available to suppress the abnormal.

result in increasingly active antibody formation. Antigens may, however, be shared by many unrelated types of cell and antibodies can be formed in response to exposure to an antigen derived from a source unrelated to the form in which it occurs in the body. 'Naturally occurring' antibodies – of which those reacting with the ABO blood cell antigens are the prime example – are probably made in this way.

In the ideal situation, a gene should be demonstrable in both its dominant and recessive forms. Suppose a gene Z has an allele z. If we can demonstrate both Z and z by means of antisera (that is, blood sera containing antibodies) we can distinguish the *genotypes* – or full genetic profiles – ZZ, Zz and zz; if, on the other hand, we can only show the presence of the dominant Z we are limited to describing a person as Z+ve or Z−ve and this inadequate genetic portrait is known as a *phenotype* (although, Z−ve is, in fact, a genotype as, by a process of elimination, it must represent zz). The genotype ZZ or Zz can be derived from the phenotype either on the basis of probability – that is, by knowing the proportional distribution in the population – or by a knowledge of the phenotypes of parents, siblings or children, the reverse process of paternity testing.

Diagnostic antigens must be stable – they must not be affected by disease, age and the like and they must not *mutate,* which is to alter their structure and their expression. If a gene is to be useful in genetic studies – particularly if these are to be used in a medico-legal context – natural mutation must be so rare as to be unaccountable. The general mutation rate in humans is of the order of 1 in 1 million gene generations; no proven example of a blood group gene mutating between two generations has ever been found.[1]

The ideal genetic test substance should be readily available and it should contain a number of systems which *segregate* independently thus increasing the number of variable and recognizable characteristics.

The red blood cells meet almost all these requirements and, as a result, testing for parentage, which forms the major part of medico-legal genetics, is virtually a matter of blood testing.

TESTING FOR PARENTAGE

Very occasionally, an allegation may be made that a child has been wrongly identified in the maternity crèche, while extraordinary instances of fabricated pregnancy followed by appropriation of an infant have been reported; there can be few other occasions in which the identity of a mother is in doubt and, for practical purposes, testing for parentage is a matter of paternity testing; it is in this context that the subject will be discussed.[2] The principal circumstances in which paternity tests are called for are in divorce proceedings and in the adjudication of affiliation orders.

In either case, the putative father is denying responsibility for a child and it is emphasized that genetic studies cannot prove paternity *conclusively*; although a very strong probability may be established (*see* p. 221), the main function of the blood testing laboratory is to exclude paternity in a man unjustly accused; this it can do with ever-increasing

---

[1] The principle that mutation can be accepted as excessively rare seems to have been agreed – *see Halsbury's Statutes of England,* 3rd ed., Vol. 40, p. 617. Excluded from paternity means excluded subject to the occurrence of mutation (Family Law Reform Act 1969, s. 25).

[2] It has been pointed out by Dodd B. E. (personal communication) that incest poses the fascinating problem in which the laboratory not only has to give evidence as to whether or not a man is excluded from paternity of his daughter's child but also whether or not he is excluded from being the father of his daughter.

efficiency.[3] It will be seen that, in practice, unless the problem is one of choosing between two or three candidates for parenthood, the man has little to lose and perhaps everything to gain from blood testing: the mother of the child has, by contrast, comparatively little expectation of advantage.

It seems that Scots law has taken little cognizance of blood tests for parentage and the statutory basis of such tests, the Family Law Reform Act 1969, applies only to England and Wales. Under s. 20(1), the courts may give a direction for the use of blood tests to see whether or not a person is excluded from paternity on application from any party to the proceedings; in practice, blood tests are generally agreed between the parties and court orders are very seldom required. Consent is necessary, the age of consent being 16 (s. 21) but, under s. 23(1), the court may draw inferences from the fact that a person has failed to take steps as directed.

There is nothing to stop such evidence being brought by agreement in Scotland but the admissibility of such evidence could be strongly challenged especially in relation to the taking of blood from a child. The law would not compel that this be done and, in 1958, Lord President Clyde was of the opinion that there should be hesitation before allowing a course to be taken which might have a serious effect on the child.[4] One would feel, however, that the truth ought to prevail – '. . . there is nothing more shocking than that injustice should be done on the basis of a legal presumption when justice can be done on the basis of fact';[5] modern serology is clearly an expression of fact.

Certain essentials must be met before the results of the tests can be admitted as evidence even in England and Wales. Firstly, specimens must be obtained as a minimum from the mother, the child and any putative father. Secondly, the specimen must be suitably identified by the parties concerned and by their legal advisers. Thirdly, declarations of consent and agreement as to the validity of the specimens must be signed together with a declaration that neither party has received a blood transfusion within the last three months. Blood tests on infants less than two months old are somewhat less satisfactory than in the adult and, ideally, a child should be at least six months old at the time of testing.

Principles of Paternity Testing
The simple principles which govern the exclusion of paternity by blood

---

[3] See, for example, the discussion by Grant A. and Bradbrook I. D. (1973) Newer Techniques in Paternity Blood Grouping. In: Mant A. K. (ed.) *Modern Trends in Forensic Medicine* – 3, London, Butterworth.

[4] Quoted in the monograph Brownlie A. R. (1965) Blood and the blood groups. *J. Forensic Sci. Soc.* **5**, 124. *See also* the same author (1966) Paternity blood tests. *J. Law Soc. Scot.*, **11**, 328.

[5] Ormrod J. in Holmes v. Holmes [1966] 1 W.L.R. 187, at p. 188.

testing can be summarized:

    a. Save in conditions of extreme rarity, generally involving deletion of genes, blood group genes and antigens are passed on 'true' by a parent to its offspring.

    b. One gene of an allelic pair is derived from each parent. Each parent has one of two genes to donate at random.

    c. A blood group antigen cannot be present in a child unless it is also present in at least one parent.

    d. If one parent possesses a homozygous allelic gene pair, then that gene *must* be conferred on all his or her offspring.

The blood group antigens are contained in a number of 'systems', each system containing a number of allelic pairs. Systems are distinguished in that they are segregated independently from each other – the more systems tested, the more likely is a wrongly accused father to be positively excluded from paternity. The 'value' of a system in this respect depends on several factors – the number of allelic pairs it contains, the relative distribution of the genes in the population and, not least important, the ease with which its component antigens can be demonstrated. This last point needs explanation. There is no true dominance or recessiveness in blood group genes; the terms relate, in effect, to the ease with which they can be demonstrated. Antigens are of different 'strengths' – i.e. they react either strongly or weakly both in the laboratory and *in vivo* as to their capacity to provoke the formation of antibodies. They are demonstrated by different methods, some of which are complex; in the nature of things, the systems which were documented earliest contain the strongest antigens and are most easily defined in the laboratory. The determination of an antigen usually requires an antibody and the necessary test antisera vary from being universally available to being extremely rare or nonexistent. It may, therefore, be beyond the technical ability of a laboratory to demonstrate some of the lesser blood group systems.

For present purposes, it is proposed to deal only with the ABO, MNS and Rhesus (CDE) systems in detail – the use of these three systems alone could eliminate 59 per cent of wrongfully accused putative fathers.

The MNS system is the most 'efficient' individual system[6] and illustrates some points which are not easily appreciated in the better-known ABO system; it will be used as the main example of testing for paternity.

Use of the MNS System in Paternity Cases
The allelic antigens originally discovered were designated M and N.

---

[6] MNS typing alone will exclude 32 per cent of wrongly accused men; the comparable figure for the ABO system is 17 per cent and for the Rhesus system 28 per cent.

Antisera are readily available to both so that the genotypes MM, MN and NN can be distinguished with ease. The simple rules described on p. 216 can now be applied:

Parents	Impossible children
MM × MM	MN, NN
MM × MN	NN
MM × NN	MM, NN
MN × NN	MM
NN × NN	MM, MN
MN × MN	None.

However, the system also contains the alleles S and s. These are 'linked' to the M and N alleles so that the genes are always transmitted in a group of two. We therefore have the following possible 'system' gene profiles: MS, Ms, NS, Ns, and these can be combined to form 10 genotypes. This greatly increases the usefulness of the system. For example, there are no impossible children from the mating MN × MN; but if it is, in fact, MsNs × MsNs then any child containing the antigen S can be eliminated as a product of the union.

The MNS system also illustrates some of the difficulties in blood testing. In the first place, anti-s is an example of a rare antibody although it is obtainable commercially. If it were not available, it would be possible to speak in terms of genotypes only when no S was demonstrable – the genotype would then be ss (see p. 213). Secondly, the antigen M may occur as a variant which does not react with anti-M;[7] the significance of this is illustrated in Fig. 16. Any such variations must be interpreted in relation to their occurrence; while all concerned should be aware of them, they cannot, as a matter of simple statistics, be regarded as valid means of discrediting a laboratory result.

The Rhesus System

The Rhesus system differs from the MNS system in that it is basically composed of three allelic pairs – Cc, Dd, Ee. The most powerful antigen is D while, in contrast, d is so weak as to be non-antigenic. In common parlance, Rhesus-positive implies the possession of the gene D and Rhesus-negative its absence. The value of the whole system is, however, much greater as the individual genes of the three pairs can be combined in 8 different ways to form 'system' genes[8] which are so closely linked that they are always transmitted as a group; although alterations in the

---

[7] Variations in the M antigen are, in fact, so rare as to be of no practical importance – over 60 000 consecutive British donors have been tested without a single example being discovered; they serve only to demonstrate the effect of such variations which can occur in other systems.

[8] I.e.: CDE, CDe, CdE, Cde, cDE, cDe, cdE, cde.

group during the formation of the sex cells are theoretically just possible, the likelihood of 'crossing over' occurring so as to cause difficulty in the medico-legal sense is so infinitesimal as to be beyond practical consideration.

MATING	MM_g		MN	
	Father		Mother	
POSSIBLE	MM	M_gM	MN	M_gN
CHILDREN	1	2	3	4

Fig. 16. Effect of a nonreacting variant of a gene. Mg is a variant of M which does not react with anti-M. Child 4 could, therefore, appear as NN and the putative could be wrongly excluded. Variants such as these are excessively rare.

The Rhesus system has become more complicated than was originally described. Almost all the antigens have variants, one of which, C^w, is sufficiently common to be regarded as a standard antigen. Simply using the single genes CC^wDEcde, the groups of 'system' genes can be paired to form 78 potential genotypes. Such, however, is the regularity of group transmission, that 98 per cent of the groups consist of either CDe, cDE or cde. 32 per cent of Britons are of the genotype CDe/cde, 16 per cent are CDe/CDe and 15 per cent cde/cde – i.e. 15 per cent are Rhesus-negative.

In practice, the Rhesus system suffers from the inability to identify the potential antigen d. Thus, it is impossible to distinguish with certainty between the common genotype CDe/cde and the rare CDe/cDe because each can be defined only as the phenotype CcDe; the genotype is only inferred on a system of probabilities. This applies otherwise than in relation to d; thus, CDE/cDe is indistinguishable, save on likelihood, from CDe/cDE. The effect on paternity testing is, however, only marginal. The important feature is that a child cannot possess D unless one or both parents do so and this applies equally to C, c, E and e, all of which can be easily identified.

The Rhesus antigens are developed *in utero* and additional importance lies in their capacity to cause haemolytic disease of the newborn Theoretically, all Rhesus antigens could cause this potentially lethal condition – C and E are not without a significant morbidity – but, in practice, the antigen D is mainly responsible. Cells from a fetus which is D+ve by reason of the gene derived from its father may pass into a mother who is D−ve. The mother reacts to the foreign antigen by form ing anti-D which then passes back to the fetus whose cells are destroyed. One medico-legally important aspect of the condition is that, nowadays, it would certainly be medically negligent to fail to identify the possibility of the condition and to take the necessary steps to protect the fetus and the mother.

The ABO System

Although it is by far the best-known and easiest system to demonstrate, the ABO system is slightly less easy to understand because, instead of one gene of a pair being available to fill the locus on the chromosome, there are three possibilities – A, B or O. There is no positive method of identifying the 'silent' gene O and it follows that the so-called blood groups A and B are phenotypes, the possible genotypes being AA, AO, BB and BO; the genotype AB is directly definable and the genotype OO is indicated by the absence of A and B. Certain absolute exclusions can be accepted in paternity testing – firstly, a person of group O cannot parent a child of group AB and, conversely, if one parent is group AB, no child can be of group O; secondly, if the genes A or B are present in a child, they *must* appear in one or both parents; on the other hand, the group mating A × B can produce children of any group provided it is actually a genotypic mating AO × BO.

Proteins of identical structure to the antigen A and B are widely distributed in nature. As a result, within a few weeks of birth, individuals 'recognize' a foreign antigen; a person of group A then produces, as a natural process, the antibody anti-B, a group B person forms anti-A, a group O person forms both anti-A and anti-B but an AB person recognizes no foreign substances and forms no antibodies. Not only does this provide a ready source of testing agents but, also, a blood group can be checked by testing the serum as opposed to the cells.

There is some practical importance in this in that the gene A can appear in a number of variant forms known as A_1 – which is the common presentation – A_2, A_3 etc. The further removed they are from A_1, the weaker are the antigens and this difference can be demonstrated in the laboratory; moreover, persons of group A_2 etc may contain anti-A_1 in their sera. These features breed true and greatly increase the value of the system in excluding or, perhaps, in providing presumptive evidence of parenthood.

Secretor Groups

The ability to secrete water soluble forms of A and B antigens into the body fluids is also determined genetically; the silent O antigen is also secreted in the form of 'H substance'. Secretion is dominant to non-secretion; thus some 76 per cent of persons secrete the antigens and 24 per cent fail to do so.[9] A further important feature is that secretors having the blood group O secrete 'H substance' and this can be demonstrated by using anti-H which occurs in certain plants.

While secretion has a minor part to play in testing for parentage, far greater medico-legal importance lies in the resultant ability to identify the blood group antigens in body fluids which either contain very few cells – e.g. saliva – or in which the cells have been fragmented – e.g. old blood or seminal stains. Thus, it may be possible to exclude – or strongly to corroborate – identity in any criminal case involving the spillage of body fluids; sexual assault provides the most obvious example.[10] The matter is discussed further at the end of this chapter.

Other Cellular Blood Groups

Many other antigenic systems are present in the blood cells. The genetic distribution of some of these shows such disparity as to render them comparatively valueless as test systems; the necessary antisera are often rare; and, occasionally, special techniques are needed for their demonstration.

The *Kell system*, which may cause haemolytic disease of the newborn as does the Rhesus system, the *Duffy system* and the *Kidd system* are widely used in paternity testing although their individual capacities to exclude wrongly-accused fathers are limited. The *Lutheran system* can also be used if antibodies are available.

Systems which have been well studied but which are not used in paternity testing because of their complexity or instability include the *P system* which, again, may be responsible for fetal death, and the *Lewis system*, the main interest of which is that all persons of the phenotype Le(a+) are 'nonsecretors'.

Serum 'Blood Groups'

In addition to the antigens bound to the surface of the red cells, the blood plasma – or serum as it is when prepared for testing – contains protein substances which also appear as genetically controlled individual variants within systems. The principles of inheritance are similar to those described for the red cells. The serum groups are usually demonstrated by electrophoresis – a variant of chromatography (*see* Chapter 26) which measures the movement on paper of different proteins under the influence of an electric potential; the Gm system is an exception.

---

[9] This is a practical division. In fact, a minor degree of secretion can be demonstrated in some 'nonsecretors' using very sensitive techniques.

[10] Note that 'nonsecretion' refers only to nonsecretion of water soluble antigens; the cellular antigens A and B are determinable irrespective of the secretor status. Total deletion of the ABO antigens is excessively rare and results in the so-called 'Bombay' blood group.

These systems include the *haptoglobins* which are concerned with the body's reaction to challenge and, as a result, differ in quantity, but *not* in quality, in disease states.

The *Gm system* is extremely complicated and is difficult to demonstrate. At least three alleles and other variants have been discovered but, no matter how the system actually functions, the principle remains that a child cannot produce a Gm factor which does not appear in the phenotype of either of its parents.

The *Gc system* is of similar type to the haptoglobins but is inherited independently.

The Enzyme Systems of the Red Blood Cells

The functions of the red cells – those of absorbing, transporting and giving up oxygen – are performed through enzyme systems which, being of protein nature, can, again, be demonstrated as genetically controlled variants. The lawyer may, therefore, be confronted with such terms as 'phosphoglucomutase' but needs to know no more than that their use in paternity testing is based on principles identical to those already described.

The Assistance available from a Major Laboratory

The value of the various systems is additive in excluding parentage; the combined use of the various systems is shown in *Table* II.

Thus, in the hands of a specialized laboratory, 9 out of 10 wrongly-accused men will expect to be excluded from paternity but these probabilities are based on the common alleles which make up the systems. The finding of an antigen of considerable rarity within the system will greatly increase the value of that particular system and, if it is discovered in both a man and a child, it opens up the possibility of identifying, as opposed to excluding, a male parent.

This aspect of paternity testing is allowed for in Section 20(2)(c) of the Family Law Reform Act which directs the laboratory performing the tests to indicate, in the event of nonexclusion, the value of the tests in determining whether a man *is* the child's father. In practice, the proportion of the population which would qualify for paternity is calculated and expressed as a percentage of the total population. Proof of paternity then becomes a matter of probability and the smaller the percentage of the population satisfying the criteria, the more likely is the man to be the father; the size of the percentage depends not only on the commonness or rarity of the antigens discovered but also on the number of systems examined. Lord Reid[11] put it that if 50 per cent of men could supply the necessary antigen, the test would be valueless in proof of paternity; if only 1 in 1000 could do so, the result would go a long way to

---

[11] In S. v. S.; W. v. Official Solicitor [1970] 3 All E.R. 107(H.L.) at p. 110.

proving the man was the father; but if the figure was 1 per cent or 10 per cent the test might go some way to making paternity probable. Even so, the courts seem reluctant to employ the principle of probability particularly when a well-established presumption is involved; in one Scottish case,[12] a statistical chance of 500 000:1 against parenthood was considered insufficient to upset an existing legal presumption of legitimacy.

Table II.

	System	Individual exclusion rate	Combined exclusion rate	
Red Cell Antigens	ABO	0·176	0·176	
	Rhesus	0·280	0·406	
	MNSs	0·321	0·597	
	Kell	0·033	0·610	
	Duffy	0·048	0·629	
	Kidd	0·045	0·645	
Serum Proteins	Gm	0·065	0·065	
	Gc	0·145	0·201	
	Hp	0·175	0·341	0·765
Red Cell Enzymes	PGM	0·145	0·145	
	6PGD	0·025	0·166	
	AK	0·045	0·204	
	ADA	0·045	0·240	
	Acid Phosphatase	0·210	0·240	
	GPT	0·190	0·514	0·890
TOTAL CHANCE OF EXCLUSION				89%

The maximum possibility of exclusion on a false paternity charge. The exclusion rate for each system is based on the gene frequencies in Great Britain. (Details kindly supplied by Dr B. E. Dodd.)

In fairness to all parties, paternity testing must be done by a specialized laboratory and, if this is impossible, the limitations imposed on the result must be clearly understood. Section 22 of the Family Law Reform Act, in fact, indicates that testing is to be undertaken only by appointed practitioners.

Ethnic Variations in Blood Groups

The genetically controlled blood group antigens would be expected to vary in incidence in different ethnic groups and this is found to be so in practice. The more stable the population the more likely are single genes to predominate, major migrations should show as gene transferences and a gene may be actually advantageous in a given environment and

[12] Sproat v. McGibney 1968 S.L.T. 33.

therefore prosper locally. Thus, the incidence of the gene O is extremely high in South America and in most island communities, while the gene B is present most commonly in central Asia, getting less frequent as one moves westward and being relatively uncommon in the Americas. Similar variations are seen in the distribution of genes of other blood cell antigens, serum groups, enzyme variants and abnormal haemoglobins.[13]

This apparently academic subject has to be mentioned because of its practical importance when considering the probability of paternity as discussed above. Racial variations must be taken into account in making any calculations and a valid assessment can be made only if large numbers of the particular relevant population have been studied. For practical purposes, Western Europe, including the United Kingdom, can be regarded as homogeneous in this context although the Basques form a markedly distinct enclave. It should be noted, however, that ethnic differences are never absolute. It is impossible to derive the race of an individual simply by analysing his blood group spectrum.

THE EXAMINATION OF STAINS

The examination of stains is a matter for the science laboratory. Nonetheless, the subject is so entwined with blood group genetics that it does not seem out of place to include a short description so as to complete the picture for the lawyer.

The 'depth' of identification of a blood stain depends very largely on its age – a fresh blood stain can be dealt with much as a specimen taken *in vivo,* whereas an old stain, in which the cellular structure has disintegrated, is greatly limited as to use and putrefactive changes may lead to erroneous results. Thus, A antigen appears to behave in certain circumstances as a B reacting substance. In one case of the author's, 10 putrefied bodies recovered from the sea were blood-grouped; 8 appeared to be of group B – an impossible result.[14]

The basic steps in the examination of a blood stain are, firstly, to prove that it is blood – a matter of either direct vision under the microscope or of a sensitive chemical test – and, secondly, to prove its human origin – a comparatively simple exercise.

The ABO group can nearly always be ascertained, even when the test has to be performed on bloodstained threads only, but the problem of degenerative change discussed above is a real one. The Rhesus antigens are probably the next most stable, while modern immuno-electrophoretic techniques are so sensitive that the serum blood groups

---

[13] The sickle cell gene, which probably protects against malaria, is very common in Africa.

[14] *See* Jenkins G. C. et al. (1972) The problem of the acquired B antigen in forensic serology. *J. Forensic Sci. Soc.* **12,** 597.

may be as useful indicators of identity as are those attached to the cells. Given a square centimetre of bloodstained material, experienced workers can often identify some 8 or 9 genetic systems; the chances of association with a given individual with reasonable probability or for excluding a suspect are very high.

The identification of other biological stains – of which semen is the most important – follow much the same lines. Recognizable spermatozoa will remain on fabric for several months and direct positive observation under the microscope is certainly the most acceptable proof of a seminal origin. The enzyme acid phosphatase is highly developed in human semen and can be differentiated from the same enzyme which may be found in vaginal fluid; the activity of the enzyme is, however, often difficult to demonstrate other than in fresh stains. The human origin of a seminal stain is seldom in doubt but can be shown with the same ease as in the case of a blood stain.

The individual identification of a seminal stain depends on the secretor state of the donor. As described above, water-soluble blood group antigens will be found in the body fluids of only approximately three-quarters of the population; even so, the correlation of a 'negative' stain with a nonsecreting suspect is not without value and increasingly sensitive testing diminishes the proportion of 'nonsecretors'. Secretion of blood groups is limited to A, B and H substances; it follows that the chances of failure to distinguish between two individuals on the basis of seminal 'grouping' are of the order of 45 per cent of secretors – the medico-legal usefulness of such testing is, therefore, virtually confined to exclusion.

Chapter 19

Unnatural Death of the Fetus and the Newborn: Abortion, Child Destruction and Infanticide or Child Murder

RECENT changes in attitudes to induced abortion have been dramatic. It was certainly regarded as one of the more serious crimes in the early medico-legal codes and it is specifically referred to in the Hippocratic Oath. Yet, today, the extent of abortion services provided is regarded as something of a measure of the community's state of civilization and the inevitable conflict of views arouses much emotion. The historical background to the present position in relation to both abortion and neonatal killing is most easily described through the statutory English law.

The basic law on abortion in England and Wales is contained in the Offences Against the Person Act 1861 which states:

Section 58. Every woman, being with child, who with intent to procure her own miscarriage, shall unlawfully administer to herself any poison, or other noxious thing, or shall unlawfully use any instrument or other means whatsoever with like intent, and whosoever, with intent to procure the miscarriage of any woman, whether she be or be not with child, shall unlawfully administer to her, or cause to be taken by her, any poison or other noxious thing, or shall unlawfully use any instrument or other means whatsoever with like intent, shall be guilty of felony.[1]

Section 59. Whosoever shall unlawfully supply or procure any poison or other noxious thing, or any instrument or thing whatsoever, knowing that the same is intended to be unlawfully used, or employed, with intent to procure the miscarriage of any woman, whether she be or be not with child, shall be guilty of a misdemeanour.

This Act has not been repealed – recent legislation has done little more than to define the word 'unlawfully'. There is no mention in the 1861 Act of therapeutic abortion which was not recognized until the passing of the Infant Life (Preservation) Act 1929. This enacted (s. 1) that child destruction is committed when any person, with intent to destroy the life of a child capable of being born alive, by any wilful act causes a child to die before it has an existence independent of its mother; provided that the prosecution must prove that the act was not done in good faith for the purpose only of preserving the mother's life. For the purposes of the Act, evidence that a woman had at any material time

---

[1] Amended to 'an offence' by the Criminal Law Act 1967, s. 12(5).

225

been pregnant for a period of 28 weeks or more shall be *prima facie* proof that she was at that time pregnant of a child capable of being born alive.

The Infant Life (Preservation) Act introduced some important legal concepts. It recognized the legal right of a child to a separate existence after the 28th week of intra-uterine development and, at the same time, established the unusual crime of child destruction. A child in the process of being born naturally cannot be the subject of criminal abortion; on the other hand, a fetus which has had no separate existence cannot be murdered. The 1929 Act, in establishing an offence which included killing a child during the process of birth, closed the door on what was, admittedly, more of a permissible defence than a practical likelihood.

The Act also introduced for the first time the statutory possibility of a legally performed abortion. Two phrases stand out. 'In good faith' are words of great importance in both permissive and prohibitory senses; they still form an essential element in the law regulating therapeutic abortion. The qualification 'for the purpose only of saving the life of the mother' is restrictive and for many years it was left to case law[2] to establish the limits within which a doctor could legally terminate a pregnancy; the Abortion Act 1967 was enacted mainly to clarify the position.

Some terms of the Infant Life (Preservation) Act may cause confusion as between medical and legal interpretation. The first involves 'viability' or 'a viable fetus'. A viable fetus to a medical practitioner is one which can be kept alive in both an intra- and extra-uterine existence; to the lawyer, it is simply a fetus which has reached 28 weeks' gestation. Similar confusion may arise in relation to a 'live birth' and a 'separate existence'. To the doctor, a live birth is represented by a child who showed signs of life at some point in the delivery; the legal definition of a separate existence insists, in addition, that it 'should have completely proceeded in a living state from the body of the mother'. Thus, it is theoretically possible to have a medical live birth of a child which has not reached the development of legal viability while the reverse situation may well arise in practice as a result of complications in delivery.

These considerations also apply to the law protecting the infant shortly after birth. The Infanticide Act 1938 provides that the offence of infanticide is committed when a woman by any wilful act or omission causes the death of her child, being under the age of 12 months, but, at the time of the act or omission, the balance of her mind was disturbed by reason of her not having fully recovered from the effect of giving birth to the child or of lactation consequent upon the birth. Thus, viability, which is of great importance in relation to child destruction, has no rele-

---

[2] The most important being R. v. Bourne [1939] 1 K.B. 687; also R. v. Newton & Stungo [1958] Crim. L.R. 469.

vance to a charge of infanticide; all that is required in the latter is that the child should have been capable of being murdered – that is, had achieved a separate existence.

When such a charge is made, it is presumed that the child was born dead unless the prosecution can show proof to the contrary; any doubts which may exist must be resolved in favour of the mother. The pathological evidence thus assumes paramount importance and will be discussed later in this Chapter. For the present, it is simply emphasized that it may be impossible, even in the presence of only early decomposition, to give positive evidence in respect of a live birth. In such cases, Section 60 of the Offences Against the Person Act allows for an alternative charge of concealment of birth. This section makes it an offence for any person to endeavour to conceal the birth of a child by secret disposition of its dead body – that is, disposition in a place where there is no normal access for the public – whether the child died before, at or after its birth; the questions of viability and separate existence are, therefore, immaterial.

The Comparative Law in Scotland
With one exception, there are no comparable statutes in Scots law, the relevant offences being subject to common law.

In general, it seems that abortion has been regarded as less of a problem in Scotland than is the case in England and this applies particularly to operations performed by medical practitioners. Despite the fact that there was no case law to support the concept of therapeutic abortion before 1967, it is doubtful if Mr Bourne would have achieved his object of clarifying the issue had he performed a 'test' abortion in Scotland because the authorities would not have prosecuted him.[3]

In both England and Scotland, a woman must be shown to have been pregnant before she can be charged with self-inflicted criminal abortion. The intention on the part of an outsider to procure an abortion is criminal in both countries – the fact that the attempt is unsuccessful is immaterial; the main difference is that it is necessary in Scotland that the woman be pregnant and it is the responsibility of the prosecution to prove that pregnancy. It would be a defence in both England and Scotland to show that the fetus was dead prior to abortion.

There is no Scottish equivalent to the English Infant Life (Preservation) Act. Some very old case law[4] covers the possibility of destruction of the fetus during the process of birth; this was regarded not as homicide but as a serious, albeit unnamed, crime but this view was later

---

[3] Gordon G. H. (1967) *The Criminal Law of Scotland*. Edinburgh, W. Green & Son, p. 383. Mr Bourne aborted a girl made pregnant as a result of rape, having informed the authorities that he was to do so; he was prosecuted and acquitted.

[4] H.M.Adv. v. M'Allum (1858) 3 Irv. 187.

disputed.[5] Smith[6] thought that, provided the child had breathed, a defence that its death took place before it was fully extruded would not be valid in Scotland. Fortunately, the need for such a charge must be excessively rare.

The Infanticide Act of 1938 is also inapplicable in Scotland; the comparable crime under Scots law is child murder. Nonetheless, it has long been appreciated that the special conditions surrounding the killing of the neonate merit leniency and, in practice, diminished responsibility is always assumed; the crime of child murder is thus reduced to one of culpable homicide. It goes almost without saying that, under both jurisdictions, the extenuating conditions can be applied only to the mother.

The Concealment of Birth (Scotland) 1809 Act is the only statute relevant to Scotland in the present context and provides that a woman may be convicted if she 'conceals her being with child during the whole period of her pregnancy and does not call for and make use of help or assistance at the birth and the child be found dead or be amissing', the presumption being that the child would have been born alive and would have lived unless it had been concealed. This enactment is, in practice, more difficult to apply than is s. 60 of the English Offences Against the Person Act, principally because the concealment must be total and must be maintained for the whole pregnancy – it must, moreover, be shown that the child was viable not only in the legal but also in the medical sense. In contrast to the situation in England a prosecution can succeed in the absence of a body.

CRIMINAL ABORTION

Infanticide or child murder, child destruction and criminal abortion are closely related, as all are ultimately referable to an unwanted pregnancy. The pattern and incidence of the basic offence of abortion – and, indirectly, of the other two – has been completely altered by the Abortion Act 1967, which applies throughout the United Kingdom with the exception of Northern Ireland. Nonetheless, the number of abortions currently sought and the legal inadmissibility of many, even under the very wide terms of the 1967 Act, result in a sufficient surplus of cases to maintain the presence of criminal abortionists. The motivation of the Act can scarcely be appreciated without an understanding of the conditions it was designed to eliminate. A short consideration of criminal abortion is, even now, appropriate.

Approximately 20 per cent of pregnancies end prematurely. The proportion of these terminated illegally before 1967 cannot, for obvious

[5] H.M.Adv. v. Scott (1892) 3 White 240.

[6] Smith S. and Fiddes F. S. (1955) *Forensic Medicine*, 10th ed., London, Churchill, p. 339.

reasons, be accurately assessed and has been estimated as being anything from 10 per cent to 70 per cent; the most widely quoted figure in the United Kingdom is 40 per cent given, with reservation, by the Inter-Departmental Committee on Abortion in 1939,[7] although more recent observers have concluded that this figure is too high.

Given the almost invariable sequence of suspicion of pregnancy, confirmation of suspicion and failure of near natural attempts at abortion – e.g. hot baths, gin or feverish equestrianism – it is to be expected that the great majority of criminal abortions are attempted at between two and four months of pregnancy. The risks escalate beyond this point and only ignorant abortionists are likely to put themselves in jeopardy. Apart from the pregnant woman herself, an abortionist is, or was, generally either of the 'Mrs Gamp' type, a member of the paramedical professions, a nurse or student or, occasionally, a registered medical practitioner – though doctors whose names have been erased from the Register should also be included. The general methods of choice used by each category will be evident from the following description (*Fig.* 17).

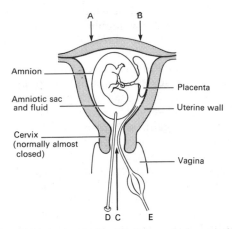

Fig. 17. Methods available to the abortionist. Drugs which cause the uterus to contract may be used (A) or direct violence may be applied to the womb (B). The cervix may be dilated by instruments or hygroscopic tampons (C) inducing the uterus to contract. The amniotic sac may be penetrated by sharp instruments (D) causing direct or indirect death of the fetus. The fetus may be separated from the uterine wall by the injection of fluids or pastes (E).

---

[7] Ministry of Health and Home Office, London, HMSO, para. 26.

Abortifacient Drugs

There are essentially three categories of drug used in attempts to procure abortion.[8]

a Purgatives and Emetics. These are used in the mistaken belief that all smooth muscle will contract if one part – the bowel – is stimulated.

b. Emmenagogues. These are substances which increase the menstrual flow. Presumably, the rationale for their use is that substances which will provoke excessive normal menstrual flow will stimulate some flow when it is inhibited by pregnancy. It is probable that many of these drugs, including the more sophisticated female hormones (oestrogenic substances) which are often used with similar intent, owe their reputation to the fact that they produce a dramatic result when inhibition of the menstrual period is due to causes other than pregnancy. The advertisement of any drugs in terms which might lead to their use to procure abortion was prohibited under the Pharmacy and Medicines Act 1941 (replaced by the Medicines Act 1968).

c. Ecbolics. These are drugs which actively promote contraction of the uterine muscle. Since most of them have a genuine pharmacological action and are therapeutically valuable, they can constitute a temptation to the medical practitioner. Two substances in this group which are well-known to the general public are lead, which is partially restricted under Schedule 1 of the Poisons Rules, and quinine which is unrestricted; both may cause severe symptoms of poisoning. The most efficient agent is ergot – which is used quite properly to ensure contraction of the uterus after delivery. Hormone preparations include pituitary extract which may, again, be rightly used to induce labour and, recently, prostaglandins have been introduced as therapeutic abortifacients particularly in the later stages of pregnancy.

The use of drugs draws attention to the interpretation of the term 'noxious thing' used in the Offences Against the Person Act. Theoretically, any substance having an unusual pharmacological effect might be regarded as noxious. For the purposes of the Act, however, it has been established that, to be relevant, the drug must be known to have abortifacient properties; otherwise it would be hard to prove intent. Moreover, the dosage must be taken into consideration lest the doctor be open to accusation every time a potential abortifacient is properly prescribed for the treatment of unrelated conditions.

---

[8] The perpetuation of this type of list might well be considered anachronistic. However, preparations, particularly of the emmenagogue variety, are still widely sold: the curious Gallic association of many of their trade names testifies to their time-worn origins (*see* David T. J. (1974) The composition and current use of abortifacients. *Med. Sci. Law* **14**, 120).

Abortion by Direct Violence

Little need be said on this other than to remark on the resistance of the fetus to direct violence. The main medico-legal implications of this 'method' of abortion are that a husband who is prepared to subject his pregnant wife to such abuse is likely to do so in the absence of pregnancy and, secondly, that severe attacks on the gravid uterus are as likely to result in rupture with death of the mother as in simple expulsion of the fetus.

Criminal Instrumentation

By far the most common form of criminal abortion involves the use of instruments of some sort. The function of these can best be understood by reference to normal pregnancy and delivery.

a. The fetus obtains its nourishment from an interwoven network of blood capillaries on the uterine wall which, at three months, is condensed into the placenta. If this connection is broken, the fetus becomes a nonviable foreign body and may be expelled. This mechanism forms the basis of the injection of pastes or of the use of the infamous enema syringe to procure abortion.

b. The fetus is maintained in a fluid medium within the amniotic sac. Drainage of this fluid results in compression of the fetus by the uterine muscle and ultimate expulsion. Any instrument which perforates the amnion may precipitate abortion and there can be few pointed objects – from quill feather pens to surgical catheters – which have not been employed for the purpose. Bundles of wax tapers have also been used.

c. Dilatation of the cervical canal initiates the normal discharge of a fetus. Artificial dilatation may, in effect, deceive the uterine muscle into believing the time for contraction to have arrived. Certain vegetable substances will absorb water and swell when placed in the cervical canal which is thereby opened. This is the mode of operation of slippery elm bark which was such a favourite of the abortionist because it was likely to leave no trace of interference.

The truly professional abortionist may, of course, combine these methods in the surgical operation of cervical dilatation and curettage or suction of the uterine cavity.

Death Following Instrumentation

An attempted abortion may fail or succeed; in either case, the woman may be unaffected, may require medical treatment or may die. A case resulting in less than fatal injury to the woman will come to light only in exceptional circumstances. But death will always be investigated and the lawyer needs an understanding of the various causative mechanisms.

Death may ensue immediately, it may occur fairly soon after the

event or it may be delayed. The practical significance of this classification is that, in the first instance, the body may well be found at the
locus; in the second, death may occur at some distance from the scene of
the abortion; while, in the third, it may even be difficult to associate the
fatality with an abortion. Deaths associated with poisoning by drugs are
not considered further at this point.

Immediate Death

a. Vagal inhibition of the heart. This is the characteristic 'death on the
couch', the abnormal sensory stimulus precipitating cardiac arrest
being contact with the inner surface of the cervical canal. As previously
discussed, the pathologist's major difficulty is that the post-mortem
diagnosis of the condition is based almost entirely on the circumstantial
evidence and on exclusion of other pathological states.

b. Air Embolism. Separation of the fetal from the maternal circulation, which is the purpose of the enema syringe, results in the opening of
blood vessels. It is possible for the receptor nozzle of the syringe to be
withdrawn from the fluid during the process of forcible douching and
air is then delivered instead of, or along with, fluid. The circulation finds
it hard to deal with large gas bubbles and death from air embolism may
result – generally in about 10 minutes which is the time taken for a lethal
concentration of bubbles to accumulate in the arteries of the heart and
brain. The amount of air needed to kill depends on the degree to which
the vital organs are embolized – 10 ml have been lethal while, in other
cases, the injection of 100 ml has been survived. Although death from
air embolism is usually rapid, cases have been reported of survival for 2
hours; the subject does not, therefore, always die where the abortion
was performed.

Moderately Delayed Death

a. Fluid Embolism. Even if air is not pumped into the circulation, the
fluid used, often containing strong soap or toxic antiseptics, can be
introduced. Death may then be fairly rapid but is as likely to be delayed
until the effects of tissue necrosis or blood haemolysis have become evident.

b. Haemorrhage. The cervical opening is small and the vaginal and cervical canals do not run in a straight line. Moreover, the majority of lay
persons are remarkably ignorant of the size and position of the pregnant
uterus. It is not surprising that many attempts at instrumentation result
in laceration not of the fetal sac alone but, additionally or alternatively,
of the vagina, of the cervix or of the uterus itself. Laceration implies
haemorrhage which may be sufficient to cause death. This does seem,
however, to be surprisingly uncommon – the woman generally seeks
medical assistance before the situation has got out of hand.

Delayed Death
a. Sepsis. Sepsis was the commonest cause of death following criminal abortion before the advent of antibiotics and the occurrence of sepsis following an abortion could be taken as a strong indication that the condition was unnatural. Three features contributed in the main to this. Firstly, the instrumentation was either unhygenic from the outset or became so during the process of procuring an abortion. Secondly, the uterus was often not cleared properly and this left a dead nidus of infection. Thirdly, the closeness of the lower bowel to an area frequently injured resulted in local sepsis or in septicaemia caused by organisms normally present in the faeces. The most dangerous of these were those causing gas gangrene and tetanus – they remain so even in the antibiotic age because of the very severe toxic effects they may exhibit and the often fulminating nature of the infection.
b. Acute renal failure. As described in Chapter 1, any condition which results in surgical shock may well have a profound effect on the kidneys. Many of the complications of criminal abortion are essentially 'shocking' and renal failure may ensue even if a woman has survived the original crisis.

The Legal Position of the Doctor in Criminal Abortion
The relationship between the doctor and his patient is under considerable strain whenever a patient is involved in criminal activity, particularly when that criminality derives from acute mental distress as must most often be the case when illegal abortion is attempted.

The position is statutory when death results. In both England and Scotland the Registrar will, by regulation, report the matter to the Coroner or to the Procurator Fiscal. At any subsequent hearing, the doctor may properly protest his right to professional secrecy but, under both jurisdictions, he must ultimately provide evidence and answer questions which are put to him.

The concept that professional confidentiality takes precedence over the disclosure of criminality in life has also been disapproved. Lord Justice Inglis[9] was quite clear – 'I care not for professional etiquette or rule; there is a rule of life and a consideration far higher than these, and that is the duty of every citizen . . . to prevent the destruction of human life'. An English *obiter dictum* which is commonly quoted is that of Avory J. (1914)[10] who stated, 'there are cases where the desire to preserve [the confidential relation which exists between the medical man and his patient] must be subordinated to the duty which is cast on every good

[9] In Roughead W. (ed.) (1906) *Trial of Dr Pritchard*, Glasgow, W. Hodge & Co., p. 283. The trial took place in 1865.

[10] Reported in: The duties of medical practitioners in cases of criminal abortion, *Br. Med. J.* (1916) 1, 206.

citizen to assist in the investigation of a serious crime'.[11] This view was challenged by the Royal College of Physicians who issued a statement in 1916 which still represents authoritative medical opinion on this question. Briefly, this statement concluded that every medical practitioner has a moral duty to respect the confidence of his patient; that, when convinced that criminal abortion has been practised on his patient, the doctor should urge her to make a statement as evidence against the person who performed the operation; that he is under no legal obligation either to so urge his patient or to press the point should she refuse; that, in any event, he should obtain good legal and medical advice before taking any action which might lead to legal proceedings; and that he should inform the Coroner should the patient die.

Times change as do attitudes. No practitioner would now be likely to report a criminal abortion in which no second party was involved. Yet there is surely sufficient violence in the world today without, by remaining silent, effectively conniving at the survival of criminals whose activities may well result in culpable homicide. The basic wrong lies not so much in the niceties of medical jurisprudence as in the fact that such cases should ever occur. It was against this background that the Abortion Act 1967 was passed.

THE ABORTION ACT 1967

The bones of the Act are contained in Section 1 which states:

(1) . . . a person shall not be guilty of an offence under the law relating to abortion when a pregnancy is terminated by a registered medical practitioner if two medical practitioners are of the opinion, formed in good faith:
    (a) that the continuance of the pregnancy would involve risk to the life of the pregnant woman, or of injury to the physical or mental health of the pregnant woman or any existing children of her family, greater than if the pregnancy were terminated; or
    (b) that there is substantial risk that if the child were born it would suffer from such physical or mental abnormalities as to be seriously handicapped.
(2) [In making a decision under Para 1 (a)] account may be taken of the pregnant woman's actual or reasonably foreseeable environment.

As has already been stressed, this is not the definitive law on abortion; indeed, Section 5 specifically retains the provisions of the Infant Life (Preservation) Act 1929 and states that 'anything done with intent to procure the miscarriage of a woman is unlawfully done unless authorized by Section 1 of this Act'. The purpose of the 1967 Act was to simplify the position in relation to therapeutic abortion. That it was never intended to be a licence for 'abortion on demand' seems clear from the

---

[11] It has been questioned whether this constitutes more than a well-informed opinion (Polson C. J. and Gee D. J. (1973) *Essentials of Forensic Medicine,* 3rd ed., Oxford, Pergamon, p. 697).

number of regulations which must be satisfied to make the operation legal. Not only must a legal abortion be carried out in a hospital of the National Health Service or in a place specifically approved for the purpose, but standardized forms must be used for recommending the abortion and for reporting that an emergency abortion has been performed – in which case, the need for two opinions is waived; a statutory form must be completed for notification of the termination of pregnancy within seven days of the event. Part II of the latter form contains a number of questions designed to improve the statistical basis of any future legislation (Abortion Regulations 1968; Abortion (Scotland) Regulations 1968).

Nevertheless, the phrasing of the Act is very open and the scope for legalized abortion is considerable – it has been argued that the risks of normal pregnancy are greater than those of early abortion and that, consequently, any termination carried out in an approved place must be legal. An increasing number of operations are being carried out in Great Britain; this trend has been noted in other countries which have followed the general format of British legislation. Over 160 000 legal terminations were notified in England and Wales during the period April 1968 – December 1970; in 1973 alone the figure was 169 360. The National Health Service cannot cope with such escalation and well over half the legal abortions in England and Wales are conducted in 'approved places'.

The situation in Scotland is illuminating. There were just under 11 000 notifications between April 1968 and December 1970; the figure for 1973 was 7498. Thus, although there has been an increase, it is not as great as has been the case in England. Moreover, only 88 abortions were carried out in approved places in Scotland in 1973. The figures indicate that, when related to population, the number of abortions carried out in National Health Service hospitals is very comparable in both countries and tend to refute the suggestion occasionally made that obviously deserving cases are being denied termination.

While a return to the situation which existed before 1967 is unthinkable, it has been argued that the Act as it stands is too lax.[12] The basis of the legislation is the almost undefinable phrase 'in good faith'. Since no prosecutions have been brought relating to contravention of the 1967

---

[12] A second Abortion (Amendment) Bill is currently before Parliament. The Bill seeks, *inter alia*, to limit 'lawful' abortion to pregnancies of less than 20 weeks duration, to those of 24 weeks or less duration in which there is a substantial risk that the child might suffer from such abnormalities as to make it seriously handicapped in life or to those in which the treatment is necessary either to save the life of the pregnant woman or to prevent grave permanent injury to her physical or mental health; there are provisions for licensing and inspection of places where abortions may be performed, where advice as to the treatment for the termination of a pregnancy is given and for pregnancy testing services. The more controversial clauses in the original Amendment Bill have been dropped.

Act, it must be assumed that the phrase is legally satisfactory. Nevertheless, the fact that one-third of the abortions performed in England are performed on foreign girls whose patronage is actively solicited and whose total stay in Great Britain is commonly of the order of three days must raise considerable doubts in the medical profession.[13] A conscience clause, excusing persons of a duty to participate in the treatment authorized, was included as Section 4 of the Act. Paradoxically, it is this element in the Act which has led to the most justifiable criticism of its operation to the effect that local prejudice tends to regionalize pockets of more stringent application.

Resistance to a very wide interpretation of the law would seem to be a natural reflection of the doctor's 'Hippocratic conscience'. Surprisingly, however, by far the greatest publicity is given to religious principles – in particular, to those regulated by Roman Catholicism. The author recently obtained an opinion from a leading Roman Catholic philosopher particularly as to the apparent priority given by the Church to the well-being of the fetus when this affected the life of the mother. He wrote:

On a subjective level, I can fully appreciate the position of the doctor or surgeon faced with the woman with serious complications which make it unlikely or impossible that her baby will come to term before she dies. He is bound to feel that [in failing to terminate the pregnancy] he has not done all he can for her and that therefore he is guilty of her death.

On an objective level, two things seem to me rather clear. The first is that this attitude, entirely admirable as it is, does somewhat presuppose that the mother's life is more important than the child's and that therefore, if the mother is to be saved, the child has to be sacrificed. But would it work the other way round? Would it be right and proper for the doctor to end the mother's life in order to give a viable child a decent chance of survival? Clearly not. You may answer that the eventuality is not in fact practical because it wouldn't arise. But if it did, no doctor would countenance it and no moralist allow it. Why? Because it would be plain murder. And that is the crucial second point. If it is plain murder in the case of the mother, why is it not in the case of the child?

Which brings us back to the dilemma. Objectively, the doctor is not entitled to kill either in order to save the other. His job is to save both. He is bound to do all in his power to save the mother, short of doing what is wrong – and killing the baby is wrong.

I would have to add that, if he still felt in conscience bound to terminate the pregnancy, I would not and could not blame him – because that is in the subjective order, and he is entitled to follow the dictates of his own conscience.

The practical importance of the last paragraph is self-evident.

This apparently irrelevant diversion into the field of conscience has

---

[13] Even so, the *Report of the Committee on the Working of the Abortion Act*, 1974 (Cmnd. 5579, HMSO), after an exhaustive inquiry, recommended very few changes. The most important were that an upper time limit for abortion of 24 weeks should be imposed (the legal presumption of viability at 28 weeks would no longer apply), that the penalties for false certification should be increased, that both certifying doctors should be required to examine the pregnant woman and that the Chief Medical Officer should be empowered to disclose to the General Medical Council information furnished to him if it appeared that there had been serious professional misconduct.

practical medico-legal significance. No conscientious objection to terminating pregnancy is allowable under the Act when the operation is necessary to save the life of, or to prevent serious permanent injury to, the woman; it is also possible that a doctor, or a medical ancillary, could be held negligent in failing to provide or arrange such treatment for lesser reasons. Whereas, in Scotland, a simple statement on oath establishes the doctor's legal position, the burden of proof of conscientious objection in England rests on the person claiming it. Irrespective of conscience, any doctor is at risk of civil action should a decision not to terminate be shown in the end to have been wrong; the most significant effect of successful actions of this type would be to force the profession into performing abortions at the dictate of any pregnant woman. Even allowing for sincere conscientious objection on the doctor's part, it would obviously be improper for him to attempt to influence his patient on any grounds other than those he believes to be in accord with current medical practice and, if necessary, he must himself act according to these principles; while the Act excuses the medical profession from participation in the treatment authorized, there is no exemption from advising a patient as to the correct medical course. On the other hand, the doctor has to appreciate that his patient too may have a strong conscience and it goes without saying that, except in relation to minors and to emergency procedures, it could amount to serious professional misconduct to procure an abortion other than with the full consent of the patient and, ideally, also of the husband.

POTENTIAL EVIDENCE FROM THE EXPERT WITNESS

Abortion
For reasons previously discussed, prosecutions for criminal abortion are unusual unless the woman dies. Should she do so, important pathological evidence may be obtained under four main headings.

Firstly, the fact of pregnancy or of delivery must be established under both English and Scots law – particularly the latter. Evidence of these may include the signs of response in the breast although they are poorly developed at the elective time of criminal abortion. Discharge or haemorrhage from the vulva may be evident. Internally, the persistence in an ovary of a corpus luteum – the hormonal response to ovulation and subsequent pregnancy – may be noted; this atrophies in some 10 days in the absence of pregnancy but persists for approximately the first 20 weeks of gestation. The major evidence, however, comes from the uterus which will still contain a fetus in the case of unsuccessful attempted abortion. Otherwise, there will almost certainly be enlargement of the organ; the normal uterus measures some $2\frac{3}{4} \times 1\frac{1}{2}$ in. (7 × 4 cm) while at three months the size is of the order of a 3-in. (8-cm) globe. Internally, the lining will be haemorrhagic and furry for a few days and a recognizable placental area may persist for 2 months. An attempt should be made to prove the presence of placental tissue microscopically. These signs are so general in nature that the pathologist can give no more than an estimate as to when delivery took place. The longer the interval, the more imprecise must be that estimate and, at 2 months, even the fact of delivery may be in doubt.

Secondly, evidence of interference will be sought. If there is any suggestion of the use of 'noxious substances', specimens of blood, bowel content and tissues will be sent for analysis. Direct violence may be evidenced by abdominal bruising. The greatest significance will, however, be attached to the finding of lacerations which are commonly in the posterior vagina, the cervix or the uterus itself. The peritoneum lining the abdominal cavity may be penetrated and injuries of any sort may be complicated by haemorrhage or by sepsis. The presence of the latter is strong, but not conclusive, evidence of unnatural abortion; the type of the infecting organisms should be established in every case not only to indicate their origin but also for possible comparison with cultures made from suspect instruments. In addition to evidence of the use of penetrating instruments, the post-mortem may also show local signs of abortion by injection. Thus, frothy soapy fluid or paste may persist within the uterus and may even be found in the abdominal cavity in the event of very unskilled use.

It is equally the responsibility of the pathologist to exclude the possibility of natural abortion. A full autopsy is necessary to exclude such conditions as nephritis, diabetes, heart disease or placental abnormalities – accidental placental haemorrhage, although generally occurring late in pregnancy, is a natural phenomenon which may closely simulate illegal interference.

Thirdly, the cause of death may have a great bearing on the case and, while the pathologist can generally make a confident assessment, it may, on occasion, be surprisingly difficult to do so. Thus, it has already been noted that vagal inhibition is essentially a post-mortem diagnosis of exclusion; haemorrhage may appear inconspicuous although copious quantities of blood have been lost elsewhere; purulent exudate involving the genitalia may, even when of apparently severe degree, be no more than of incidental significance.

Embolic modes of death may involve extra interpretative and technical skills. The production of apparent bubbles in the cerebral circulation is a common artefact induced by removal of the skull at post-mortem dissection; the competent pathologist is, however, aware of this and well able to distinguish such a localized abnormality from the full-blown picture of fatal air embolism with characteristic churning of the blood in the chambers of the heart. Most pastes used in abortion contain a fatty base; should such pastes be embolized to the lungs or brain, their presence should be demonstrable by special microscopic techniques. An expert chemical and spectrographic examination of the blood might well be of value in death supposed to be due to the introduction of toxic solutions by syringe.

Finally, evidence as to whether an abortion was self-induced or was the result of interference by an outside party can seldom be given unequivocally on the basis of the post-mortem examination alone. The pathologist will be led by the general assumption that the greater the injury produced, the more likely was it to have resulted from the woman's own efforts. It is of course possible that an abortionist may be very unskilled – only practice makes perfect; but it is far less likely that a woman, even given some special knowledge, will perform a clean surgical operation upon herself.

The 'patient' of the competent abortionist is likely to die only from those conditions which are unpredictable – vagal shock and embolism. It is in these cases that the circumstantial evidence – the place of death, the presence or absence of equipment, etc. – becomes so important and dictates the need for a visit by the pathologist to the scene. Even then, the wide variations in pathological processes must be taken into consideration and exceptions to general rules must, if within reason, sometimes be admitted as possibilities.

Concealment of Birth or of Pregnancy
Only the mother may be available for expert medical examination in cases involving these unusual charges and proof of recent delivery will depend largely on the clinical findings. The child is likely to have been close to or at full term and manifest enlargement of the uterus may well be found together with evidence of recent stretching of the abdomen – the typical recent red 'striae gravidarum'. The uterus remains easily palpable for about 10 days after giving birth and the cervix may be flabby and/or torn. A typical bloody discharge, the lochia, persists for some 3 days to be replaced by a more normal appearing post-partum discharge which lasts for a further week; microscopy of this may prove its nature. Evidence of tearing of the perineum can be of great value – it need not necessarily occur and tears could conceivably be due to causes other than the passage of the fetus; but this is the most likely cause and the extent of laceration may suggest the maturity of the child.

Some time can elapse in cases of concealment – or of child murder – before the need for examination becomes apparent. There will, then, be wide variation in the findings as some women return to normal much faster or slower than the average; it is generally accepted that positive proof of delivery, sufficient to satisfy the Court, will be difficult to obtain in the living person after a lapse of 8–10 days.

In the event that the body of the infant is discovered, its examination will follow the lines indicated below, in the sections Child Destruction and Child Murder, but it should be noted that there is a presumption of a live birth in the Scottish offence of concealment of pregnancy.

Child Destruction

The main medical evidence peculiar to this charge concerns the legal viability of the child – has it or has it not achieved the 28th week of intra-uterine life? The evidence is based on two main sets of observations – the general appearances of the fetus and the presence of centres of ossification in various bones.

By the 28th week, the fetus will have developed easily recognizable external sex organs but the testes are not descended into the scrotum; it will have head and body hair together with eyebrows and eyelashes; the skin will be developed and creased; and the nails will almost have reached the ends of the digits. The length from crown to heel is classically 14 in. (35 cm). This is based on the formula that, after the fourth month, the length of the fetus in inches is twice the month of gestation (or five times in centimetres). There will be significant variations about this mean – at 7 months the possible scatter is likely to lie between 13 and 15 in. The weight at this point is generally between 2½ and 3½ lb (1·1 and 1·6 kg).

Centres of ossification have been explained in Chapter 1. Many centres appear early in fetal life and are of little legal significance. Those which appear at or around the critical period include:

20th week:	calcaneus bone of heel;
24th week:	manubrium (upper end) of breast bone;
28th week:	talus bone of heel, first segment of the sternum (breast bone) proper;
32nd week:	last segment of breast bone;
At term:	lower end of femur (thigh bone); cuboid bone of the foot, upper end of tibia (shin bone).

In general it is the presence of ossification centres which has the greatest significance; the negative evidence of their absence is less valuable (*Plate* 15).

Child Murder or Infanticide

The great majority of instances of child murder or infanticide occur during the first 24 hours of the infant's life. The basic pathological problem is, therefore, to distinguish between wilful killing and stillbirth, which has been defined on p. 72. Since it is for the prosecution to prove

PLATE 1

a, Tattoo disclosed beneath a layer of carbonization. The figure illustrates also the difficulties of interpretation – the design was positively recognized by relatives as being that of a peacock; it certainly does not appear so to the author.

b, An unusual example of cadaveric spasm. The amputated hand of an airline passenger is firmly grasping the seat-belt (there has been post-mortem burning).

PLATE 2

a, Post-mortem injuries caused by land crabs.

b, Transverse section through the heart of a young man who died while playing football. There is massive hypertrophy of the left ventricle (the scale is in centimetres) and the heart weighed 1 kg.

PLATE 3

a, The stages in coronary atherosclerosis. The artery (A) is almost normal; there is a minor degree of thickening at '4–5 o'clock'. At B there is some 70 per cent restriction of the lumen by atheroma; note how this is generally asymmetric. At C, there has been haemorrhage into such an atheromatous plaque which has burst. Coronary thrombosis with total occlusion of the lumen is illustrated at D.

b, Imprint of centre of steering wheel on the chest of a car driver.

PLATE 4

a, Irregular lacerations of generally similar type caused by battering with bottles.

b, Typical self-inflicted injuries. Apparently made with the intention of implicating a lover who had jilted her.

PLATE 5

Post-mortem instruments have been placed in two stab wounds to show the direction of thrusts.

PLATE 6

A shotgun lies in the doorway of a room, well separated from the body. The conditions clearly indicate homicide.

PLATE 7

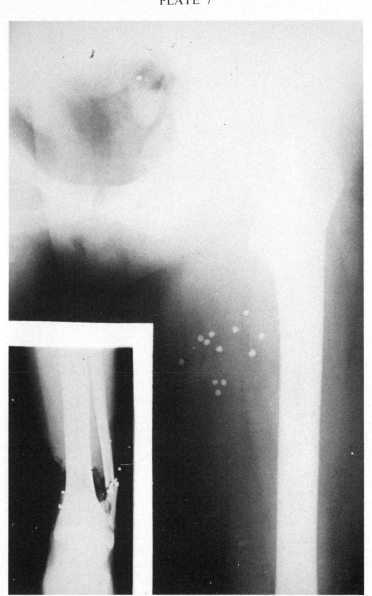

Both barrels of a shotgun were discharged during a marital altercation. One shot was aimed at and disrupted the heart. Pellets from the other can be seen in the left groin and left ankle; the victim must have been kneeling at the time she was shot.

PLATE 8

The hands of the passenger in a light aircraft show linear lacerations. It was subsequently established that part of the duties of this man was to pay out an aerial
from the rear of the cockpit. The injuries indicate that the apparently inexplicable accident was due to the aerial catching in trees during low flying.

PLATE 9

a, The head of a passenger in a car accident is uninjured save for a laceration of the chin.

b, The force has been transmitted through the jaw bone to the base of the skull which is completely divided (in between arrows).

PLATE 10

X-ray of larynx. The left superior cornu of the thyroid cartilage is fractured (arrowed).

PLATE 11

Strangulation by ligature. The conditions at the locus clearly raise the possibility of suicide or accident. There were few signs of asphyxia at the post mortem and death was attributed to vagal inhibition of the heart.

PLATE 12

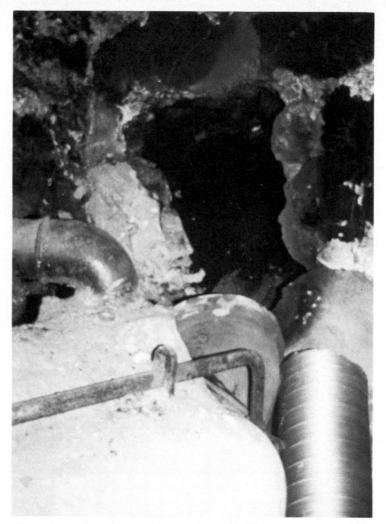

Conditions in a cellar where a night watchman died from carbon monoxide poisoning. The boiler was alight but the flue had been disconnected for replacement. The deceased's blood alcohol was 260 mg/100 ml.

PLATE 13

a, Suicidal electrocution. The leads have been removed from beneath Sellotaping. The precise pattern of burning is shown beneath the upper tape.

b, Chest radiograph from a case of certified pneumoconiosis in a coal miner (early Category 3).

PLATE 14

The illustrations show a Barr body at '11 o'clock' in a nucleus from the buccal
surface of a normal female (1a); a negative cell from a male is shown at 1b. Section 2a is from a similar male cell stained with quinacrene and shows a brightly
fluorescent Y body; 2b is the equivalent from a female and shows no Y body.
(Illustrations by courtesy of Professor H. J. Evans, Western General Hospital,
Edinburgh.)

PLATE 15

X-ray of an infant found dead in a rubbish tip. Note particularly (arrowed) the centre of ossification at the lower end of the femur indicating full-term maturity and the two centres in the heel showing legal viability.

PLATE 16

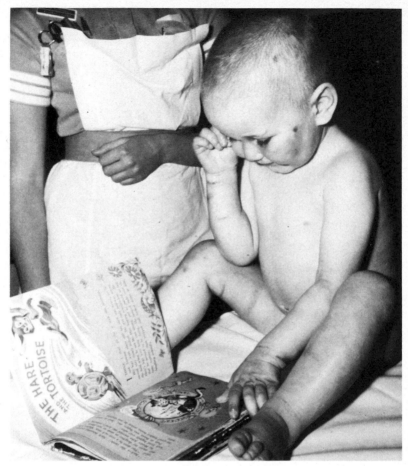

Typical appearances of a 'battered child'.

PLATE 17

Rape. There is exceptional violence indicated by the damage to the face and right arm.

PLATE 18

Rape – scratch injuries on the chest of the assailant indicating determined resistance. A typical 'love bite' is seen at the front of the left shoulder; this was unrelated to the incident.

PLATE 19

a, Outline of the frontal sinuses; the chances of any two people having precisely the same outline are negligible. (Radiographs by courtesy of Professor Eric Samuel, University of Edinburgh.)

b, X-ray appearances of the pituitary fossa in three individuals; the possible differences are legion. (Radiographs by courtesy of Professor Eric Samuel, University of Edinburgh.)

PLATE 20

Unusual appearances due to the explosion of bullets in the pocket of an armed guard during a fire. (Reproduced by courtesy of Dr P. J. Stevens.)

a live birth, the medical evidence divides logically into two main categories – firstly, as to whether the child was, in fact, born alive and
achieved a separate existence and, secondly, as to indications of an unnatural death.

Evidence of a live birth simply in the sense of full extrusion from the
mother is almost impossible to give from a pathological examination
but it may well be possible to assert that a live birth was, at least, improbable. Thus, it is unusual for an immature infant of less than 7
months' gestation to be born live; monstrous abnormalities of various
sorts – in particular anencephaly (lack of a brain) – may be incompatible
with life and the pathologist can generally give a firm opinion; macera-
tion is certain evidence of this type as it constitutes *aseptic* degeneration
of the fetal tissues following death in utero.

Positive evidence of a separate existence, however, may well be
derived from the post-mortem examination.

Major interest centres on the condition of the lungs which, as described in Chapter 1, are not only without function in utero but are relatively isolated from the general blood circulation. Fetal lungs are,
therefore, virtually solid organs, homogeneous in consistency and
colour. The effect of reflex inspiration of air at birth is to expand the
lungs, a process which, in turn, initiates the true pulmonary respiratory
blood circulation; both these processes take time – a matter of minutes –
and, until they are fully established, the lungs may vary from place to
place as to the degree of aeration and of vascularization. Thus, as the
lungs fill the chest cavity they change in colour from purple to mottled
pink and they increase in weight. These general changes can be further
demonstrated by the so-called hydrostatic test or by microscopy.

The basis of the hydrostatic test is that an organ which contains air
will float in water whereas one that does not will sink. Since aeration
may be irregular, the lungs must be tested one by one, then lobe by lobe,
and finally, and if necessary, piece by piece.

It is customary to decry the hydrostatic test. It appears to the author
to be a good practical test which has suffered from being given too great
a 'scientific' significance as a single observation; this has resulted in the
elaboration of theoretical objections which would be invalid if the post-
mortem findings were taken as a composite whole. It is true, for
example, that a child could have a separate existence and then develop
disease of the lungs of such a type as to make them sink in water; but it
has been pointed out that such disease would constitute a natural cause
of death and despite a 'false' result no harm would be done because the
charge of infanticide would rightly fail. The occurrence of a spurious
flotation of the lungs is a far more important, and a more practical, objection to the test. It might arise in two ways. Firstly, there is the possibility of artificial mouth-to-mouth respiration having been given. It is

said that satisfactory aeration of the fetal lung by this means is difficult to achieve and that, even if it is effective, the pulmonary circulation would not be started – the appearances of the lungs would, therefore, be different from those of normal breathing. It could, however, be a difficult pathological decision to make. Secondly, there is a very real problem of putrefaction and aeration of the lungs by gas forming bacteria. Compression of the lung tissue, which fails to remove inspired air but does discharge putrefactive gases, has been recommended to distinguish the ,two but the author has little experience of the value of the manœuvre. It is a matter in the main of common sense and looking at the overall picture – if there is putrefaction of the lungs there will be putrefaction elsewhere, but the near impossibility of diagnosing a separate existence from the pulmonary findings in the presence of even early decomposition is stressed by all authorities. The most objective differentiation is to be made through microscopy; there is little histological similarity between freshly aerated and markedly putrefied lungs but the appearances of aeration *and* putrefaction may be very confusing. Some of the microscopic changes which indicate that normal breathing has occurred are subtle while others depend upon survival for some time; there is no space for their detailed discussion here and the interested reader is referred to the classic article by Osborn.[14]

Although the condition of the lungs has been discussed in detail, 'some other signs of a separate existence' must also be sought. Thus, the presence of gulped air in the stomach and intestine has been suggested as being valid evidence; anoxic convulsions are not, however, evidence of life and this sign could only be acceptable when combined with evidence of aeration of the lungs. Presence of food in the stomach or bowel would, of course, be evidence of a separate existence but this would imply long-term survival. The main evidence of this degree of survival is to be found in the umbilical cord which characteristically shows an inflammatory disposal reaction at the abdominal wall approximately 2 days after birth. The cord is shed on the 5th or 6th day but the time may be longer or shorter; the umbilical scar is healed in 10–12 days.

There remains the evidence to be drawn as to whether the infant's death was, in fact, due to 'some wilful act or omission'. There are very few limits to the way in which an infant may be murdered – widespread generalized violence, suffocation in its many forms, strangling, including the use of the readily available umbilical cord, drowning and wounding by one method or another are the commonest methods of infanticide. The pathology of all is described elsewhere and needs no repetition here.

It should, however, be stressed that the differentiation of homicide

¹⁴ Osborn G. R. (1953) Pathology of the lung in stillbirth and neonatal death. In: Simpson K. (ed.) *Modern Trends in Forensic Medicine*, London, Butterworth, Ch. 2.

from accident or from natural disease is exceptionally difficult in the newborn period. Thus, the distinction between death due to natural asphyxia of central origin and that due to the application of a pillow to the face may be impossible, while frightened mothers can and do suffocate their infants accidentally; intracranial haemorrhage due to natural birth trauma may be indistinguishable from that due to deliberate violence, precipitate labour does occur and newborn infants *can* slip through the hands to the floor; an infant *may* drown in its own amniotic fluid; the umbilical cord *does* sometimes entangle with the child's neck. So much depends in each case on the circumstantial evidence and, again, it is the total picture which counts; it would be a brave pathologist who was convinced he could correctly diagnose every newborn death on his unsupported post-mortem findings alone.

Nothing has been said about infanticide by omission, and it is the experience of most authorities that deliberate killing of babies by abandonment alone is surprisingly rare. A large proportion of embarrassing dead newborn infants are, however, hidden and this is irrespective of whether death was due to natural or unnatural causes. Discovery is frequently delayed and in many instances changes due to putrefaction or animal scavengers may be so severe that the pathologist can do no more than state that there is no way of proving a separate existence. The possible procedures then include a charge of concealment of birth or, far more often, the issue of a certificate of stillbirth.

Chapter 20

Injury and Death in Infancy and Childhood

ALTHOUGH only a small proportion of deaths in infants and children are of criminal origin, many of them are obscure and may give rise to suspicion. Both lawyers and doctors may find the pathological, sociological and criminological aspects more complex than appears at first sight.

NATURAL DEATH IN CHILDHOOD

Natural death in the first 2 or 3 days of life is especially important as it is in this phase that child murder is most probable. The proportion of 'neonatal deaths'[1] which arise in the first 24 hours of life is high, varying between 30 per cent and 40 per cent largely according to the medical skills available; a further 15 per cent occur between 24 and 48 hours after delivery. Thus, approximately half of all such deaths take place within the first 2 days of life. There is a very close association with prematurity – a premature infant being defined as one with a birth weight of less than 2500 g (5¼ lb). Over 50 per cent of all stillbirths and neonatal deaths occur in premature babies and the smaller the infant, the less are its chances of survival. Only some 1 in 20 or 30 babies weighing less than 1250 g (2¾ lb) will survive for 28 days despite the fact that approximately half are born alive – generally to die within a few hours. It requires only a small increase in birth weight to improve the prospects of survival very markedly and, within the weight bracket 1500–2000 g (3⅓–4½ lb), nearly three-quarters should survive given modern medical attention.

Lack of oxygen resulting from damage to the placenta or cord is a common cause of stillbirth but the signs of hypoxia (*see* Chapter 13) are found in only some 10 per cent of neonatal deaths due to natural causes. Indeed, an autopsy indication of oxygen starvation in a mature infant should give pause for thought. However, deaths due to birth trauma make up what is probably the most important group from the medicolegal aspect because they may be difficult to distinguish from homicidal injury. These are rare in well-conducted obstetric practice and probably

---

[1] The 'neonatal' period is defined as the first 28 days of extra-uterine life.

account for less than 5 per cent of deaths which follow live birth. Prematurity plays its part here too – the brain of a small baby being particularly susceptible – but, obviously, the unusually large infant is also at risk. Although subdural haemorrhage is rare in fetal fatalities taken as a whole (it has a general incidence of about 4 per cent), it is an almost invariable finding in death due to birth injury; since this lesion also results from homicidal injury to the infant's skull, its forensic significance needs no emphasis. In the end result, the true interpretation of a fatal injury discovered in this period may depend upon the combined evidence of the obstetrician, the pathologist and the police authority.[2]

Following the immediate postnatal period, the majority of infant deaths are the result either of infection or of congenital abnormalities. The former are being rapidly eliminated as a result of improved antenatal and postnatal care; syphilis, for example, used to be a prominent cause of neonatal death but is by now virtually nonexistent. Congenital defects which may result in sudden death of the neonate are confined in practice to the cardiovascular and central nervous systems and to biochemical abnormalities which are not apparent on ordinary postmortem dissection.

Congenital abnormalities of the cardiovascular system are mainly associated with failure of the heart to establish its four chambers with normal relationships – if, for example, the interventricular septum (see p. 17) is inadequately developed, one is left with the classic 'hole in the heart' baby. Alternatively, the distinction between systemic and pulmonary circulations may not be achieved or the intra-uterine cardiac anatomy (see p. 18) may persist into extra-uterine life.

The main abnormalities of the central nervous system include anencephaly – that is, absence or partial absence of the brain – which often results in stillbirth. Otherwise, there may be obstruction to the normal flow of cerebrospinal fluid which results in hydrocephalus ('water on the brain'), or the protective skeletal covering of the spinal cord may develop inadequately which leads to herniation of the spinal cord or of its surrounding membranes – so-called 'spina bifida'.

Anatomic abnormalities of all sorts account for at least 15 per cent of neonatal deaths.

Biochemical defects may be concerned with the metabolism of carbohydrates, of proteins or of fats; when they occur in the neonate they are known as 'inborn errors of metabolism'. Some of these – for example, phenylketonuria – may cause severe and irreparable damage including

---

[2] The figures quoted for natural death are based on those kindly provided to the author by Dr J. C. H. Dunlop who analysed the records of the Simpson Memorial Maternity Pavilion, Edinburgh. They therefore represent the experience of a major obstetric unit which has ideal facilities but, at the same time, accepts many cases which are referred because of their difficulty.

injury to the brain.

Both environmental and genetic factors may play a part in the causation of congenital disease.

Environmental factors may interfere with the development of the fetus by reason of a specific insult, the end result depending greatly upon the actual time of the adverse stimulus. Basically, the more primitive the tissue at the time of attack, the more profound will be the effect; hence, infection in the mother – particularly by the rubella (or German measles) virus – or X-irradiation will have maximal effect in the first 3 months of pregnancy. By contrast, the effect of environmental factors which act upon the developed fetus as opposed to the developing embryo, will increase *pari passu* with growth; in such conditions, of which Rhesus incompatibility is perhaps the prime example, premature birth may be a positive advantage.

Congenital disease may also be genetically dictated by a familial influence – i.e. it is a hereditary disease – or it may result from abnormal division and apportioning of the sex cell chromosomes. The latter may, perhaps, be induced. The influence of irradiation on gene mutation is, at present, of undecided significance – but maternal age is probably the most important factor which determines chromosomal abnormality; mongolism, for example, is some fifteen times more common in the children of mothers aged 40 and over than in the general child-bearing population.

The inheritance of genes has been described in Chapter 18 where the concept of penetrance – that is, the ability of a gene to demonstrate itself in practice – was also discussed. A familial abnormality of low penetrance will appear clinically only if the total hereditary environment is particularly propitious. In such circumstances, the abnormality is likely to recur in subsequent pregnancies; as a statistical example, 10 per cent of families with one child suffering from spina bifida will have a recurrence.

A major modern medico-legal interest therefore centres on the application of the Abortion Act 1967, s.1(1)(b) (*see* Chapter 19). What, in effect, are the chances of accurately predicting – and preventing – the birth of a seriously handicapped child?

Pre-natal Diagnosis of Congenital Defects

Much current research is being undertaken in this field. The available methods are divisible into so-called noninvasive techniques and those which involve penetration of the fetal environment – the amniotic sac.

Of the noninvasive methods, the use of X-rays to examine the fetus is certainly contra-indicated and studies by ultrasonic scanning have not been proved to be innocuous. Estimation of the levels of α-feto protein in the serum of the mother may demonstrate severe defects of the fetal central nervous system before 20 weeks' pregnancy but, at present, the technique is at the research stage and a proportion of cases will be missed. Invasive techniques which involve the withdrawal of amniotic fluid from the fetal sac (*see Fig.* 17) are more promising. The fluid obtained can be used for:

a. direct diagnosis, by biochemical analyses, of open lesions of the fetal central nervous system – in particular, anencephaly and spina bifida;

b. culture of cells from the amniotic fluid to detect chromosomal abnormalities – which can be identified after 10–20 days in tissue culture – or to demonstrate inborn errors of metabolism which may entail culture for 6 weeks before adequate enzyme assays can be made.

All these techniques have their difficulties. Firstly, there is a 10 per cent failure rate in obtaining fluid in the early – and, therefore, useful – stage of pregnancy and this may necessitate repeated amniocentesis (puncture of the sac). Secondly, every amniocentesis carries with it the risk of miscarriage which follows the procedure in about 1 per cent of cases, and elective abortion, if proven to be advisable, must be performed rather later in pregnancy than is desirable. Thirdly, and perhaps of greatest medico-legal importance, neither positive nor negative accuracy can be guaranteed; although the diagnosis of central nervous system lesions and of chromosome abnormalities is about 95 per cent correct in skilled hands, enzymatic testing still has some way to go before achieving such accuracy.

The medico-legal problems posed include the possibility of actions for negligence in the event of an error of diagnosis and, perhaps, a subsequent action for damages on the part of a deformed fetus for an enforced inadequate life;[3] it is doubtful if any obstetric department could accept such a threatening situation and a single successful action might put a halt to a promising field of laboratory diagnosis. It is submitted that this would have a disastrous effect for the many pregnancies which might be correctly managed despite an occasional failure. It is fair to point out, however, that opposing views have been expressed largely because of the fear of extending selective abortion to a general policy of fetal destruction on eugenic grounds. Amniocentesis is a procedure which demands from the diagnostic subject a full understanding of all its hazards whether these be actual or implied. Consent of a special

---

[3] In fact, the Law Commission (*Working Paper No. 47*, 1973) have recommended that, whereas the mother might well have a case for negligence if the doctor failed to warn her of the likelihood that the child would be born disabled, the child itself should not have a right of action against the doctor because the disablement was inevitable. *See Br. Med. J.* (1973) **1**, 244, and (1974) **3**, 695.

nature is needed; a suitable form of consent is reproduced at Appendix L.

Good sense must also protect the genetic counsellor, who, with or without the benefit of amniocentesis, can only advise as to the wisdom of childbearing on the basis of probabilities. Any likelihood of success-ful litigation following incorrect advice to continue with a pregnancy would make the counsellor's position intolerable.

Sudden Death in Infancy
Many studies indicate that the number of 'cot deaths' is decreasing. This trend may be more apparent than real as much depends on definition and on available diagnostic resources. This particular type of sudden natural death still poses a baffling problem to the forensic pathologist. Briefly, the condition presents as an apparently healthy child being put to bed by unsuspecting parents and being found dead either at the next feed or at normal waking time. The process may be extremely rapid; in a case examined by the author, an apparently healthy infant was placed in its carrycot on the back seat of a car – it was found to be dead at the end of a 40-minute journey.

Cases may occur between the ages of 2 weeks and 2 years – the main incidence being at 3–4 months. They are reported all over the world but always have a marked seasonal association, the great majority of deaths being in the colder months. There is a rather indefinite association with the lower socio-economic groups but no type of family is immune. Esti-mates of the total number of deaths must, by the nature of the con-dition, be very inaccurate but have been put as high as 25 000 per year in the United States and 3000 per year in England and Wales.

The search for a 'cause' of cot deaths has been world-wide and inten-sive, yet no satisfactory answer has been reached. Many explanations – ranging from trace metal deficiency to allergy to cow's milk – have been proposed but no theory stands up to critical analysis. Much attention is currently being paid to 'sleep apnoea' – a periodic failure to breathe during sleep which occurs in adults and may be exaggerated in infancy – but such a physiological death cannot be proved by normal autopsy techniques. Acute viral infections have been suspected and viruses may, indeed, be isolated from the lungs; the problem of whether the organ-isms are causative of death or are present in a purely incidental role remains. The difficulty of interpretation lies in the merciful shortage of control cases – that is, infants of a similar age killed accidentally – which can be examined in parallel. It is possible that there is no common cause but rather a common presentation of a number of abnormal states which provide no anatomical evidence of their origin.[4]

[4] A most valuable exposition of the various aspects of 'cot-death' is to be found in Robinson R. R. (ed.) (1974) *SIDS, 1974*, Toronto, Canadian Foundation for the Study of Infant Deaths.

The fact remains that 'cot deaths' certainly occur and their medico-legal significance is twofold. Firstly, they are natural deaths for which no blame can be attached; this is of great importance to the subsequent medico-legal investigation which should be so designed as to cause minimum distress to parents who are already distraught. It is a mark of humane progress that the autopsy diagnosis of 'Suddẹn Infant Death Syndrome' is now accepted throughout the United Kingdom and the need for public inquests in England and Wales has been virtually eliminated. The second point of importance is the reverse of this – that post-mortem dissection is essential in every case to eliminate the possibility of unlawful killing. It is frequently stated that natural death nearly always occurs in the early hours of the morning and that cot deaths occurring at other times should arouse suspicion, if not of homicide, then of a demonstrable, specific pathological condition. In point of fact, this is not the author's personal experience but, nevertheless, it is significant that 4 of the first 74 'cot deaths' admitted to the current Edinburgh study of the condition were found to be unnatural in origin. This fact cannot, of course, be taken as providing an 'incidence' but it does underline the need for full medical investigation of all unexplained deaths.[5]

ACCIDENTAL DEATH IN CHILDHOOD

Many forms of accidental death which are likely to occur in childhood are discussed in specific terms under the various headings in this book. These deaths do, however, form a special group, firstly, because there is a volume of legislation aimed at protection of the very young and, as a consequence, an offence may have been committed despite the undisputed fact that death was accidental while, secondly, the most common defence against a charge of infanticide, child murder or homicide of a young person is to suggest that the fatal injury resulted from an accident – the pathological distinction is of major importance and may be very difficult to make.

Many accidental deaths in this age group are asphyxial in nature and, of these, death from burning is comparatively common. Infants and children may be left unattended and be killed as a fire engulfs a whole house or hotel. More commonly, children accidentally pour boiling liquids from the stove on to themselves as a result of curiosity or they are exposed to an unguarded fire from which their clothes are accidentally lit. It is an offence for any person over the age of 16 having charge of a

---

[5] Without wishing to complicate the situation unduly, the possibility must be included of true cot deaths occurring in infants who have been *accidentally* injured during life – the Edinburgh series of cases contains one such instance.

person under the age of 12 (or 7 in Scotland) to allow the child to be burned or scalded by reason of being in a room containing an open fire grate or any heating appliance insufficiently protected to guard against the risk of the child being injured.[6]

The same Acts[7] also refer to the relationship of acute alcoholism and suffocation by overlaying in bed, criminal charges being possible if a child under 3 years old has been overlaid by a person aged more than 16 years who was under the influence of drink; even in the absence of drunkenness, true accidental overlaying may occur, particularly in the appalling housing conditions which still persist in many major cities. Asphyxial deaths in sleeping accommodation – be it crib, pram, cot or parents' bed – pose special problems. At one time, many 'cot deaths' were ascribed to asphyxia resulting from suffocation in bedding and the like. Such views have become markedly less common due to the intensive study given to the condition, to the desire to spare the parents' feelings of guilt and to real doubt as to whether such a condition can occur; the subject has been discussed in Chapter 13. It need only be reiterated here that accidental asphyxia in infancy must be accepted as a cause of death with caution; it may be difficult, if not impossible, to distinguish pathologically between a baby which has been accidentally trapped face down on its pillow and one which has been held in that position in such a way as to leave no mark on the back of the head or body; cot deaths themselves pose the same basic problem. Similar difficulties surround the occasional case in which an infant is strangled by its restraining harness; only rarely can the pathologist do other than describe the cause of death leaving the circumstantial evidence to indicate the way in which it arose.

Accidental drowning in children may, of course, occur amongst the older age group while at play. Drowning in infancy happens not uncommonly in the bath and, when accidental, death is often due to vagal inhibition of the heart – the baby slips backwards and water contacts the nasopharynx and larynx; as in adults, the finding of the conventional signs of drowning following death in the bath should arouse suspicion.

Asphyxia of central nervous system origin is usually a result of drug overdosage and is a tragically common cause of accidental death in young children. The subject is discussed in greater detail in Chapter 22.

Death due to accidental injury may cause very great forensic difficulties when occurring in infancy and early childhood. Infant deaths due to road traffic accidents are relatively rare due mainly, one suspects, to the improbability of drivers being drunk when transporting the baby.

---

[6] Children and Young Persons (Amendment) Act 1952, s.8; Children and Young Persons (Scotland) Act 1937, s. 22. Should death or serious injury result, the penalty on summary conviction is a fine not exceeding £10!

[7] Section 1(2)(b) of the 1933 English and s. 12(2)(b) of the Scottish Acts.

In older infancy and early childhood, automobile tragedies occur through inadvertent opening of car doors; child safety locks provide problems of their own, particularly in relation to rescue from a post-crash fire, and the importance of adequate harness restraint for children in the rear of cars deserves greater appreciation. Death due to cervical spinal fracture is also common in children subjected to quite minor deceleration trauma while standing unrestrained in vehicles. The frequency of pedestrian deaths in childhood needs no emphasis; they are doubly distressing in their emotional effects not only on the bereaved parents but also on the driver who, especially where this age group is concerned, may well have been blameless. Children may fall down the stairs or out of windows; again, the distinction between accident and homicide must depend very largely on the circumstantial evidence.

Perhaps the most difficult diagnostic area in infant death concerns the isolated head injury.

Such injuries are often explained as 'the baby slipped off my shoulder while I tried to turn on the light', or 'I fell down the stairs with the baby in my arms'. There is no doubt that such accidents do occur and it may be impossible to distinguish the resultant injuries from those caused by deliberate dropping of the baby from comparable positions purely through the pathological findings. Commonly, however, false explanations of this type are used to cloak deliberate injury of a different type – homicidal head injuries in infancy are frequently caused by direct manual violence or by swinging the child by the feet against a wall or other solid object. Certain features may help to distinguish these injuries in the post-mortem dissection. Firstly, there is the degree of injury which may be greatly in excess of that likely from the given explanation. Secondly, the position and external appearances of the injury may give rise to suspicion. Thus, a blow from the hand may leave no external mark and the resulting deep bruising and fracture may be markedly localized to one side of the head whereas injuries due to a fall, which are uncomplicated by bruising of the shoulder or arm, are far more likely to be vertical in presentation. The most important cause for suspicion is the unexpected finding of a head injury in a death purported to be natural – the great majority of genuine accidental injuries will be reported immediately to the doctor.

DELIBERATE INJURY IN INFANCY AND CHILDHOOD

There remains for discussion one important condition which is far more common than is generally suspected and is becoming more prevalent[8] –

---

[8] Some 2 per cent of infant deaths between the ages of 4 weeks and 1 year are due to premeditated violence (*Memorandum of the Standing Medical Advisory Committee for the Central Health Service Council* (1970). London, DHSS).

that is, the 'battered baby syndrome' which should, less emotionally, be referred to as 'repetitive nonaccidental injury in childhood'. The term 'battered child' was chosen deliberately for its impact by Kempe to whom must be given the major credit for bringing the subject to public notice.[9]

Nonaccidental Injury in Childhood

From approximately 1945, a syndrome describing head injury and multiple limb fractures in children[10] was regarded as a clinical entity; only in the mid-1950s was it realized that these children were suffering from repeated injury inflicted by those responsible for their care – almost invariably including one or both parents. Children frequently come to autopsy as a result of such treatment but the main bulk of sufferers present as clinical and sociological problems; one of the most disturbing features is that violence breeds violence – a high proportion of those who deliberately injure their children were themselves the objects of similar assault. Some 4500 children are 'battered' each year in Great Britain; between 10 per cent and 17 per cent of these will die, while 30 per cent will become permanently handicapped from brain damage.[11]

The clinicosocial expression of the condition is difficult to summarize but, in general, the following may be found:

a. the family is often inadequate, maladjusted, immature and under social stress.

b. the child is usually aged less than 4 years and about half the cases, both fatal and non-fatal, are reported in the first year of life.

c. there is frequently a delay in, or failure of, reporting the injuries to the medical practitioner and a false explanation of their cause is then given.

d. the commonest injuries are bruises and fractures, the latter being predominantly of the chest cage (especially the back), long bones and skull. Burns and bite marks are sometimes seen and severe injury to the abdominal viscera may occasionally be present. Injuries to the inside of the lips or the gums and dislocation of the teeth are almost diagnostic. Bizarre variations include deliberate poisoning or immersion. The child nearly always

---

[9] See the original paper: Kempe C. H. et al. (1962) The battered child syndrome. J. Am. Med. Assoc. **181,** 17. A major collection of modern monographs on the subject is contained in Franklin A. W. (ed.) (1975) Concerning Child Abuse, Edinburgh, Churchill Livingstone.

[10] Caffey J. (1946) Multiple fractures in the long bones of infants suffering from chronic subdural hematoma. Am. J. Roentgenol. **56,** 163.

[11] A guide to management of non-accidental injury in children. Prepared by a Working Party in the Department of Child Health, University of Newcastle-upon-Tyne. Br. Med. J. (1973) **4,** 657.

shows evidence of emotional and, sometimes physical deprivation (*Plate* 16).
  e. Perhaps the most important diagnostic feature is that the injuries
  have been caused at different times.

These clinical signs will be mirrored in fatal cases at post-mortem dissection, which must include a full X-ray study as a routine – the plates
are invaluable not only as evidence of injury and its dating but also in
assessing the possibility of bone disease as a causative or contributory
factor. The examination should also include a microscopic study of the
wounds in an attempt to establish their various ages. Death is frequently
due to some terminal excessive injury resulting in cerebral or abdominal
haemorrhage; a more difficult situation arises when it is effectively due
to a combination of malnutrition and neglect which may be wilful or
due merely to intellectual inadequacy.

Nonaccidental childhood injury raises some questions of medical
confidentiality. Ultimate responsibility for the safety of children lies
with the local Director of Social Services – but doctors are likely to see
the injured baby first and the medical profession cannot abnegate its ob-
ligations for eliminating a condition which, in mortality and morbidity
alone, is a serious problem for society. Since the doctor's responsibility
is to the patient, who is, in this case, the child, there can be no ethical
contra-indication to reporting the case but such reports should be made
in the first instance to the Department of Social Services (or the children's department of the Area Health Services) – who have a clear 'right
to know' – rather than to the police. An alternative might be to arrange
for admission to a paediatric hospital with the express purpose of protecting the patient;[12] the wide consultation which is regarded as of such
importance in the management of the children[13] can probably be best
arranged from such a unit.[14]

There are other practical problems in relation to repetitive nonaccidental childhood injury which lie in the sphere of criminology. The predisposing conditions must be dealt with correctly and, in fatal cases, the
pathological examination has its role to play in fully defining the nature
and the sequence of the injuries discovered. This may affect the outcome
of any criminal trial. A murderous attack on a child can seldom be
excused on medical grounds; by contrast, the establishment of a true
'battered baby syndrome', which is widely accepted as the outcome of a
psychosocial disorder, may rightly result in conviction for culpable

---

[12] Tunbridge Wells Study Group on nonaccidental injury to children. (1973) *Br. Med. J.*
4, 96.

[13] *Report of the Committee of Inquiry into the Care and Supervision provided in relation to
Maria Colwell* (1974). London, HMSO.

[14] *See also* Arthur L. J. H. et al. (1976) Nonaccidental injury in children: What we do in
Derby, *Br. Med. J.* **1**, 1363, for an account of the team approach.

homicide or manslaughter rather than murder and be followed by equally enlightened sentencing. The view is gaining ground that rehabilitation of the family is more important to society than is its punishment and that battering parents need help rather than condemnation.[15] This may, however, be too great a simplification. There would seem to be two essentially different groups involved. On the one hand, there are those unstable parents who, in a perpetual state of exasperated inability to cope with family life, resort to violence as the only apparent escape from such pressures; these persons are surely to be treated as social invalids. On the other hand, parents who subject their children to deliberate torture by seating them on electric fires, burning them with cigarettes and the like cannot be deserving of public sympathy. The pathologist makes a further contribution to criminology in distinguishing between these two types of injury.

Deliberate injury to children is a social evil which cannot be solved by unilateral action – be it on the part of the medical profession, the social workers or the police. It is a problem which emphasizes particularly well the interdependence of forensic and community services in the protection of the individual.

[15] Deliberate injury to children. (1973) *Br. Med. J.* **3**, 61.

Chapter 21

Sexual Offences

EXPERT medical evidence will be called in relation to a number of offences associated with sexual activity, among which the following will be discussed in some detail:

a. Rape.
b. Inflicting clandestine injury on a woman.
c. Indecent assault.
d. Lewd, indecent or libidinous practices.
e. Indecency with children.
f. Homosexual offences.
g. Incest.

The extent and value of such evidence will vary according to the charges laid.

THE LAW

The majority of sexual offences are defined in England and Wales by the Sexual Offences Acts 1956 to 1976. There is a slight medico-legal interest in the Indecency with Children Act 1960. Homosexual practices conducted between consenting adults in privacy are no longer regarded as criminal by virtue of the Sexual Offences Act 1967. Exceptionally, charges of assault with intent to commit rape could still be brought under the Offences Against the Person Act 1861, s. 38.

In Scotland, the more serious sexual offences are dealt with at common law. Otherwise, the earlier enactments of the Criminal Law Amendment Acts 1885 to 1928 are consolidated in the Sexual Offences (Scotland) Act 1976.

AGE AND CONSENT IN SEXUAL OFFENCES

Largely as a result of the recommendations of the Heilbron Committee,[1] rape has been redefined in England and Wales. A man commits

---

[1] *Report of the Advisory Group on the Law of Rape* (1975). Cmnd. 6352. London, HMSO.

rape if he has unlawful sexual intercourse with a woman who at the time of the intercourse does not consent to it and, at the time, he knows that she does not consent to the intercourse or he is reckless as to whether she consents (Sexual Offences (Amendment) Act 1976, s. 1). In Scotland, rape is a crime at common law defined as 'the carnal knowledge of a female by a male person obtained by overcoming her will'.[2] It follows that, so long as there is no consent, the age of the victim is immaterial to a charge of rape; age, however, becomes important in the event of apparent consent by a young person.

Irrespective of consent, intercourse with a girl under the age of 16 is unlawful. In England and Wales, there is no defence on the basis of mistaking the victim's age in the case of a girl under the age of 13.[3] In Scotland, the Sexual Offences (Scotland) Act, s. 3, specifies the offences of having or attempting to have intercourse with a girl under the age of 13 (the comparable common law age for constructive rape is 12 years); while the question of error as to age might be raised as a defence in common law, there is, again, no such possibility when charges are brought under the Act.

The age of the victim between 13 and 16 years is significant under both jurisdictions. In England, having or attempting to have intercourse with a girl above the age of 13 and under 16 years constitutes the offence of having or attempting to have unlawful sexual intercourse, rather than rape. Section 4 of the 1976 Act defines a similar offence in Scotland. Under both codes it is a defence for a man under the age of 24, who has not been previously charged with a like offence, to claim he had reasonable cause to believe that the girl was aged 16 or over.[4]

In England, a boy aged less than 14 years is presumed incapable of committing rape and this presumption is irrebuttable; such a boy could, however, be convicted of indecent assault. No such presumption exists in Scots law.

Irrespective of age, consent to sexual intercourse is considered impossible in the case of a mental defective as defined by the Mental Health Act 1959 or the Mental Health (Scotland) Act 1960. The situation is similar to that of a normal girl below the age of 16. It is a defence that the accused did not know or could not reasonably suspect that a girl was a defective and any consent given, although invalid in law, would

---

[2] The authority for Scots law quoted in this chapter is almost entirely from Gordon G. H. (1967) *The Criminal Law of Scotland*, Edinburgh, W. Green & Sons.

[3] Sexual Offences Act 1956, s. 5.

[4] In the event of a man 'marrying' a girl below the age of 16, it is a defence throughout Great Britain, irrespective of the man's age or of the number of convictions, that he had reasonable cause to suppose his wife was over 16 years old at the time of marriage (Age of Marriage Act 1929; Marriage Act 1949; Sexual Offences (Scotland) Act 1976). A similar exception is made in connection with the offence of indecent assault.

certainly mitigate the offence. The situation in Scotland would be covered by the 1960 Act, s. 96 which defines the offence of having intercourse with a defective – a clear indication that such an action need not necessarily amount to rape. The subtle distinction between mental defect and mental illness in this context is unlikely to have any effect on the outcome of a charge.

Age and consent are relevant also in the offence of indecent assault – an offence which falls short of rape generally because of absence of penetration of the vulva, although this may not necessarily be the reason (*see H.M.Adv. v. Logan, below*). Under the 1956 Act it is an offence in England and Wales to commit an indecent assault on a man or woman.[5] Children under 16 cannot give legal consent and, therefore, indecent assault on them must always be an offence; there is specific statutory support for this generalization.[6] The potential defence of error as to age by a young man is not available against a charge of indecent assault, unless it should arise in association with 'marriage'.

An actual assault is necessary to establish a charge of indecent assault and, to cover those cases in which no assault was alleged, the Indecency with Children Act 1960 was applied to England and Wales; under the Act, it is an offence for a person to commit an act of gross indecency with or towards a child under the age of 14. In Scotland, these cases are loosely referred to as 'lewd and libidinous practices' which are an offence at common law when associated with children below the age of puberty (12 years in relation to girls). Between the ages of 12 and 16, the offence is defined in the Sexual Offences (Scotland) Act 1976, s. 5; consent is no defence nor is error as to age.

Age is important in relation to homosexual offences under the Sexual Offences Act 1967, in which an adult is defined as any person more than 21 years of age. A boy aged less than 14 cannot be charged with buggery though he can be charged with indecent assault. The 1967 Act does not apply in Scotland where the more serious homosexual offences are dealt with at common law; in theory, though probably not in practice, there is no limitation as to age. Gross indecency between males is covered by Section 7 of the Sexual Offences (Scotland) Act 1976; a consenting child cannot be held guilty of such an offence.

MEDICAL EVIDENCE IN ALLEGED RAPE

The medical evidence to be obtained in a case of alleged rape can be directed to answering the questions implied in the wording of the definitions – was there sexual intercourse, was there lack of consent and, if so, what was done by the man to overcome the woman's will? The evidence

[5] As compared with rape which can only be perpetrated by a man on a woman.
[6] Sexual Offences Act 1956, s. 14; Sexual Offences (Scotland) Act 1976, s. 5.

may be derived from a medical examination both of the victim and of the accused.

Unlawful Sexual Intercourse

Unlawfulness in relation to age and mental state has been discussed above. After the age of legal consent, unlawful sexual intercourse is generally defined as intercourse out of wedlock and, from this, it has been extrapolated that a man cannot be charged with the rape of his wife unless there is a legal separation order in force.[7] The archaic nature of such a presumption and its consequent dubiety is beautifully argued by Gordon with particular respect to Scotland.[8] If there is such a thing as 'irrevocable privilege' for a husband, it is anomalous to suggest that he could be charged with assault in circumstances which, outside marriage, would constitute rape, yet there is no doubt that such a charge would be valid in England.[9] Medical evidence of sexual offence might, therefore, be called even within the confines of marriage.

Sexual intercourse is defined as intercourse intended to be within the vagina; by an extraordinary process of reasoning, a man cannot rape a woman in a deviate fashion. The medical examiner may well have little difficulty in saying positively that sexual intercourse has taken place when a previously virginal hymen has been recently penetrated, particularly if this has been accompanied by some force. The external genitalia are often bruised or swollen and obvious lacerations of the hymen, together with bleeding, may well be present, the main problem being to differentiate the latter from menstrual efflux. Difficulties arise when such typical signs are lacking. The absence of lacerations may be due to failure to achieve the intention but do not necessarily exclude penetration even when previous intercourse can be discounted; the hymen may be naturally lax and sufficiently patent to admit a male organ or it may have been rendered so by the use of tampons or by masturbation. The certain sign of penetration is the finding of spermatozoa in the deeper portion of the vagina. It has been stated that recognizable spermatozoa can be found 3 days or more after intercourse and that morphologically perfect specimens with tails are present up to 16 hours after deposition.[10] In the author's experience, such survival is the exception rather than the rule; while being abundant at 2 hours, perfect forms are

[7] R. v. Clarke (1949) 33 Cr. App. R. 216.

[8] *The Criminal Law of Scotland* (1967), p. 830, quoting, in particular, Willis J. in R. v. Clarence [1888] 22 Q.B.D. 23, 33.

[9] R. v. Miller [1954] 2 Q.B. 282.

[10] David A. and Wilson E. (1974) The persistence of seminal constituents in the human vagina. *Forensic Sci.* **3,** 45. It is, perhaps, worth noting that these figures were obtained from studies following normal intramarital intercourse; see the very different results, in keeping with the author's, reported by Sharpe N. (1963) The significance of spermatozoa in victims of sexual offences, *Can. Med. Assoc. J.* **89,** 513.

rare at 12 hours, the usual finding at that time being of 'scanty bodies indistinguishable from degenerating spermatozoal heads'. In any event, the taking of adequate swabs from within the vagina is an essential step in the examination of the suspected victim, certainly within 24 hours of the alleged offence. It is the positive finding which is of evidential value; a failure to identify spermatozoa is of little consequence as, in law, emission is not essential to sexual intercourse.

The difficulties facing the medical examiner have not yet been exhausted. Full penetration is not required to constitute rape, sexual intercourse being held to mean 'a degree of penetration of the vulva by the penis'; quite clearly, the doctor cannot, and should not be expected to, provide positive evidence on this point on the basis of a simple physical examination. Again, however, a search for spermatozoa may be of very great value; superficial swabs should be taken from the area between the labia in addition to those taken deeply as a positive finding in them would, save in exceptional circumstances, be very good evidence of intercourse within the legal definition.

The examination of the suspect for evidence of sexual intercourse is generally unrewarding. The glans is very seldom found to be injured beyond what might be anticipated following legal sexual intercourse. Attempts to identify the woman's secretor substance on the male penis – somewhat after the fashion in the examination of bite marks (see Chapter 29) – would theoretically be useful, particularly in cases involving multiple potential assailants, but have proved disappointing in the author's experience. Others have suggested a search for cells from the vaginal epithelium, which have fairly individual staining properties, but the time during which they will be recognizable must be limited. During the process of the examination evidence of venereal disease may come to light and, in the event that the victim subsequently develops a similar disease, this might be useful supporting evidence. The alternative proposition, though less probable, might also hold good, the former state of chastity of the victim being no bar to a charge of rape.

The Use of Force or Fear
Lack of consent is essential to the ordinary case of rape and evidence of the use of force is strong, though not essential, corroboration of such a state – perhaps it is of particular relevance in relation to Scots law.

The ultimate evidence of force is the death of the victim.[11] A careful pathological assessment of the mode of dying is then essential both to the prosecution and to the defence. However, the remainder of this section will be confined to uncomplicated rape.

[11] In England, the Homicide Act 1957, s. 1, abolished the concept of 'constructive malice' whereby the victim's death as part of the process of rape would have amounted to murder. In Scotland, death during rape would be murder only if the cause of death was unrelated to the act of rape (see The Criminal Law of Scotland, p. 691).

It is commonly stated that the victim's resistance must be 'to the utmost'. In practice, this absolute term must be interpreted in a relative fashion; the important feature is lack of consent or unwillingness to take part throughout the act (*Plate* 17). The medical examiner is often in great difficulty on this point, it being surprising how little tangible evidence of force or resistance may be found either in the victim or in the assailant – particularly if several men have been involved. The author has seen a case in which the vulval damage to the girl was such that an urgent hospital appointment was arranged, yet the most which could be discovered in the accused was a small abrasion over one eye. In another instance, two young men were convicted of rape; no injuries were found in either and those in the victim could only be described as 'no more than could be anticipated as a result of aggressive lovemaking'.

Many potential injuries in the victim are prevented by the interposition of clothing, and examination of the clothes is an essential part of the complete medical inspection. All doctors will be aware of the possibility of artefacts induced by the accuser herself but real difficulty occurs surprisingly seldom. An association with blood or seminal stains is evidence of genuineness but it is particularly important to examine with care the precise relationship between stains and tears as these may demonstrate anomalies as to timing; the scientific investigation of clothing is a matter for the laboratory but the doctor must be allowed to make his own assessment at the time of examination.

Injury to the accused may be minimal for the same reason. There may be a gross disparity in size between victim and rapist and, as indicated above, less injury will be anticipated if there is more than one assailant (*Plate* 18). An element of subjectivity is almost inescapable and the medical evidence as to a struggle seldom carries more weight than does that derived from the circumstances.

Resistance to rape may be modified by fear, say, of reprisals against a third party, and there can be little or no medical evidence to be drawn on this score – other than a dubious inference from the lack of injury. There seems to be some difference in the English and Scots law on this point. In the former jurisdiction, a charge of rape would still stand under this type of duress. Scots law would, however, require threats of immediate harm rather than of future action; the Sexual Offences (Scotland) Act 1976, s. 2(1) prescribes a specific offence of procuring or attempting to procure by threats a woman to have unlawful sexual intercourse. Medical evidence might, however, be sought in the event that the will of the female is said to have been overcome by drugs – of which alcohol must be by far the commonest. In practice, the medical examiner would be unlikely to be able to do more than take the necessary samples for laboratory analyses. The law is, again, of interest and importance. It is an offence under the Sexual Offences Act 1956, s. 4, 'to administer any drug, matter or thing to a woman with intent to stupify or overpower so as thereby to enable any person to have unlawful sexual intercourse with her'; there is a similar provision in the Sexual Offences (Scotland) Act 1976, s. 2(1)(c). It is accepted under common law in Scotland that rape itself can be committed by drugging a woman so that she becomes incapable of resisting the accused – drugging, in that it constitutes a means of overcoming the will of the victim is, in effect, a loose form of force. Only alcohol can have any real relevance and the important points would seem to be, firstly, that the woman must be plied with drink *in order* to overcome her resistance – the mere process of 'softening up' by excessive social drinking would be insufficient to substantiate a charge of rape[12] – and, secondly, that the woman must be deprived of the ability to consent or refuse consent to intercourse.

It is not rape in Scotland to have intercourse with a woman who is insensible through alcoholism of her own making or who is asleep[13] – if such a thing be possible. The reason given is that since the helplessly intoxicated woman is incapable of consenting or refusing consent, there can be no rape because rape involves intercourse against the woman's will.[14] Such cases provide examples of the Scottish offence of inflicting clandestine injury to a woman; they would probably constitute rape in England due to the absence of positive consent, the alternative of indecent assault being precluded by the act of intercourse. Medical evidence would certainly be called but since there was, by definition, no resistance and previous virginity would be unlikely, the evidence would probably be limited in practice to the demonstration of spermatozoa in the vagina.

Intercourse by Fraud
Examples of rape by fraud include impersonation of the woman's husband, an offence defined as rape in both the Sexual Offences Act 1956, s. 1(2) and in the Sexual Offences (Scotland) Act 1976, s. 2(2). Obtaining intercourse by pretending to be giving medical treatment has been regarded as rape in England[15] but would probably be regarded as only fraud in Scotland. Again, the medical evidence would be likely to be limited to demonstration of emission in such cases.

Scientific Evidence of a Medical Nature in Rape
During the medical examination, the doctor will seek and retain certain specimens for laboratory study and analyses; these may be of nonhuman or of human biological nature.

[12] H.M.Adv. v. Logan 1936 J.C. 100.

[13] H.M.Adv. v. Sweenie (1858) 3 Irv. 109.

[14] H.M.Adv. v. Grainger and Rae 1932 J.C. 40. The author regards this as something of a circular argument.

[15] R. v. Flattery [1877] 2 Q.B.D. 410.

The former need not be dealt with here as they will lie in the province of the forensic science laboratory – obvious examples would be the retention of any loose fibres, grass or seeds about the person or clothing which might provide rebutting or corroborative evidence of circumstantial detail.

Although the biological specimens will probably be examined in a science laboratory, the interpretation of results may well fall to the medical witness. Those which may most often be of value include:

a. Blood stains and seminal stains from the clothing of both male and female. Seminal stains can be grouped on the ABO system in secretors while blood may well be fresh enough to demonstrate additional group antigens, 'serum groups' and specific enzyme systems. For these investigations to be of maximal value, blood samples must also be obtained from the female and from a suspect when this is possible. If the bloods are of different groups, the distribution of the stains between the couple may be of evidential value. The use of the precise antigenic groups of both blood and semen to exclude or incriminate a suspect follows the pattern indicated in the section on paternity testing (*see* Chapter 18). Apparent seminal stains will also be examined for the presence of spermatozoa which may remain recognisable for long periods – up to six months – on fabric; admixture with other body fluids may, however, result in their early disappearance.

b. Pubic hair combings from both victim and accused. The presence of foreign hair will at least show proximity. Hair known to be from the two principals – i.e. obtained by plucking – should also be available for comparison.

c. Nail scrapings. To be examined for blood or tissue from the other party.

d. Any potential bite marks should be examined for the presence of saliva as described in Chapter 29. The use of similar preparations from the glans penis has been discussed above.

The nature of consent on the part of the person being examined is important (*see also* Chapter 30). All current textbooks of Forensic Medicine are categoric that an examination without consent is a potential assault and of, at least, doubtful evidential value. In cases of rape, there is little difficulty as to the woman because she will generally appreciate that an examination is an essential adjunct to her accusation; even so, it is well that the doctor should specifically warn the girl of the intimate nature of the examination as this may, albeit surprisingly, not be understood, particularly when the prime complainants are the girl's parents. It is also important to emphasize that there is no confidentiality as regards the findings. The problem is more complex in the case of the suspect, to whom the advantage of examination may be in doubt. Simpson[16] states, 'the voluntary nature [of the examination] must be made clear before commencing'. Glaister,[17] who must be regarded as the Scottish authority, advises that 'it is not sufficient that the person to be examined offers no resistance or objection, for that may result solely from ignorance of his or her rights. The proper procedure is to inform the accused, in the presence of a third party, that the examiner has been asked by the authorities to make an examination, but that he can only do so after obtaining consent, which can be withheld, and that he will report the results of his examination whatever they may be'. No one would deny that the taking of blood or even the removal of pubic hair requires consent as the person examined sustains injury in the process – this principle will apply equally to the female. But a medical examination involves no injury and increasing regard is being given to the interests both of the victim and of the public – particularly in relation to evidence which may be ephemeral. This is especially so in Scotland where it is extremely probable that an examination undertaken without consent but on the authority of a Sheriff's warrant would be regarded as a fair procedure.[18] The amount of force which might properly be used in making an examination under warrant is, however, still in dispute. The proper course would seem to be for the doctor to insure himself against a charge of unethical practice by requesting the Crown to seek a warrant on his behalf and to obtain the advice of the Procurator Fiscal on any subsequent points of difficulty; it would then be for the Court to decide on the admissibility of the evidence.

Charges against Practitioners
Charges of rape, of attempted rape or, more commonly, of indecent assault are not infrequently made against doctors and dentists in the course of their practice. The more serious charges almost invariably result from delusions, possibly wishful, arising under anaesthesia; dentists are, therefore, particularly at risk when they operate and anaesthetize single-handed while the practice of 'horizontal dentistry' is psychologically predisposing to sexual fantasy on the part of the patient. The general medical examination would go far to exclude the possibility of rape but, in the event of deliberate premeditated fabrication, the 'patient' would be likely to inflict damage on her clothing and person. An interesting situation could arise in the event of the charges being substantially true. It would clearly be rape to give a woman an anaes-

[16] In *Forensic Medicine*, 7th ed., p. 196.
[17] In *Medical Jurisprudence and Toxicology*, 13th ed., p. 56.
[18] *See* H.M.Adv. v. Hay, discussed in Chapter 29, and H.M.Adv. v. Milford 1973 S.L.T. 12.

thetic in order to have intercourse; on the other hand, Gordon[19] suggests that it is not rape to drug a woman for a lawful purpose, such as to give an anaesthetic for an operation, and afterwards to have sexual intercourse – *Grainger and Rae* would presumably apply.

The doctor is particularly open to charges of indecent assault – some of which arise from a genuine misunderstanding of the nature of an intended examination. It was once a truism that a doctor should not allow himself to be isolated with a female patient; such are the present economic conditions, however, that the counsel of chaperoning at all times cannot always be followed. It would, however, be foolhardy for a doctor to undertake an examination of the genitalia or even of the breasts in the absence of a female witness.

Medical Evidence in Attempted Rape or Indecent Assault

The examination of a victim of assault with attempt to commit rape would follow the lines of investigation of any case of assault. Medical evidence would be called to assess the severity of the assault and this might derive from an examination of both parties.

Indecent assault, which is not a specific offence in Scotland, may be perpetrated homosexually or heterosexually by either sex; it is unlikely to be accompanied by great violence and medical evidence becomes of decreasing value as the element of assault diminishes. The least traumatic offence is the commission of lewd or libidinous practice for which no physical contact is required. It may well be that the medical examination which is often required in such cases does more psychological harm to the very young girls who are involved than does the occurrence itself; the offence is limited to practices against girls under 16[20] and boys under 14 years,[21] the only alternative in the case of offended adults being a charge of what is loosely known as 'indecent exposure'.

INCEST

Incestuous relationships differ in England and Scotland. In England, the Sexual Offences Act 1956 makes it an offence for a man to have intercourse with his mother, sister, daughter, grand-daughter or half-sister; there may, of course, be further charges if the female is aged below 16 years. Similar relationships with the sexes reversed are also forbidden but a girl must be over 16 years old to be guilty of incest. Scots law is based on the Incest Act 1567, this being the only relevant statute not repealed in the 1976 Act; the Act is based on Biblical Law.[22] Thus, in

---

[19] p. 828.

[20] Sexual Offences (Scotland) Act 1976, s. 5.

[21] The common law age of puberty.

[22] Lev. 18:6–18. But the express prohibitions therein are regarded as examples of degrees

Scotland, relationships between uncle and niece are also incestuous and, where the relationship is of direct descent, the prohibition does not stop at grandparent level. Half-blood relationships are treated in Scotland in the same way as full relationships. Biblical prohibitions based on affinity have been greatly modified by statute law (Criminal Procedure (Scotland) Act 1938; Marriage Enabling Act 1960) so that, now, incest by affinity relates only to parents and children-in-law and step-parents and step-children. Marriages with adopted children are forbidden in both England and Scotland but extramarital sexual relationships are not incestuous.[23] There is an interesting difference in the two jurisdictions in that, whereas English law specifically includes relationships not traced through lawful wedlock there can, in general, be no incest between bastard relations in Scotland – though common law would probably regard mother/bastard son and father/bastard daughter sexual relationships as criminal.

The conditions for proof of incest are the same as those for rape – there must be penetration but this need only be vulval. Medical and medico-scientific evidence in incest is largely confined to establishing the fact of intercourse in the female and either not excluding or excluding the suspect male. Cases seldom come to light immediately and it may well be that pregnancy provides the evidence of intercourse. In addition, the relationships might be tested as described in Chapter 18. Both parties are equally guilty of the crime but, in practice, the female is very rarely prosecuted. Deviate intercourse cannot be incest.

HOMOSEXUAL OFFENCES

Homosexual relationships between consenting women do not constitute an offence.

In England, sodomy is a form of buggery and consists of connection per anum with any other person; the term is slightly more restrictive in Scotland and refers to unnatural carnal connection between men.

Buggery is an offence in England under the Sexual Offences Act 1956, s. 12, but the Sexual Offences Act 1967, s. 1, provides that it is not so when performed in private by consenting parties who have both attained the age of 21. Merchant seamen and members of the armed forces have no such licence. Sodomy in Scotland is regarded with greater severity. It is a separate common law crime; gross indecency between males, irrespective of whether penetration has taken place, is proscribed in the Sexual Offences (Scotland) Act 1976, s. 7. The permissive clause of the English Act of 1967 has no application in Scotland; nevertheless,

of forbidden relationship – the Law of Scotland is, therefore, more strict as regards incest than is the Old Testament.

[23] H.M.Adv. v. R.M. 1969 J.C. 52.

the Lord Advocate has directed that no prosecutions are to be taken up in Scotland for gross indecency in private.

Proof of penetration of the anus is needed to establish unnatural carnal connection but proof of emission is not required. As in rape, therefore, the examining doctor may be in great difficulty in the event of incomplete penetration but, in practice, serious resistance by the passive partner is unlikely to occur – full distention of the anus is probable. The signs likely to be discovered depend, therefore, on the habituation of the passive partner. In the case of a first offender, tenderness, oedema and, perhaps, laceration or bruising will be present around the anus. The orifice of the habitual passive sodomist by contrast becomes dilated and smooth, the sphincter is lax and, of greatest importance, loses its elasticity; the surrounding skin may become horny and may also show scars from earlier lacerations. The presence of traces of lubricant may provide suggestive evidence and the finding of spermatozoa on swabs prepared either from within the canal or from the anal mucosa will prove the act almost beyond dispute. But it must be admitted that, in many cases, there will be insufficient evidence for the doctor to reach a firm conclusion that unnatural intercourse has occurred. The pathologist examining a dead man may have difficulty in distinguishing true sodomy from the effects of post-mortem change; cases are often seen, particularly in young persons, where an apparently grossly patulous anus could only be ascribed to a post-mortem phenomenon.

The examination of the active partner is unlikely to provide much firm evidence. Certainly, the glans may be damaged – but this is not proof of anal connection; remnants of faeces or lubricant may be present beneath the foreskin in the unlikely event of a suspect not having washed himself before examination. In practice, convictions are more likely on a charge of gross indecency than on a charge of sodomy.

TRANSVESTISM AND TRANSSEXUALISM

Although by no means an offence, transvestism – that is, changing into clothes of the other sex – or transsexualism – a psychiatric change which includes attempting to simulate the sexual appearances of the other sex – are of forensic significance on occasion. The close association of transvestism with the sexual asphyxias is discussed in Chapter 13; the problems of transsexualism and marriage are discussed in Chapter 17. Extremely sophisticated measures to alter the sexual characteristics of the body may be undertaken and have even caused considerable difficulty in the identification of mass casualties.[24]

---

[24] See Stevens P. J. (1970) Fatal Civil Aircraft Accidents, Bristol, Wright, p. 149.

INTERCOURSE WITH ANIMALS

The English offence of buggery includes bestiality which can be committed by either a man or a woman with an animal.[25] Bestiality consists of intercourse per vaginam although Gordon (at p. 836) believes that it can also be committed per anum. It is a common law crime in Scotland to have 'unnatural carnal connection' with an animal; it is doubtful if a woman could be so charged.

The offence is committed when there is penetration; emission is not essential. Veterinary evidence would be important if a small animal was used but the only medical evidence likely to be led in most cases would relate either to the presence of human sperm in an animal or to demonstrating an animal origin of sperm in the human vagina. Spermatozoa differ in size and shape according to species;[26] some cells are, however, very similar to the human and the origin of stains and material on diagnostic swabs would probably be most easily demonstrable by serological methods (see p. 49). Most acts of bestiality are conducted in privacy and there can, therefore, be little forensic medical experience of the offence; but the emphasis on bestiality in 'hard' pornography suggests that the subject may exert a surprising fascination.

[25] Sexual Offences Act 1956, s. 12.

[26] A readily available illustration is to be found in Smith S. and Fiddes F. S. (1955) *Forensic Medicine*, 10th ed., London, Churchill, p. 305.

Chapter 22

Poisons and Poisoning

POISONING is of two main types – that which affects large sections of the community and that which involves individuals only. Environmental and industrial poisoning are the main components of the former category; the number of deaths and the extent of disability directly attributable to poisoning of the community reaches serious levels in most industrialized countries – their limitation is often a matter of legislation. Individual intoxication may be accidental, iatrogenic, suicidal or homicidal. While the last has certainly the greatest medico-legal significance, it is now rare compared with some decades ago; far more individuals die from accident or suicide.

ENVIRONMENTAL POISONING

Basically, environmental poisoning results either from the effects of smoke pollutants in the air or from the presence of specific substances or elements in the surroundings as a whole. The major contributors to the former are coal fires and motor car exhausts.

The production of factory smoke is controlled through the activities of the Alkali and Clean Air Inspectorate and contributes surprisingly little to the total smoke pollution of the urban atmosphere. Most pollution comes from domestic coal fires the products of which, when reacting with a simple fog in windless conditions, produce the classical London 'pea-souper'. If the fog is not dispersed, there is a massive build-up of smoke particles and of the gas sulphur dioxide. Mortality and morbidity are related closely to the combined concentration of these substances, the majority of deaths occurring in those already suffering from disease of the lungs or heart.

The most effective way of controlling this type of poisoning is through the limitation of smoke – it is doubtful if sulphur dioxide, which is the main industrial atmospheric contaminant, is harmful by itself. Local authorities are now empowered to regulate smoke production in their area[1] and it is a matter of general observation that the incidence of 'pea-soupers' has steadily declined; concurrently, there has

---

[1] Clean Air Act 1956 and 1968.

268

been a reduction in the associated cardiopulmonary diseases which can, therefore, be regarded as controllable by legislation.

The effects of motor car exhausts stem from several factors. Depending on the efficiency of the engine, the exhaust gases contain between 2 per cent and 10 per cent carbon monoxide and this is reflected in the carboxyhaemoglobin levels in persons such as policemen on traffic duty. Although the levels reached – of the order of 5–6 per cent – will not cause deterioration in function, the condition is of minor medico-legal importance in that it has been claimed that carbon monoxide derived from smoking – and, therefore, also from other environmental sources – is to some extent responsible for the development of coronary heart disease;[2] it is thought, however, that this view would get little general support. Other important forms of carbon monoxide poisoning are discussed later in this section but, in the present context, the main significance of the gas when derived from motor car exhausts lies in its potential as a cause of vehicular accidents, especially in a synergistic role; this has been discussed in Chapter 10.

The hydrocarbons liberated in exhaust gases due to incomplete combustion of the fuel are more important from the environmental aspect. The interaction of sunlight and exhaust vapour produces an atmosphere which is irritating to the nose and eyes – the characteristic 'smog' of the western USA. Unlike the British fog, 'smog' has little permanent effect on human beings but has been reported as being damaging to crops.

Motor car exhaust gases also contain lead, which forms a link with the second aspect of environmental pollution – that is, pollution by specific elements. Apart from radioactive pollution (discussed in Chapter 27), the outstandingly significant substance in this class is lead. Lead poisoning is, in the main, a matter of industrial medicine but outbreaks of subclinical poisoning occur at an environmental level particularly in areas close to lead works. Lead present in the soil, as well as that present in the air, then constitutes a significant part of the health hazard and children, who are more susceptible to the metal, are at greatest risk.[3] The contribution of motor cars to this risk is not clear. Certainly there is more lead in the atmosphere of urban streets than there is in country areas but absorption into the body is not proportionately increased; nevertheless, all industrial countries are legislating to reduce the amount of lead in motor car fuels.[4]

---

[2] See, for example, Wald N. et al. (1973) Association between atherosclerotic disease and carboxyhaemoglobin levels in tobacco smokers, *Br. Med. J.* **1**, 761.

[3] A lead level of 40–50 μg/100 ml blood in a child is regarded as requiring investigation whereas the level at which an industrial worker is considered in danger of developing lead poisoning is 80 μg/100 ml.

[4] In the United Kingdom, petrol may contain no more lead than 0·45 g/litre.

INDUSTRIAL POISONING

Industrial poisons may be absorbed through the skin, they may be ingested or they may be inhaled; inhalation is by far the most important source not only on physiological grounds but also because it is largely outwith the control of the individual. Much of the preventive legislation is, therefore, concentrated on the maintenance of a pure atmosphere.

Industrial poisons are given threshold limit values (TLV) which are expressed as the airborne concentration of the given substance to which it is believed that nearly all workers may be repeatedly exposed without ill-effects. Such values, which are expressed either in weight per cubic metre or in parts per million, are to some extent artificial and are well compared with the 30 mph speed limits on roads – not all accidents will be prevented by such a limit but it is an arbitrary standard below which it is impracticable to go; in industry, the TLV represents the level which is estimated as likely to be injurious if exceeded.

When dust or fumes of a potentially dangerous character are present to an extent which exceeds this limit, then all practicable measures must be taken to protect the persons employed against their inhalation.[5] The Act stipulates all practicable measures, not merely some, and practicality refers only to the technical possibilities within the limits of current knowledge – cost, for example, does not enter into the definition. The measures taken may include substitution either of the offending substance or of a particularly dangerous process; they may take the form of purely passive prevention as by the use of masks and hoods; active elimination by extraction is, however, incomparably the best means of preventing industrial poisoning and it must be used, ideally sited as close to the source as possible, when the conditions make it practicable. It scarcely needs emphasis that the extraction cannot be haphazard and care must be taken to ensure that contamination of the local community is kept to a minimum. The Factories Act also deals with the possibility of ingestion of industrial poisons; s. 64 prohibits the eating of meals where a toxic process is carried out.

The early identification of cases of poisoning forms one check on the lack of efficiency[6] of a factory's preventive methods. It is for this reason that a number of conditions (listed in Appendix K) are scheduled as Notifiable Diseases – notifiable, that is, to the Chief Inspector of Factories. These diseases must be distinguished from Prescribed Diseases (see p. 181); it is true that nearly all Notifiable Diseases are also Prescribed but the method and purpose of reporting are different. Many of the notifiable conditions are specific; others – for example, 'toxic anae-

[5] Factories Act 1961, s. 63.
[6] Efficiency is positively identified by monitoring or measuring the atmosphere at regular intervals.

mia' – are usefully nonspecific in that they open possibilities for clinical notification of dangerous conditions before they are specifically defined by regulation.

Poisoning in industry is a vast subject which is constantly changing in emphasis and growing in extent – for example, increasing attention[7] is now being given to the possibility that vinyl chloride, which is basic to the manufacture of essential plastics, may predispose to cancer of the liver (see Appendix I, Addendum). The subject will, therefore, be dealt with only in general terms, attention being drawn to the main categories of hazard.

Firstly, there is poisoning by heavy metals of which, as has been seen, lead is the outstanding example; industrial processes involving lead are subject to several statutes and regulations additional to the Social Security and Factories Acts.[8] Section 74 of the Factories Act also limits the employment of women and young persons in lead manufacturing processes and Section 82 orders the notification of any case of lead poisoning contracted while painting a building.[9] Industrial intoxication by lead is almost entirely a matter of inhalation although ingestion is also considered hazardous. The main danger of lead lies in its cumulative effect; industrial cases are all examples of chronic intoxication – colic, joint-pain, anaemia, muscle paralyses and generalized brain dysfunction (encephalopathy) may result and are probably due to the fact that lead is basically a poison to enzymes.

Other metallic poisons which are dangerous mainly by way of inspiration include beryllium and cadmium, which are intensely harmful to the lungs, and manganese and mercury, chronic poisoning from both of which causes extensive abnormality of the central nervous system – the latter metal giving origin to the term 'mad as a hatter'. The effects of chronic metallic poisoning may be delayed for many years; much responsibility rests on the medical profession in establishing a cause-and-effect relationship.

The second major group of industrial poisons consists of the hydrocarbons, of both aromatic and of aliphatic type. Again, intoxication is generally by inhalation but absorption through the skin plays a significant part in many cases.

Poisonous aromatic hydrocarbons include benzene itself – which, in its chronic form, causes an anaemia of very specific type; nitrobenzene – which may be acutely fatal if splashed on the skin; nitroglycerin – again absorbed rapidly through the skin and capable of causing a fatal fall in

[7] Some 35 pages are devoted to the problem in Proc. R. Soc. Med. (1976) 69 (No. 4).

[8] The Alkali etc. Works Regulation Act 1906, for example, deals with the control of fumes from lead smelting works.

[9] All building operations are now subject to the Factories Act and its associated legislation.

blood pressure; and trinitrotoluene, which was responsible for a large number of industrial deaths in both World Wars, the outstanding features being cyanosis, anaemia and, occasionally, toxic jaundice – jaundice, or yellowness, being a visible indication of liver failure.

Aliphatic hydrocarbons may be dangerous industrial chemicals when halogenated – that is, combined with chlorine or bromine. The simplest of these compounds – methyl chloride and methyl bromide, which can be used as refrigerants or, in the case of the latter, as a fire extinguisher – are acutely poisonous to the brain. Otherwise, the common characteristic of this group of poisons is their action on the liver and, to a lesser extent, the kidney. Halogenated hydrocarbons are used principally as cleaning agents or industrial solvents. Most have a narcotic action and the least toxic can be used as anaesthetics. Carbon tetrachloride, tetrachlorethane and, especially, dichlorethane are severely damaging to the liver and are the main sources of industrial toxic jaundice. Tetrachlorethane was a serious cause of illness in early aircraft workers when it was used to tighten the fabric of aeroplanes. The variations in toxicity of the halogenated hydrocarbons offer wide opportunities for substitution and, as a result, the extent of the industrial hazard is diminishing.

Finally, attention is drawn to the potential association of cancer with some industrial processes. Many of these conditions are of historic interest – for example, the 'mule spinner's' cancer induced by chronic friction between the skin and clothing impregnated with mineral oil. Others, as discussed above in relation to vinyl chloride, are only beginning to appear. For an association with occupation to be clear, a cancer must, generally, be of a fairly rare type; it is possible that some common tumours are related to specific substances – the association of carcinoma of the lung with asbestosis and smoking is an example (see p. 185) – but, for the purposes of the Social Security Act, it may be difficult to show that they 'do not constitute a risk to the whole population'. Examples of unusual cancers which are prescribed include carcinoma of the nasal membrane in workers exposed to nickel fumes (disease No. 37) or to wood dust (disease No. 45); mesothelioma (disease No. 44) is sufficiently rare to be firmly attributable to asbestosis. Disease No. 39, cancer of the bladder, is interesting as the most common industrial association of this tumour is with workers in aniline factories; the condition is, in fact, due to the presence as an impurity of the prescribed substance naphthylamine. The association of angiosarcoma of the liver with vinyl chloride monomer has already been mentioned.

AGRICULTURAL POISONS

Agricultural poisoning merits isolation from other industrial hazards because, apart from potential effects on the workers, there may well be secondary ecological effects; the community as a whole may also be at risk if a toxic substance is distributed widely in the environment or is incorporated in foodstuffs. Excluding manifest abuses such as using defoliation as a weapon of war, potential agricultural poisons may be either of the insecticide, the fungicide or the herbicide groups.[10] To be effective, these agents must be toxic; the art of their production and use lies in limiting that toxicity to the species it is intended to destroy.

Control of the problems of nonspecificity lies in the Notification of Pesticides Scheme 1955 under which expert advisory committees have been established to regulate the introduction of new agricultural chemicals. Trials of such substances must be notified to the appropriate Ministry, whose expert advisory committees must be provided with full details of a proposed pesticide – including its justification for use, its toxic properties and its potential residual effects in foodstuffs; particular importance is placed on possible harm to the human users and consumers of treated crops, to livestock and to wildlife. Products so notified are given trials clearance – usually for a limited period – which may involve destruction of all treated material until the remaining safety measures have been taken. Following trials, there is usually a period of limited clearance during which regulated sales may be permitted; if this is passed satisfactorily, a provisional commercial clearance is granted which allows the product to be marketed commercially for a defined period. If the exhaustive inquiries demanded during these phases have indicated that the product is safe to use[11] and is free from serious ecological ill-effects, a full commercial clearance may be given subject to recommendations as to labelling, as to the method of treatment and the choice of crops and as to the protection of man, livestock and wildlife. The advisory panels keep any chemical under review and may vary the regulations in the light of any fresh evidence which accrues during normal use.

In addition to this monitoring system, several statutory controls are imposed. Those chemicals which are most toxic to the user are specified under the Agriculture (Poisonous Substances) Act 1952;[12] a main danger of the specified chemicals is that, in addition to inhalation, entry to the body through the skin is a common method of poisoning. The Act is, therefore, very much concerned with the provision of protective

---

[10] Rodenticides will not be discussed at this point.

[11] Note that a chemical may be poisonous but, when used in a specific way taking normal precautions, it may not necessarily be hazardous – paraquat is a prime example of such a substance (see below).

[12] These are the dinitrophenol compounds; endrin; the organophosphorus compounds; fluoroacetic acid compounds; organomercury sprays; arsenic; the organotin compounds; nicotine; and sulphuric acid.

clothing. Other chemicals, which constitute a hazard if improperly used, are listed in the Farm and Garden Chemicals Act 1967; the main purpose of this Act is to ensure that toxic chemicals are adequately labelled and carry appropriate warnings. Less specifically, certain chemicals which may be used as insecticides or herbicides are subject to the Poisons Rules made under the Poisons Act 1972; the Act is described in greater detail in Chapter 23.[13]

In assessing the poisonous properties of an agricultural chemical, due note must be taken of the advantages offered. Some of the organochlorines are theoretically if not actually poisonous;[14] but the massive benefits to mankind resulting from the widespread reduction of insect-borne diseases, including malaria, infinitely outweigh any such considerations. Similarly, paraquat (see below) has revolutionized the agricultural economy of many developing countries; an occasional suicide in such areas must be accepted as a price to pay for the community benefit. Certain insecticides or herbicides will, however, be specifically mentioned in view of their current medico-legal interest on other than industrial grounds.

The most important group among the insecticides is probably that of the organophosphorus compounds which can enter the body through the inspired air, the skin or even the eye. They owe their profound effect to altering the normal mode of action of the nerves on the muscle masses and to antagonizing the effects of the sympathetic nervous system. The most common preparation, parathion, has been used homicidally; because the action of the organophosphates is essentially physiological, the detection of such cases presents a formidable forensic challenge.

Nicotine is a common fungicide which, when concentrated, is a powerful poison; it enters the body through either the lungs or the skin. The author has been concerned with two deaths in children which could only be attributed to contamination with a nicotine spray.

The herbicide currently causing greatest public concern is paraquat. This remarkable substance is immediately destroyed on contact with the ground – used normally it is, therefore, remarkably safe and highly efficient. Unfortunately, and possibly directly associated with the publicity given to individual cases, it has become a frequent medium for suicide in farming communities; accidental poisoning is also common and there have been at least three convictions for murder by its use in the

---

[13] Numerous Acts have been passed with the intention of preserving the ecology in general or specific species of wildlife. These include the Protection of Animals Acts 1911 to 1927; the Rivers (Prevention of Pollution) Acts 1951 to 1961; the Animals (Cruel Poisons) Act 1962; the Protection of Birds Acts 1954 to 1967; and Control of Pollution Act 1974.

[14] In fact, the Research Committee on Toxic Chemicals reported in 1970 that no evidence had been produced of risks to man resulting from the use of DDT or Dieldrin when these were applied properly nor when occurring as residues in a normal diet. Other members of the group – e.g. Aldrin – might be more hazardous.

United Kingdom. Death from paraquat poisoning is singularly un-pleasant and, currently, there is no proven antidote.[15] Its major action is on the lungs; the pathological appearances are so unusual that fatal poisoning can be diagnosed without recourse to the toxicologist.

One other slightly bizarre medico-legal aspect of chemical agriculture deserves mention – crop spraying is that type of aviation which has the highest mortality. This is related almost solely to the difficult flying conditions; actual poisoning of pilots by their chemical cargo is extremely rare, though minor effects, such as those of the organophosphates on the eyes, could be very dangerous in this situation.

IATROGENIC AND SUICIDAL POISONING

These forms of poisoning are interlinked and can be discussed under one heading.

Very large numbers of new medicinal compounds, which are of increasing complexity both as to their multiplicity of content and as to the effects of the individual drugs contained, appear regularly on the market; doctors are under constant pressure to try new remedies; and, in the conditions of an overworked practice, there is a positive economy of surgery time to be gained by prescribing drugs in such quantity as will serve the patient for a considerable period. Accidental poisoning can occur, therefore, in the normal process of medical practice and, in essence, mishaps can be put down to one of four sources of error:

a. overprescribing the quantity of a single drug;
b. the cumulative effects of drugs;
c. adverse reactions on bodily systems other than that being treated;
d. drug interactions with one another or with articles of diet.

The statutory defence against the majority of these mishaps is provided by the Medicines Act 1968 which is described in Chapter 23. The Act, *inter alia,* authorizes the establishment of a Medicines Commission.[16] The Commission, which now consists of a chairman and thirteen members, advises the licensing authorities and, to this end, appoints Committees which are charged with overseeing the safety, quality or efficiency of medicines and with promoting the collection and investigation of information relating to adverse reactions to drugs on which such advice will be based.[17] The most relevant of the Committees so far established is the Committee on the Safety of Medicines.[18] This Committee meets monthly to review the position of drugs on trial and

---

[15] Paraquat is now restricted as to sale save in its weak, granulated form.

[16] The Medicines Commission and Committees Regulations 1970.

[17] Medicines Act 1968, s. 4(2) and 4(3).

[18] The Medicines (Committee on Safety of Medicines) Order 1970.

has a subcommittèe to consider notifications of adverse drug reactions which have been made by practitioners. When satisfied that a hazard may exist, the Committee, on its own authority, dispatches warning notices drawing the attention of practitioners to areas of danger. All manufacturers of drugs are now required to circulate data sheets in association with advertisements sent direct to practitioners (Medicines Act 1968, s. 96); these data sheets must give all reasonable information as to dosage, effect, contra-indications, adverse reactions and the like. Much of the information is published annually by the Association of the British Pharmaceutical Industry as a Data Sheet Compendium which is issued free to doctors. There is, therefore, now ample opportunity for doctors to appreciate the hazards of drug therapy and failure to heed the many warnings given is likely to be construed by the courts as negligence.

It is unusual for a drug to act on only one system – for example, a high proportion of those usually prescribed for disorders of the central nervous system also have a profound effect on the heart and blood vessels; the danger here is that the prescribing doctor may fail to make himself aware of the patient's total condition. Occasionally, drugs may have serious side effects in humans which did not show up in preliminary animal testing. Unexpected cumulative effects may arise if the patient's capacity for metabolism or excretion of a drug is reduced by disease, say, of the liver or kidney which has passed unnoticed. Drug interactions are extremely common – they may be complementary or antagonistic, the effects may be dangerous or, on occasion, may be desirable; in many instances, a known effect can be counterbalanced by modifications of the dose. Occasionally, a catastrophe may occur because of unawareness on the part of the practitioner, but the most common cause of adverse interactions results from the use by patients of drugs remaining from a previous prescription – repeated self-medication may be dangerous if the patient is by then receiving another drug for another complaint.

This introduces the concept of iatrogenic poisoning, i.e. overprescribing which may be unintentional as, for example, when a doctor prescribes two preparations each of which contains an element of the same drug. But the far greater problem lies in semi-elective overprescribing forced by pressure of work; a not uncommon pattern is of a large primary issue followed by repeated prescriptions without adequate confirmation of the patient's need. This can scarcely be regarded as professional negligence but, as a direct result, there are few households in which an excess of potentially dangerous medicines is not to be found; while some persons would take their own lives no matter how carefully their prescriptions were regulated, there is little doubt that a degree of responsibility for many deaths due to suicidal or accidental poisoning must be laid at the door of the National Health Service. The pattern of suicidal poisoning varies over the years but, at present, it is universal experience that the great majority of cases stem from the misuse of the barbiturate group of drugs. There can be no misuse without availability and, since these drugs are obtainable on prescription only – although not otherwise controlled (p. 286) – it is clear that the majority of supplies must derive from legal prescriptions. Some three persons die in Great Britain each day as a result of suicidal barbiturate poisoning; the virtually innocuous nitrazepam is therapeutically as effective as barbiturates, and strenuous efforts have been made to outlaw barbiturates from treatment schedules in much the same way as was successfully accomplished in some localities in respect of amphetamines. Present indications are, however, that the medical profession is unwilling to take the lead in this movement.[19] It is problematical whether all or even the majority of fatal barbiturate poisonings are, in fact, suicidal; some may be accidental and the relationship with alcoholism is discussed in Chapter 25. Apart from barbiturates, the 'tranquillizers' as a heterogeneous group also account for a large number of suicides – again, these drugs must nearly always be obtained on prescription.

One difficulty in establishing the cause of death in drug poisoning lies in the great variation in post-mortem tissue levels which have been reported in fatal cases; this problem is discussed more fully in Chapter 26. Certainly, there are obvious features which may make one person more susceptible to a drug than another – the route of absorption and the presentation of the drug (i.e. how it is dissolved or otherwise compounded) may be of significance; an unwell patient is likely to be less tolerant of a given poison than is one who is fully fit – a fact which emphasizes the importance of a full autopsy to assess the real significance of drugs in the mode of death; by and large, children and old persons are more susceptible to poisons than are those in the middle age range. But very often these features will not, in themselves, explain apparently anomalous findings and both the pathologist and the toxicologist are dependent to a large extent on the circumstantial evidence; certainly, attempts to estimate the dose taken which are based on a single post-mortem tissue analysis are liable to very wide error.

Other common suicidal poisonings relate to substances which are generally available. Aspirin has perhaps passed its peak as a successful medium – it remains a common means of attempted poisoning but many cases survive with modern treatment; paracetamol is to some extent replacing aspirin and its use again leads to the suspicion that it is publicity which determines vogues in suicide. The author has been surprised at the number of deaths due to lysol or similar corrosive

[19] *Daily Telegraph*, 11 July, 1975, p. 7.

poisoning which still occur – these seem to be confined to the elderly. Other suicidal poisonings are rare and their individual nature often indicates severe mental derangement; many cases of suicidal paraquat poisoning exhibit this feature.

There remains carbon monoxide poisoning which, some ten years ago, was as common a method of suicide as was barbiturate poisoning. It has always been rare in the United States where domestic gas supplies are almost universally of natural origin; the introduction of natural gas into British homes has, similarly, reduced the incidence of carbon monoxide suicides to negligible numbers. Such cases as occur are largely associated with motor car exhaust fumes. Generally, some method of increasing the certainty of success – e.g. by passing a tube from the exhaust to the interior of the car – is used. In the absence of such apparatus, the distinction between suicide and accident may be very difficult to make; in fact, poisoning by exhaust fumes from motor cars is probably more often accidental than suicidal.

ACCIDENTAL POISONING

Accidental poisoning is of considerable medico-legal significance firstly because of its commonness and, secondly, because of the not infrequent difficulty met in distinguishing it from suicide or homicide. It is best discussed in two phases – as related to children and to adults.

Children are most often poisoned by reason of genuine mistake. Perhaps the most dangerous factor lies in the similarity between some medicinal tablets and some widely advertised brands of sweets. Alternatively, poisonous berries growing naturally may be mistaken for fruits seen more commonly in the greengrocer's shop. Children may also be victims of their natural inquisitiveness – there is a strong urge to discover what is so pleasant about the 'sweets' kept beside the parents' beds. The prevention of accidental poisoning in children is a matter, first, of adequate security of containers,[20] medicine cupboards, cleaning closets, garden sheds and the like, coupled with adequate surveillance when in an unusual environment – as, for example, on infrequent picnic outings. The determination and agility of children is well known; locks are essential wherever potentially poisonous substances are stored.

Accidental poisoning in adults is, again, of dual origin. Firstly, there are incidents involving errors of perception – the dose of a drug is misread due to age or ill health, medicines are poured out in the dark or when half-asleep; such errors are potentiated by the effects of alcohol. It may be very difficult to distinguish genuine error from a deliberate act. Secondly, there is involuntary error – the taking of poison in the belief

---

[20] See Br. Med. J. (1976) 1, 604 for a description of compulsory (with reference to paediatric presentation) or voluntary (adult presentation) use of child-resistant containers.

that it is an innocuous substance. As in the case of children, this may occur in nature or in the home. Common examples in the former situation include the eating of the poisonous fungus *Amanita* in mistake for the edible mushroom *Agaricus* or the use of aconite root instead of horse-radish. Poisoning due to involuntary error in the home is almost always a matter of improper labelling – the frequency with which intensely poisonous substances are stored in open areas in beer or lemonade bottles while these still retain their original labels is astounding. Once again, the possibility of deliberate substitution has to be considered.

Carbon monoxide is a very common agent of accidental poisoning which may, on occasion, give rise to unusual findings at the scene of death. The subject has been discussed in detail in Chapter 13. The diagnosis often depends upon awareness of the possibility; curious mistakes, such as attributing death to food poisoning rather than to carbon monoxide, have resulted from inadequate post-mortem examination.

HOMICIDAL POISONING

The pattern of homicidal poisoning also seems to have changed over the years. Not only have the types of poison used altered, but the condition as a whole appears to have become very uncommon. Amongst other factors, the direction of social change is such as to reduce the overall need for the disposal of wives or husbands; when a poisoning occurs it is often found to have unusual background features such as a motivation on eugenic grounds.

Other than at common law, poisoning is covered in Scots law by the quiescent Criminal Law (Scotland) Act 1829, s. 2, which refers to the administration of 'any deadly poison or other noxious substance or thing with intent thereby . . . to murder or disable . . . or to do some other grievous bodily harm'. The English Offences Against the Person Act 1861 is even more stringent and deals with attempts to murder by a 'poison or other destructive thing' (s. 11 and 14), with causing grievous bodily harm by poisoning (s. 23) and even goes so far as to specify an intention to annoy (s. 24). No distinction is made under either jurisdiction between a drug and a poison; both may be noxious things but, as regards the former, the dose given is relevant to the definition as is its mode of presentation – that is, for example, whether or not the substance is in the form of a reputable pharmaceutical preparation. There is no attempt to specify a noxious substance; it is the intention of the user in individual cases which is of paramount importance.

Very occasionally, homicidal poisoning may be associated with medical treatment, when the injurious substance may be introduced by injection. In the vast majority of cases, however, such poisons are administered by mouth and the victim must suffer to some extent from symptoms of gastro-enteritis; the great majority of poisons used with intent to murder will cause vomiting with or without diarrhoea. This is particularly true of the well-known irritant metallic poisons, of which arsenic is the most infamous, and of phosphorus.[21] Nevertheless, natural food poisoning (*see below*) or diarrhoea and vomiting due to virus disease or to psychiatric causes are far more common than is homicidal poisoning. The practitioner may well be excused for failing to diagnose such a case at first glance but when his suspicions are aroused he is faced with an ethical dilemma. He must have the interests of his patient as his main concern; yet, to take action which might be interpreted publicly as implying suspicion of foul play could result in serious charges in the event that it was ill founded.

The doctor in this position should continue to treat his patient but should take extra precautions against the time when his evidence may be needed in court. Thus, particularly careful notes ought to be made of statements, of relevant times and of the specific points which are considered unusual. The normal specimens of vomit and faeces should be taken and labelled accurately, there would seem to be no reason why a toxicological analysis should not be arranged in parallel with bacteriological examinations provided confidentiality is assured. Ideally, specimens of food might be obtained and sent for similar analysis but this could be extremely difficult to achieve if a homicidal attempt were really being made. The ultimate test is to remove the patient to hospital and, in practice, this is what will usually happen in the conditions of a National Health Service. By the time a practitioner is sufficiently concerned to suspect poisoning, he will have been already anxious to obtain improved conditions for his patient on purely medical grounds; this will be particularly so if he finds, as may well happen, that he has been called in late to the case.

If attempted homicidal poisoning is proved to the satisfaction of both the practitioner and the hospital consultant, then it would be right for a confidential report to be made to a senior police officer; few doctors would, however, like to do so without the support of their defence or protection society. In the event of a death which arouses suspicion, the doctor's duty is clear and unequivocal – the case must be reported to the Fiscal or to the Coroner; this applies also following deaths due to natural poisoning.

---

[21] Many of the poisons used in the famous cases of the past were incorporated in rodenticides – thallium is, perhaps, the most modern example; no rat poison may now contain strychnine and the use of monofluoroacetic acid in rat control is mainly restricted to use in ships or sewers (Poisons Rules 1972, para. 6(1), Thirteenth Schedule). Rat poisons are now largely compounded of biological substances but acquired resistance may dictate a return to chemical control.

NATURAL POISONING

Food Poisoning

Food poisoning as a cause of accidental death has been already mentioned as has its importance in the differential diagnosis of homicidal poisoning. This is probably its main forensic significance although actions for tort or delict might well be brought against suppliers, restaurants and the like when damage is suffered; conceivably, criminal charges could be brought in the event of death.

Acute poisoning may result from the ingestion of either living virulent bacteria or of toxins or toxic principles which, in turn, can derive from bacteria or may be normal components of the foodstuff. An important distinction is that bacteria, unless present in the form of resistant spores, are killed by heat; toxins, however, may be thermostable particularly when they are mixed with or are part of the food.

Strictly speaking, bacterial food poisoning will include any disease transmitted through food or water or by a food handler – for example, typhoid fever, cholera or dysentery either of bacterial or of amoebic (protozoal) type. However, while a few other bacteria may cause very similar symptoms, the term is virtually confined to infection by organisms of the *Salmonella* group, virulent *Staphylococci* or *Clostridium welchii* – an organism which also causes gas gangrene. *Salmonellae* are essentially parasites of animals and may pre-exist in the foodstuff or be introduced by contamination; the food shows no evidence of putrefaction and symptoms may be due to the presence of preformed toxin or to proliferation of the bacteria in the human host. *Staphylococci*, on the other hand, are nearly always introduced from a human carrier during the processing of food such as icecream or bakery products. In either case, the symptoms of abdominal pain, vomiting and diarrhoea may closely simulate those of acute metallic poisoning. *Cl. welchii* typically contaminates raw meat, poultry or stews; outbreaks of food poisoning in institutions are often due to this organism.

Botulism is the classic food poisoning due to the presence of preformed bacterial toxin. The organism (*Cl. botulinum*) lives in soil and can, therefore, be transmitted in vegetables; it grows only in the absence of oxygen and will flourish in canned or bottled foodstuffs. Home bottling of vegetables is probably the least uncommon source of the condition but meat products are also implicated. The disease is generally of great severity and is often fatal; it causes paralysis of the central nervous system and the usual symptoms of food poisoning are absent. Cases are very rare in the United Kingdom.

Poisoning resulting from the nature of the food may come from either vegetables or animals. The fungi, which are most likely to be eaten in error, are the best known of the very many vegetables which have poisonous properties. Fungi of the genus *Amanita*, eaten in mistake for the common mushroom *Agaricus*, contain toxins which may cause severe gastro-intestinal upset with accompanying surgical shock or, through the action of the alkaloid muscarine, may interfere with the nervous stimulation of the muscles. The toxic principles of some fungi are hallucinogenic. The most dangerous fungus, *A. phalloides*, is toxic even having been cooked. On the other hand, many fungi apart from the common field mushroom are palatable and nontoxic.

Animal foods which are toxic in the absence of bacterial contamination mostly derive from fish.[22] The poisonous principle is neurotoxic and is concentrated maximally in the gonads and the liver at spawning time.

Poisonous fungi and poisonous fish are used both homicidally and suicidally in primitive societies.

Poisons Naturally Injected
Many animal species inject venom either as a defence mechanism or as a means of immobilizing their prey. Of these, snakes are by far the most important both medically and in the forensic context.

There are two main families of venomous snake – the *Viperidae*, which are all poisonous, and the *Colubridae,* many of which are non-poisonous but which include the very dangerous cobras and kraits. Venom is injected reflexly through the fangs when the snake strikes or bites. All venoms contain a mixture of toxic principles but, in general, the colubride venom is neurotoxic and kills rapidly due to paralysis while that of the viperidae acts on the blood and kills slowly by destroying the red cells and altering the clotting mechanisms. Tragedies have occurred in mistaking the staggering gait and slurred speech of the victim of cobra bite for drunkenness.

Snake venoms are not of equal potency nor is each injection equally efficient; but the concentration of the dose depends upon the body weight and it follows that snake bite, or any other venomous injection is more dangerous in the case of children than in adults. The prognosis is also greatly influenced by the availability of efficient treatment.

The treatment of snake bite is both general and specific. It is the latter, in the form of antivenin therapy, which causes most medico-legal concern. Horses can be immunized against snake venom and thus provide antisera for the treatment of humans. The most specific antisera will be the most efficacious but their use depends upon accurate identification of the specific snake; in practice, therefore, the doctor is often

---

[22] The dangers of most shellfish and molluscs stem not only from their primary toxicity at certain times of the year – perhaps due to the presence of commensals – but also from their lifestyle of scavengers and their frequent contamination with disease-producing organisms.

forced to use a less efficient, 'wide spectrum' antivenin. At the same time, there is always a risk of severe reaction by the patient to the 'horse' components of the injection (*see* p. 82). There may well be a therapeutic dilemma. Little doubt would be raised in areas in which poisonous snakes abounded – provided the patient was seen within eight hours of being bitten, antivenin would be given without hesitation. At the other extreme, the only poisonous snake which exists in Great Britain, *V. berus*, injects a venom which is only slightly toxic – it has accordingly been concluded that its bite is less dangerous than is the use of the available antivenin.[23] The decision could be a hard one in the case of a small child; if antiserum was given, test dosing followed by very careful administration and desensitization (e.g. by the use of adrenalin) would be mandatory. It is believed that snake bite kills some 40 000 persons annually throughout the world, the most dangerous areas being Asia, Central America and Australia. Most Asian practitioners would probably agree, however, that a number of otherwise violent deaths are incorrectly attributed to snake bite.

The sting of the scorpion, which does not live outside the subtropics, is perhaps the second most common serious envenomation on a worldwide basis; at the very least, the sting is intensely painful while the venom of certain species is as dangerous as is that of some snakes. Dangerously poisonous spiders are far less common than is generally supposed. The most serious bite is that of the species *Latrodectus* – the 'black widow' – which tends to lurk on rustic latrine seats. Antivenins are available for both scorpion sting and spider bite and, again, the seriousness of the prognosis is inversely proportional to the body weight of the person attacked.

Few insect stings are completely free from danger, particularly if they are multiple. The sheer pain may induce a vagal type of shock while unduly sensitive persons may die from an antigen/antibody reaction. Between 1962 and 1971, there were 44 deaths due to bee and wasp stings in England and Wales; about 40 comparable deaths occur annually in the USA.

---

[23] Royal Society of Tropical Medicine and Hygiene (1962) Notes on the treatment of snake bite. *Trans. R. Soc. Trop. Med. Hyg.* **56,** 93.

Chapter 23

The Law Relating to Drugs and Poisons

THE law relating to environmental and industrial poisoning is a wide subject very largely beyond the control of the individual. The purpose of this section is to outline only the statutory control of poisons and drugs which are dispensed through the pharmaceutical and medical professions.

Thus limited, there are few relevant enactments of importance. The current Pharmacy and Poisons Act 1933 is in the process of replacement by the Poisons Act 1972 and the Medicines Act 1968.[1] The first of these is concerned entirely with nonmedicinal poisons and, in the main, regulates the storage of poisons and their sale and supply to the public and to the health professions. The second large Act is, as its name indicates, related to medicinal drugs; it covers many administrative aspects of advertisement and sale and essentially regulates the standards of pharmaceutical practice. The Misuse of Drugs Act 1971 deals with only a limited list of drugs; nevertheless, it is that part of drug legislation which most closely concerns the individual doctor, the law enforcement officer and the drug taker.

SALE OF NONMEDICINAL POISONS TO THE PUBLIC

The Poisons Act 1972 takes over the main functions of the 1933 Act in so far as nonmedicinal poisons are concerned. It provides for:

i. the registration of sellers of poisons;
ii. the categorization of poisons in relation to how they may be sold or supplied;
iii. the drawing-up of Poisons Rules and their review. The latest Poisons Rules were drawn up in 1972 under the 1933 Act and are currently in force.

---

[1] Although both these Acts have reached the Statute Book, surprisingly few regulations to be made under them have passed the stage of consultation. Much of this discussion is, of necessity, a matter of history and/or speculation.

The last two provisions are amongst the functions of the Poisons Board which advises the Secretaries of State on both aspects.[2] The *Poisons List* is divided into two Parts. Part I poisons may be sold only by pharmacists from registered premises; Part II poisons may be sold only by pharmacists or, from specified premises, by persons who are approved by the local authority as listed sellers of Part II poisons. The Poisons Board has authority to recommend the precise listing of poisons but, in general, Part II poisons are those to which it is reasonable for the public to have adequate access – they thus include those substances which, although poisonous if misused, are in everyday household use.

All listed poisons must be sold in containers which show the name of the poison and the proportion contained in any mixture, the word 'Poison' and the name and address of the seller. Those Part I poisons which are included in the First Schedule of the Poisons Rules (*see below*) are restricted in that the purchaser must either be known to the seller or must provide a certificate signed either by a householder known to the pharmacist or by a police officer in charge of a Station; full details of the sale must be entered in a book kept for the purpose and the purchaser must sign the entry. The permissive sections of the old 1933 Act, whereby there was no interference with the sale of listed poisons to doctors, dentists, veterinary surgeons etc., no longer have any relevance.

The Act empowers the Secretaries of State, after consultation with the Poisons Board, to draw up *Poisons Rules*. Many of these Rules are expressed as Schedules, some of which are of extremely limited application – the existing Schedule 13, for example, deals with the restriction of the supply of strychnine to authorized mole-catchers, while others, such as Schedule 3, lead to relaxation of the regulations if the poison is present below a stated concentration or is supplied in a particular form. Schedules 1 and 4 are, however, of considerable importance in forensic medicine as they stand at present.

Schedule 1 includes, *inter alia*, all the poisons which are intended for the treatment of human or animal disease, but these will be removed when regulations are made under Part III of the Medicines Act; the important restriction imposed on a doctor who supplies a Schedule 1 poison to keep a record of having done so will disappear.

Schedule 4 was drawn up with the intention of ensuring medical supervision of certain drugs which could be misused, had a critical dosage or possessed a potentially high grade of toxicity. The Schedule is

<hr>

[2] The Poisons Board consists of 5 members appointed by the interested Government Departments, the Government Chemist, 5 persons approved by the Pharmaceutical Society of Great Britain, 4 members appointed by echelons of the medical profession, 1 by the Royal Institute of Chemistry and any additional members thought necessary.

currently divided into Parts A and B, the distinction being that Part B substances are not, at the same time, Schedule 1 poisons. Schedule 4 drugs can be supplied to members of the general public only on a prescription signed by a doctor, dentist or veterinary surgeon.[3] If the drug concerned is in Part A, the prescription must be in writing (including typewriting); it must show the name and address of the prescriber unless it is written on a National Health Service prescription form; it must also include the name and address of the patient, the total amount of the drug to be dispensed and the dose to be taken. For private prescriptions, the prescriber may indicate the number of times the prescription may be repeated together with the interval between the repetitions. Schedule 4 and its associated regulations are of major importance because they represent the only form of control exercised over the distribution of the barbiturate group of drugs. Schedule 4 will, presumably, be replaced by regulations due to be made under s. 58 of the Medicines Act (*see below*); the draft of these regulations indicates that the requirements for prescription may be even less restrictive.

THE MEDICINES ACT 1968[4]

This massive Act is concerned, in the main, with the regulation of the manufacture and supply of medicinal products, which are defined (s. 130) as any substances (not being instruments, apparatus or appliances) which are manufactured, sold, supplied, imported or exported for use by being administered to human beings or animals for a medicinal purpose or which are ingredients of a substance or article used for medicinal purposes. A 'medicinal purpose' implies treatment or prevention of disease, diagnosis, contraception, induction of anaesthesia or interference with a normal physiological function in either a negative or positive fashion.

Part II of the Act introduces licences and certificates relating to the sale, wholesale and manufacture of medicinal products with general exceptions from the restrictive regulations for doctors, dentists, veterinary practitioners and pharmacists; clinical trials on patients and medicinal tests on animals are also controlled (ss. 31 and 32). Part III deals with the sale of medicinal products and the designation of some on a general sales list which authorizes their sale otherwise than by a pharmacist; products not so classified can only be sold in a registered pharmacy. Again, there are the usual professional exceptions. Section 58

---

[3] Prescriptions signed by dentists or veterinary surgeons must state 'for dental treatment only' or 'for animal treatment only' respectively. The veterinary prescription must show the name of the person to whom the drug is to be delivered.

[4] This Act repeals the Pharmacy and Medicines Act 1941, the Therapeutic Substances Act 1956 and the greater part of the Pharmacy and Poisons Act 1933.

provides for the making of regulations to specify products which may be supplied to the general public only on the prescription of a medical practitioner, dentist or veterinary surgeon.[5] Part IV defines pharmacists and pharmacies and their registration. Part V deals with the labelling, packaging and identification of medicinal products and Part VI lays down criteria on the important subject of advertising – particular attention is paid to the problems of false or misleading advertisements and representations.

It is evident that, while the Act defines a number of offences, all of which may come within the ambit of the lawyer, very few of these involve directly the doctor or the dentist – indeed they are specifically excluded from the majority of the provisions; a detailed discussion is, therefore, beyond the scope of a text on forensic medicine. Apart from orders which may be made under Section 58, only Part I – the administration of the Act – is apposite in that it establishes the Medicines Commission which, in turn, has the power to recommend to the Minister the setting up of committees with particular responsibility for the safety and efficacy of medicinal drugs. These functions have already been discussed.

DRUG ABUSE

The Misuse of Drugs Act 1971 is one of the most important current statutes in relation of medical jurisprudence – which can be loosely defined as 'the legal aspects of medical practice'. The 1971 Act repeals the Drugs (Prevention of Misuse) Act 1964 and the Dangerous Drugs Acts 1965 and 1967. The major regulations in pursuance of the Act are the Misuse of Drugs Regulations 1973 (S.I. 1973 No. 797), the Misuse of Drugs (Safe Custody) Regulations 1973 (S.I. 1973 No. 798) and the Misuse of Drugs (Notification of and Supply to Addicts) Regulations 1973 (S.I. 1973 No. 799).

The 1971 Act does four main things:

  a. it establishes an Advisory Council on the Misuse of Drugs;
  b. it classifies certain drugs as Controlled Drugs;
  c. it takes steps to regulate doctors who are deemed unsuitable to prescribe or administer controlled Drugs (ss. 12 and 13);

---

[5] There is an interesting change of emphasis in the 1933 and 1968 Acts. Thus, every medicine is now, effectively, a Part I poison unless it is specifically listed in the general sales list. 'Prescription only drugs' are classified not so much on their content as on the reason for their use and method of administration. All drugs which must be given by injection are classed as 'prescription only' and, in general, these can only be given by qualified persons – the major exception is insulin which can, of course, be self administered.

d. it empowers the Advisory Council to advise on the establishment of centres for treatment, rehabilitation and aftercare of persons affected by the misuse of drugs.

The Act is, therefore, far more than simply repressive in type and represents a great advance in social legislation over the statutes it repeals.

The Advisory Council, as presently constituted, consists of not less than 20 persons with wide and recent experience in the specialties of medicine, dentistry, veterinary medicine, pharmacy, pharmaceutical manufacturing, chemistry and social work involving the misuse of drugs. The remit of the Council has the very great advantage of flexibility. It must monitor the national situation in regard to drug abuse and can advise on measures to be taken in the light of changing circumstances. Drugs can, therefore, be controlled rapidly; alternatively, drugs which seem at any time to have ceased to be a problem can be released from restriction. Equally important functions of the Advisory Council include the promotion of cooperation between all the social services involved in the eradication of drug abuse and the education of the public – and especially the younger public – as to the dangers of the misuse of drugs.

Historically, dangerous drugs have been equated with narcotic drugs – as evidenced by the establishment of Narcotics Bureaux and Commissions in many countries. The pharmaceutical industry has, however, made such advances in recent years in the production of drugs which have powerful effects outwith their intended therapeutic roles that drug abuse has escaped from its previous confines. Stimulants, hallucinogens and the like may be just as dangerous or antisocial as are the narcotics, particularly when they are used as mixtures; it is this trend which Section 2 of the Act is designed to combat. Under this Section and its resultant regulations, certain drugs are listed as 'controlled'. Controlled drugs are classified into classes A, B and C, the classes being determined by the punishment specified for the offences of their production, supply and possession. The penalties are greatest in the case of Class A and least in the case of Class C drugs[6] and, in all cases, are more severe in relation to production and supply than as to possession. It is a logical consequence that, in practice, the most harmful drugs are placed in Class A. A distinction is made, however, in the case of drugs which are both harmful and have negligible therapeutic application; these drugs are listed in Schedule 4 of the 1973 Regulations. Whereas numerous professional persons – including doctors, dentists, etc. – may legally possess controlled drugs for the purpose of carrying on their profession,

---

[6] Rather surprisingly, the only difference between Class A and Class B drugs relates to the punishment for possession of a controlled drug (Schedule 4).

a special licence is needed for the possession of those in Schedule 4.[7]
The lawful supply of controlled drugs is carefully regulated. A prescription given by a doctor must be in ink or otherwise indelible and be written in the prescriber's own hand and signed and dated by him; it must state the name and address of the person to be treated and of the prescriber unless it is written on a National Health Service prescription form; and the dose of the controlled drug must be written in both words and figures. Repeat prescriptions are not permitted and, should it be the intention to dispense the prescription by instalments, the total amount of controlled drug to be given in each instalment and the intervals to be observed must be stated. The pharmacist must either know the signature of the prescriber or must have no reason to doubt its genuineness. These restrictions are intended to detect or discourage forgery and to prevent the stockpiling of controlled drugs by individuals (*Fig.* 18).

The 1973 Regulations also introduced new requirements for recording the supply and administration of controlled drugs. Unless the drugs are supplied to a patient on prescription, an entry must be made in a bound register of receipt and supply of all drugs in Classes A and B and of all those in Schedule 4 of the Regulations. A doctor must keep such a register and must produce this for inspection on request when so directed in writing by the Secretary of State. Controlled drugs must be kept in locked containers which can only be opened by the person legally in possession but there are relaxations in respect of many Class B and Class C drugs. It has been stated that a locked car would not be considered a locked receptacle for the purposes of the Regulations.

The Misuse of Drugs Act includes statutory controls over the rights of doctors to prescribe and possess drugs. Under s. 12, the Secretary of State may direct that a doctor who has been convicted of an offence under the Act[8] shall be prohibited from possessing or prescribing controlled drugs; such a direction is operative once it has been served on the practitioner to whom it applies but can be cancelled or suspended at any time.

Sections 13 and 14 are of more practical concern to the lawyer. Under the former, the Secretary of State may prohibit a practitioner from possessing or prescribing controlled drugs either if the doctor prescribes controlled drugs to an addict without notifying the case as required or if he contravenes the Regulations which state that heroin and cocaine can only be prescribed under licence unless it be for treatment of organic disease or injury; a prohibition may also result if the Secretary of State is of the opinion that the practitioner has been prescribing controlled

---

[7] This is not stated positively but would appear to be so by a process of deductive reasoning – it is certainly the policy adopted by inspectors appointed under s. 23 of the Act.

[8] Or certain offences in connection with the Customs and Excise Act 1952.

Fig. 18. Typical prescriptions for controlled drugs in the National Health Service (*left*) and in private practice (*right*).

drugs in an irresponsible fashion. Section 14 describes the necessary procedure.

In the first instance, the case is referred to a Tribunal[9] who may find that there is no reason for a direction of prohibition to be made; in that case, the practitioner is so informed. Should the Tribunal find against the practitioner, a recommendation is made to the Secretary of State indicating those controlled drugs which he should be forbidden to possess or prescribe. The proceedings before the Tribunal are private, unless a public hearing is requested by the respondent, and the practitioner may be legally represented. An appeal against the findings of a Tribunal is referred to an Advisory Body which consists of a Queen's Counsel as Chairman, a medical (or dental or veterinary) practitioner in Government employ and a further member appointed by the respondent's profession; legal representation is again allowed. The Advisory Body may recommend a direction of prohibition either accepting or modifying the advice of the Tribunal, it may refer the case back to the Tribunal or another Tribunal, or it may advise that no further proceedings be taken.

A further disciplinary power exists when there appears to be considerable urgency over the need to suspend a practitioner's right to supply controlled drugs (Section 15). In these circumstances, the Secretary of State refers the case to a professional panel which consists of three members of the respondent's profession. In the event that the panel advises the need, the Secretary of State may issue a direction of temporary prohibition for a period of 6 weeks but must, at the same time, refer the case to a Tribunal. The temporary prohibition may be extended, subject to the agreement of the Tribunal, for periods of 28 days.

This control of a doctor's or dentist's practice by statute is a departure from the established regulation of professional conduct by the General Medical or Dental Councils (see Chapter 30); the seriousness of this step is reflected in the intricacy of the procedure. Nevertheless, it is noteworthy that, with the exception of the legal Chairmen, the respondent's case is still tried entirely by his peers.

A final word is needed concerning the Misuse of Drugs (Notification of and Supply to Addicts) Regulations 1973, which are of additional medico-legal significance in that they constitute a new statutory relaxation of the general principles relating to professional confidentiality. A person is to be regarded as an addict under the Regulations if he has, as a result of repeated administration, become so dependent on a drug that he has an overpowering desire for the administration of it to be continued. If a doctor has reasonable grounds for considering a patient he attends to be addicted to one of the drugs specified in the Regulations, he must notify the Chief Medical Officer at the Home Office (who is also

[9] The Tribunal consists of a lawyer of at least seven years standing as Chairman and four members from the medical (or dental or veterinary as appropriate) profession.

responsible for Scottish notifications) of the patient's particulars. Only one notification is required from a group practice or from a hospital but renotification is required yearly. As noted above, the doctor who fails to notify an addict yet continues to treat him makes himself liable to severe professional restriction.

Chapter 24

Drug Addiction*

FOR centuries most groups in society have used drugs whether for their pleasurable and relaxing effects, for communicating with the spirits, for religious reasons or simply to make possible prolonged physical exertion in the face of hunger and other adversities. Present-day society is no exception but, in addition to a wider range of drugs (in the generally accepted sense of the word) than ever before, it has to contend with the interrelated problems of cigarette smoking, dependence on alcohol, overeating and gambling. The 'rules' governing the use of a drug are determined by the society concerned and its use outwith these rules is best termed 'abuse' or 'misuse'. It is implicit in any definition of misuse that the drug is being taken apart from medical need and there will often be difficulty in deciding where use ends and misuse begins. The borderline may be controversial even when the drug is being prescribed by a doctor. The nightly use of sleeping capsules for months or years by middle-aged women (a common occurrence) would be regarded as legitimate by some physicians and misuse by others; likewise, the consumption of tranquillizing drugs by young women who would otherwise have difficulty in coping with daily living is debatable practice.

The repeated use of some drugs leads to the individual becoming compelled to continue taking the drug. The amount taken may have to be increased to obtain the effect produced by the initial dose because of the development of tolerance. Psychological and physical dependence on the drug soon occurs and its sudden discontinuance leads to a complex sequence of withdrawal symptoms. Not every misused drug will produce all these features or the same combination of them, but they are to many the hallmarks of 'addiction' and were incorporated in early definitions of the term.

Addiction used to be distinguished from 'habituation', which was a less serious state. Though the habituated individual might have the desire to continue taking the drug the element of compulsion to do so was absent; there was little or no tendency to increase the dose, no physical dependence and no ill-effects on stopping the drug.

However, 'habituation' has fallen into disuse and although 'addiction'

---

* By A. T. Proudfoot, BSc, M B, ChB, FRCPE.

is an unsatisfactory term because it has been used over the years with such various meanings, it is so much part of the vocabulary that it is unlikely to be dropped. Some definition is necessary if only from a legislative standpoint. The Misuse of Drugs (Notification of and Supply to Addicts) Regulations 1973 designates an individual an addict 'if, and only if, he has as a result of repeated administration become so dependent upon the drug that he has an overpowering desire for the administration of it to be continued'. In the context of these Regulations the term 'drug' refers only to compounds such as cocaine and a dozen or so opiates listed in a schedule to the Regulations. This definition is unsatisfactory in as far as it may be difficult to decide when an 'overpowering desire' for continuance of the drug exists.

THE DRUGS INVOLVED

Many compounds have been misused over the ages but it is only in recent decades, with the advent of a rapidly expanding pharmaceutical industry, that the number of drugs having some property attractive to misusers has mushroomed. In general, drugs are taken to alter mood, thought or perception. The effect of any drug varies from one individual to another and depends on several factors including the pharmacological properties of the drug, the personality of the consumer, his feelings and surroundings at the time of taking it and his preconceptions about its effects. The effects may also be enhanced or diminished by other drugs taken simultaneously.

Drugs may be taken in several ways. Sniffing ('snorting') and inhalation are really only suitable for vapours but occasionally solid drugs in powdered or crystalline form or in solution are taken this way. Absorption into the blood stream via this route is unreliable and the quantities of drug reaching the brain and the subsequent 'experience' are correspondingly unpredictable. Likewise, drugs taken by mouth may not produce an effect suffiently intense to satisfy many addicts although this route may provide background intoxication on which to superimpose other drug effects. Such methods tend to be used by those who are experimenting or are relatively inexperienced in the abuse of drugs. 'Skin-popping', the injection of a solution of a drug under the skin, goes some way to magnify the effects of the drug because absorption is faster and more complete than after ingestion. It does not, however, have the impact of direct injection into the blood stream ('mainlining') and for this reason – and because of the development of tolerance – it is not widely used by 'hard-core' addicts trying to recapture the intensity of earlier experiences with drugs.

The main drugs which are misused fall into three groups: those which stimulate, those which have a depressant effect and those which alter the senses, particularly perception (sometimes referred to as hallucinogens or psychedelics).

Stimulants

Cocaine, amphetamine and amphetamine-related compounds are the major constituents of this group. Cocaine is derived from the leaves of the coca plant, *Erythroxylon coca*, which is found in Peru and Bolivia. For centuries the natives of Peru have chewed coca leaves or drunk infusions of them partly for religious reasons but also so that they could work more readily in hostile environments. Coca exhilarates, increasing both physical and mental energy and, in addition, induces a sense of detachment from reality. The use of coca spread and cocaine was isolated from the leaves towards the end of the nineteenth century.

Cocaine may be inhaled as a snuff ('snow') or injected. The drug is rapidly broken down in the body and the 'flash' which addicts prize so highly and which can become the *raison d'être* wears off quickly. For this reason repeated doses are often taken at short intervals (even as frequently as every ten minutes) to prolong the flash, and very large amounts may be taken in the course of a day.

Amphetamine and its related compounds (commonly referred to as 'speed'), methylamphetamine, dextro-amphetamine, diethylproprion, phenmetrazine and methylphenidate were extensively used in the 1950s for a variety of purposes. Because of their stimulant and appetite-suppressing properties, they soon found a place in the treatment of depression and obesity. Like cocaine they make the individual more self-assured, lively and talkative and help to keep him awake but irritability, restlessness and impairment of judgement and reasoning supervene if the drugs are taken in excess. Ideas of persecution, delusions and hallucinations may also occur and lead to irrational behaviour, features which characterize a severe psychotic state that may follow chronic consumption of large doses. Some addicts find the hyperexcitability induced by these drugs unpleasant and prefer to take them in conjunction with a depressant drug, e.g. cocaine with heroin or amphetamine with a barbiturate.

Death from misuse of amphetamine is uncommon. A recent paper states that the medical literature contains reports of 43 deaths (mainly from cerebral haemorrhage or disturbance of heart rhythm) over a period of 35 years. Both cocaine and amphetamine, however, induce marked psychological dependence. Withdrawal is characterized by depression and listlessness which may lead to attempts at suicide or to restarting the drugs. Prolonged sleep and considerable increase in appetite are usual.

The number of prescriptions for amphetamines is steadily falling because some family doctors, being aware of the problems of misuse, have simply stopped prescribing them. Indeed, with rare exceptions, there is probably no place for these drugs in modern medicine. During 1967 and 1968 there was a vogue for using an ethical intravenous preparation of amphetamine. The number of ampoules manufactured rose from 3000 in the first quarter of 1967 to 206 000 in the second quarter of 1968. Two doctors were said to be responsible for two-thirds of this demand. The extent of the problem was identified at an early stage and concerted action by the pharmaceutical and medical professions promptly and drastically reduced the availability of this preparation.

Depressants
The main drugs in this group are the opiates (heroin, morphine, pethidine, methadone) and the barbiturates (of which there are numerous varieties).

Opium (the dried juice from the unripe poppy-seed capsule) has been known for many centuries and in some societies was used socially as is alcohol today. It has been used medicinally for just as long; the beneficial effects of opium and its derivatives were well recognized at a time when most 'drugs' were at best ineffective. Even today there are no more potent drugs than opiates for the relief of pain and induction of euphoria. It is these very properties that make them so desirable to the addict and make the medical profession jealously defend its right to prescribe them.

Opium may be smoked – though this is now not common in Great Britain – and, in the early nineteenth century, there was a vogue for the ingestion of a liquid extract, laudanum. Morphine and heroin (diamorphine) were soon isolated from opium and these are currently the most popular opiates, while pethidine and methadone are synthetic compounds with similar properties. Opiates are now usually mainlined, the 'fix' being prepared by dissolving the tablets in some water, gently heating, filtering, then drawing the solution into a syringe. Not everyone experimenting with these drugs finds them pleasurable. Nausea and vomiting are common with early use but they are usually followed by a feeling of calm detachment and invulnerability.

Dependence on opium is not a new phenomenon but it is only in recent years that the size of the problem has increased in Great Britain. Until about 1960, there were approximately 450 addicts known to the Home Office. The majority were middle-aged or elderly people who had been given opiates in the course of a serious disease and whom it was impossible to take off the drugs once the illness ended ('therapeutic addicts'). Doctors, their wives and others working in related professions also comprised a substantial number of the addicts at that time (so-called 'professional addicts'). After 1960, however, the number began to rise steeply, reaching a plateau of about 3000 in 1972. The rise was in the number of nontherapeutic, nonprofessional addicts and was largely confined to those between the ages of 20 and 35 years. The increase in number of addicts below the age of 20 was less marked but was still a grave cause for concern. It is virtually certain that official statistics underestimate the extent of the problem but there is no other source providing an overall view.

The opiate misuse situation has improved since 1968; the number of new heroin addicts notified has fallen considerably and so too has the number of addicts under the age of 20. In addition some heroin addicts have been switched to methadone as part of treatment programmes. Convictions for offences involving heroin also seem to have stabilized or slightly fallen, though those for morphine and methadone have increased.

Opiates rapidly induce profound psychological and physical dependence but, because of tolerance, the 'buzz' which the user obtains declines and he may find himself having to continue the drugs just to feel normal rather than to become elated. Sudden withdrawal of opiates without substituting other drugs leads to the well-known syndrome of 'cold turkey'. Running eyes and nose, sneezing, gooseflesh, feeling of cold, restlessness, muscle aches and pains are followed by nausea, vomiting and diarrhoea with abdominal cramps. These symptoms may last several days unless controlled by other drugs and, as the addict knows only too well, they may be instantly relieved by a further fix.

Barbiturates were, until the 1960s, the drugs identified with the middle-aged and elderly and shunned by the younger generation. They are synthetic compounds, among the most popular of which are pentobarbitone (*Nembutal*), sodium amylobarbitone (*Sodium amytal*) and a mixture of the latter with quinalbarbitone known as *Tuinal*. These drugs have been used widely in recent decades for inducing sleep. In 1965, 17·2 million prescriptions were issued for them in England and Wales. The number of people in the community who use hypnotics regularly over long periods is larger than one would suspect. In 1966, a survey of barbiturate prescribing in a London general practice revealed that 2 per cent of patients had been receiving barbiturates for longer than a year. Other studies have confirmed this proportion as being dependent on sleeping pills of all varieties but mainly barbiturates. The regular users are predominantly middle-aged or elderly women but serious dependence is uncommon.

Misuse of barbiturates by young people came to light in the late 1960s and differed from regular use by older generation in that the barbiturate was mainlined rather than taken orally. Serious misuse apart, these drugs are readily obtained in public houses and from other black market sources by youngsters experimenting with drugs. At current prices it is considerably less expensive to become drunk on barbiturates than on alcohol.

The size of the barbiturate market is largely the result of overprescribing by doctors. Fortunately recent years have seen a decline in barbiturate prescribing though this has been compensated to some extent by an increase in prescribing of nonbarbiturate hypnotics. Social pressure is therefore still being brought to bear on doctors to supply sleeping tablets because, with one exception (methaqualone, mainly as contained in *Mandrax*), more recent preparations have not held attractions for misusers. Expert committees have been examining barbiturate use for some time but it has not been possible to reach agreement on control of prescribing. Groups of doctors have already taken the initiative and refuse to prescribe barbiturates for night sedation and there is a growing body of opinion that, with the exception of phenobarbitone which is used in the control of epilepsy, there is probably no place for barbiturate hypnotics in present-day medicine. The hazards of barbiturate misuse will be discussed later; they produce marked psychological and physical dependence and tolerance. Sudden withdrawal can lead to a serious illness lasting several days and comprising convulsions, agitation, confusion, tremor and auditory and visual hallucinations.

Drugs altering the Senses
The main drugs in this group are cannabis and lysergic acid diethylamide (LSD). Others such as mescaline, DMT and STP (serenity, tranquillity and peace) are much less frequently used. None of these drugs has found a clearly defined place in medicine and any use is thereby misuse. They are sometimes referred to as 'hallucinogens' but this term is misleading since they rarely cause hallucinations but merely distort what is actually present, albeit frequently in a vivid manner. To call them 'psychedelics' is also unsatisfactory.

Like opium, cannabis, which is derived from the leaves and flowering top of the Indian hemp plant, has been used by some societies for very many centuries. Nor is its use in the United Kingdom a new phenomenon though it is now probably the most commonly misused drug. Some reflection of its widespread use is to be found in the number of convictions for offences involving cannabis which were relatively infrequent until 1959 when they began to increase and reached 14 119 in 1973. In Britain, the more potent hashish (the resin exuded by the plant) is preferred to marihuana (the leaves) and is usually smoked mixed with tobacco though, in other civilizations, it was frequently eaten.

The effects of cannabis vary so considerably from one individual to another that it is difficult to detail them. Some are unaffected by it while others experience excitement, contentment, greater power of concentration and breadth of thought and sociability. Time passes more slowly, colours and sounds become more vivid than normal and the individual floats in and out of a joyful, dreamlike state in which every thought or image may be grotesquely distorted. Laughing without reason is common in the early stages and, later, memory, reasoning and coordination may be impaired until restlessness gives way to drowsiness. The only physical effects are a persistent cough or bloodshot eyes.

Cannabis users maintain that the drug is not addictive and that its long-term use is harmless. There is no doubt that moderate use impairs efficiency at work and school and heavy use may render the individual incapable of work. Whilst no serious physical symptoms follow abstinence and many can stop smoking without difficulty, there are a small number of individuals who may become psychologically dependent. There is also some evidence that tolerance to cannabis (and the reverse) occurs and overseas reports suggest the development of psychotic illnesses similar to schizophrenia[1] with prolonged heavy use. Even single exposures have been said to produce panic attacks with paranoia[1] and it is also claimed that psychotic illnesses after cannabis are much slower to clear once the drug is withdrawn than are those due to amphetamines. The existence of cannabis psychosis has been questioned but the evidence for the safety or otherwise of long-term cannabis use remains sufficiently scanty for the debate to continue for some years.

LSD ('acid') and its perception-distorting properties were discovered in 1943. Its effects are similar to those produced by mescaline but the amount required to evoke them is considerably smaller. The capacity of a minute quantity of LSD taken by mouth to induce a delirious state with vivid, distorted and fantastic visions is one of the most remarkable features of the drug. Hearing and appreciation of music may be enhanced. The company and surroundings in which it is taken determine to a large extent how pleasant or otherwise the 'trip' will be. One might have expected emotionally labile, insecure individuals to react to the point of panic in the face of such experiences but this is not common. On occasions, however, some 'trippers' prefer to have one of their number not to take the drug but act as 'guide' to comfort and reassure when necessary. Bad trips characterized by acute anxiety, panic, terror or ideas of persecution are infrequent.

There is no physical dependence on LSD but the rewards of the trip may be so gratifying that the desire to take it again is very strong. For this reason psychological dependence occurs in a small minority of users.

PATTERNS OF ADDICTION
Discussion of drug addiction is, more than most other topics, guaran-

---

[1] *See* Chapter 28 for a description of these terms.

teed to arouse heated argument and produce strong polarization of views. Unfortunately the opinions held are not always based on facts, since often the facts are either not available or are distorted by the preconceived views of those who collect them. Much of what has been written about drug-taking is based on surveys of schoolchildren, students and those addicts coming to medical or legal notice. Almost certainly, none of these groups is representative of the whole drug-taking population and, while study of them has yielded much useful information, it would be foolish to extrapolate from them to drug-takers in general. It is difficult, however, to see how this deficiency in our knowledge can be remedied. For as long as drug-taking remains illegal, users, particularly those taking cannabis or other 'soft' drugs (the vast majority), will not openly discuss the subject. Probably the nearest one will get to an overall view of the misuse of drugs is that reported by researchers working within the drug-taking community and having the confidence of addicts. Even then the difficulties are formidable: a typical cross-section is probably impossible to obtain and study groups can only readily be formed by accumulating contacts over a prolonged period of time. The personalities of some of those under study may make them exaggerate or play down their activities.

Present knowledge suggests that early experience with drugs is probably on an intermittent basis and is confined to smoking cannabis or to taking small quantities of amphetamine, barbiturates, Mandrax or mild tranquillizers, often in conjunction with alcohol, at parties. Such sporadic use may stimulate some individuals to seek to repeat the experience on a more regular basis. Cannabis is the drug most commonly taken first and the one which is used most widely but probably only a small proportion of users confine themselves to this drug alone. LSD and amphetamines are the most popular other drugs but it should be appreciated that the great majority of cannabis smokers also use tobacco and alcohol. LSD is not used frequently by cannabis users, the trip being regarded by many as a special event.

Smoking cannabis has for some time been regarded as the first rung on the ladder to addiction to opiates and cocaine, although the evidence for this is slim. Cannabis smoking is generally a group activity and so much of the response to the drug is determined by the behaviour of one's fellow smokers that it has been suggested that it is a social rather than a chemical experience. Moreover, many students and so-called 'middle-class bohemians' take care to time their use of cannabis so that its effects will not interfere with work, study and other responsibilities. These groups often dissociate themselves from the injection of drugs, but 'fixers' may be attracted to such gatherings and pressurize others into experimenting with heroin and other more dangerous drugs. There is evidence, however, which suggests that those who experiment with

injecting drugs probably only do so a few times and it is a small minority
that adopts this method regularly.

A survey of 60 male addicts attending a treatment centre revealed that
all had used cannabis, amphetamines and nonbarbiturate sedatives at
some time in the past. Between two-thirds and three-quarters of them
had taken hallucinogens, barbiturates, heroin and methadone, but only
half cocaine. The pattern of daily use in the month prior to study was
considerably different, however, with only a third using barbiturates,
amphetamines, heroin or methadone. Most addicts tend, therefore, to
use selected drugs on a regular basis though anything may be tried if
needs dictate or if others are available. The concomitant use of alcohol
and tobacco is usual.

The group of addicts mainlining drugs regularly, particularly opiates,
has been written about extensively and further discussion of the 'junkie'
and his total preoccupation with the acquisition and use of drugs is unnecessary. Some mainliners manage to stop these drugs and cope with
the withdrawal symptoms on their own initiative or with medical help
but, of those who come to legal or medical attention, some 30 per cent or
more are still taking opiates 4–7 years later. Recent studies of US servicemen in Vietnam revealed a high incidence of narcotic addiction but
only a small proportion of these addicts continued using drugs during
the first year of repatriation. Although it is clearly too early to be entirely satisfied about these figures, they are, at least, encouraging.

Characteristics, Background and Lifestyle of Addicts
The great majority of those who misuse drugs are between the ages of 20
and 35 and men outnumber women by about three to one. Whereas
addiction to opiates and cocaine is largely confined to London and, to a
lesser extent, other large cities, the use of cannabis is probably much
more widespread. One community study suggested that students and
'middle-class bohemians' were more likely to confine their drug-using
to cannabis whereas a wider and more dangerous range of drugs, with
injecting, was more likely to be utilized by low-status unemployed or
manual workers. Most early experiences with drugs are the result of
curiosity, pressure from peers, abnormal personality or simply a search
for excitement, pleasure or relief from anxiety. It must be emphasized,
however, that social disintegration is not inevitable with the regular use
of drugs. Many habitual cannabis users function entirely satisfactorily
in the community, and even some opiate addicts are maintained on a
relatively small dose which fluctuates but little and either enables the individual to lead a stable and useful life or does not prevent him from
doing so.

Most addicts are of average or above-average intelligence yet,
whether because of immaturity, impulsiveness, liability to sudden

swings of mood or some other factor, they do not reach the levels of achievement that society expects. Their performance at school may be poor, truancy is frequent and they tend to leave at an early age, often only to drift from one job to another. Their personalities and their relative inability to cope with stress are important factors in producing dependence on drugs. Illness in the home is not uncommon and the family background tends to be disturbed in that many of them are illegitimate, have an institutional upbringing or come from homes broken because of the loss of one or another parent – usually the father. Even if the family is apparently intact, the disharmony between parents may be such that the home environment is no less detrimental than if the family were dissolved. Perhaps not surprisingly, addicts are frequently involved in delinquency even before starting on drugs.

A recent study of the lifestyles of addicts revealed four main types. Junkies' lives were characterized by a poor work record and considerable involvement in criminal and other activities associated with the addict subculture. On the other hand, those who have been termed 'stables' did not associate with addict groups and had a legitimate income from regular employment; involvement in crime was rare in this group. 'Two-worlders', as the term suggests, seemed to bridge the gap between the conventional and addict populations, in that individuals in this class associated with other addicts and become involved in criminal activities despite having incomes from regular employment. The last group, 'loners', were solitary people, cut off from both the addict and conventional societies. They were not involved in crime and were usually unemployed and dependent upon the state for financial support.

Addiction and Crime
About 70 per cent of addicts attending drug treatment centres have received a court conviction at some time in the past and it has often been questioned whether this high incidence can be attributed to drug dependence. The evidence is conflicting. Of 60 consecutive new male attenders at a London treatment centre almost half had been convicted before starting drugs and 90 per cent subsequent to drug use. Larceny, motoring and violence offences are common before and after drug use, with drug offences comprising an important proportion once dependence is established. Convictions after drug use were no more frequent in those whose first conviction antedated drug use than among the others convicted for the first time after starting on drugs.

Likewise, 60 per cent of a group of female addicts in prison were first convicted prior to addiction. A high proportion went on to commit further offences over the next few years and, in the majority, this paralleled continued drug use. It has been suggested, therefore, that addiction does not lead to crime but that both activities merely reflect the abnormal personality and disturbed social backgrounds of the individuals concerned. Not infrequently the father, or more commonly a sibling, of an addict may have been convicted for some crime. This, together with parental loss, tends to be commoner in those addicts whose criminal activities antedate their use of drugs.

While the majority of offences committed by addicts involve drugs or damage to property, several studies have shown an increase in the incidence of violent offences and offenders after drug use. Moreover, in one report, the nature of the offences became more serious involving, among other crimes, assault, offences with weapons, bodily harm and robbing with violence. There is no evidence that women not previously involved in prostitution become so after starting drugs.

THE MEDICAL HAZARDS OF DRUG MISUSE

The misuse of any drug carries risk to health. Most adverse effects, however, are relatively mild and may depend more on the personality of the user and his emotional reaction to the drug than on the toxic effects of the drug itself. Thus, some individuals may be unable to cope with the expected effects of a 'normal' dose and become sufficiently alarmed and disturbed in their behaviour to refer themselves to hospital or be taken there by friends. More commonly, arrival at casualty departments is the result of an emergency ambulance call or because they attract the attention of the police. Others end up in the same situation by having misjudged the amount of drug they have taken.

Despite the regional variations that may exist in patterns of drug misuse, some idea of the more common problems can be obtained from a report of 252 adult admissions (189 individuals) to an Edinburgh hospital during 1971 and 1972 because of adverse reactions to drugs taken 'for kicks'. Only 45 per cent required some form of medical care and all but 8 per cent were discharged within 24 hours. Because half the drugs involved were either barbiturates (some taken intravenously) or Mandrax, serious impairment of consciousness was present on 30 occasions. Fortunately none of these patients died and, with one exception, all were conscious within 12 hours. Bad trips after LSD are a common cause of referral to hospital.

There is no doubt that one of the major risks of drug misuse is accidental overdosage. With stimulant drugs, as indicated earlier, death is uncommon. On the other hand overdosage with depressant drugs may result in deep coma, possible obstruction of the respiratory passages, gradual failure of respiration, shock and death. If such patients reach hospital alive these problems can generally be dealt with effectively and mortality is low.

Some deaths associated with heroin misuse are due to accidental overdosage resulting from the variable potency of 'street' drugs which, depending on the ease of availability, may be adulterated to a greater or lesser extent with other materials such as milk sugars, talc and quinine. These additives in themselves may cause serious problems when injected intravenously. Fortunately, an antidote to opiates exists and most of the life-endangering effects of an opiate overdose can be dramatically reversed within seconds. No such antidote, however, is available for the treatment of barbiturate overdosage nor can the popularly misused varieties be eliminated from the body more rapidly by using artificial kidneys or other techniques. There is no alternative at present but to maintain the airway and respiration as indicated, if necessary using mechanical aids, until such time as the body degrades and eliminates the barbiturates and the patient returns to consciousness. The duration of coma may be several days and complications such as respiratory infections add considerably to the risks. It is no coincidence that barbiturates have been implicated in the deaths of a substantial number of addicts.

Many of the other important medical complications of addiction are primarily attributable to the injection of drugs. At every stage the preparation of the fix is totally lacking in sterility; the drug is frequently in a form never meant for injection, the water in which it is dissolved may at best be obtained from a tap or at worst from a public lavatory and the equipment used to hold the solution and strain it may be no more than socially clean. The same comment could be applied to many of the syringes and needles used. It will be obvious, therefore, that bacterial and virus infections are common and may be transmitted from one person to another because of sharing of 'gear'. Most of the bacterial infections occur at injection sites with abscess formation, skin ulceration and inflammation along the course of veins resulting in the formation of clot on the abnormal vein lining (thrombosis) and obliteration of the channel.

Infection on the heart valves and abscesses in the lungs may also occur and, although the multiplication of bacteria in the blood stream may potentially cause infection anywhere, there is a particular predilection for joints. A specific virus infection of the liver with jaundice (hepatitis) is not uncommon and may be transmitted from one individual to another by infected needles.

As the veins on the arms and hands become obliterated from repeated use and infection, those in the legs are usually next to be attacked but eventually no vein, regardless of its situation, is sacrosanct. It is not unknown for those on the breasts, tongue, penis and around the anus and vagina to be used by desperate addicts. Extremely dexterous as many are in injecting tiny veins, occasionally an artery is 'hit', leading to thrombosis and gangrene of the fingers or feet; amputation may be necessary.

Although death from accidental overdosage and infection is common, suicide is several times more frequent among addicts than in the general population. A review of 66 Holloway addicts after 5 years showed that 10 (15 per cent) were dead at an average age of just over 22 years. Another study of 108 opiate addicts 6–7 years after notification showed a mortality of at least 18 per cent (some could not be traced).

However much one tries to place the problem of addiction to opiates and barbiturates in perspective, the seriousness of the illnesses to which mainliners are prone and their apparently high mortality to some extent clarify the anxiety of many concerning the possibility of escalation from so-called 'soft' drugs such as cannabis.

CONTROL OF DRUGS

For as long as drugs have been used, measures to control their use or availability have been advocated or introduced. In the fourteenth century an Arab ruler extracted the teeth of those guilty of chewing cannabis; coca was denounced by the Catholic Church in the sixteenth century and peyotl by the Inquisition a few decades later. James VI of Scotland on ascending the English throne increased the tax on tobacco by some 4000 per cent in the hope of reducing its use. There is little evidence, however, that these measures met with any more success than did the prohibition of alcohol in the United States earlier this century.

As far as the United Kingdom is concerned, morphine and heroin addiction were the subject of review by the Rolleston Committee (1926) whose recommendations were incorporated into the current legislation on dangerous drugs. There was little activity from then until 1958 when the Brain Committee was convened to consider whether any change in legislation or facilities should be made in view of the increased number of potentially addictive drugs used to relieve pain and of developments in the treatment of drug addiction. It was concluded that the problem of addiction in Great Britain was very small, that special treatment centres and registration of addicts were unnecessary and that extension of statutory powers to control new drugs was not needed at the time. The recommendation that addiction be regarded as an expression of mental disorder rather than a form of criminal behaviour is still accepted and has been of paramount importance in determining attitudes and in fashioning legislation on drugs.

Between 1959 and 1964, however, the drug misuse situation changed sufficiently for the Brain Committee to be reconvened in order to consider whether its earlier advice should be revised. The total number of known addicts had risen by about 300 and the number of heroin addicts had increased fivefold. Cocaine addiction had also increased and concern was expressed at the trend towards much younger addicts. The problem was found to be largely confined to London and the main source of drugs was overprescribing by six doctors, one of whom was alleged to have prescribed about 600 000 tablets of heroin for addicts during 1962. Two others had written single prescriptions for 1000 tablets. The Committee now accepted the need for control measures and recommended that heroin and cocaine for addicts should only be prescribed by the medical staff of special treatment centres which were to be established. Notification of addicts was also advised. Overall, most of the earlier decisions were reversed and the new recommendations formed the basis for various items of legislation up to and including the Misuse of Drugs Act 1971 and its subsequent regulations which came into effect in 1973.

The desirability and effectiveness of legal control of drugs have been often questioned but are difficult to assess. Official statistics, including the number of addicts notified to the Home Office and convictions for drugs offences, are generally considered to underestimate seriously the extent of drug misuse. This is partly supported by the results of a study of 66 people from the south of England who were convicted for their first drug offence between 1967 and 1970 and were followed-up after 3 years. Only 18 had been reconvicted for a drug offence but it was learned from other sources that 49 (74 per cent) were still taking drugs, usually having restarted them within 6 months of their first conviction. Moreover, the pattern of subsequent drug-taking was more serious than would have appeared from the drug involved in the first offence. Whereas only 1 of the original convictions involved opiates, 22 individuals later used these drugs and, of 33 cannabis offenders, 10 were taking opiates and 11 were injecting some drug. Conviction for a drug offence therefore appears to have little deterrant effect and criminal statistics are a poor index not only of the extent but also of the pattern of drug misuse.

Chapter 25

Medico-legal Aspects of Alcohol

THE greatest social significance of alcohol rests on its being a drug of dependence. It has been estimated that there are some 90 000 alcoholics in Great Britain and the position is particularly serious in Scotland. Alcohol is a cortical depressant. Since it is the higher and the most recently evolved brain functions which are first affected by depressants, the immediate effect of a dose of alcohol is to inhibit those cerebral functions which are associated with orderly community behaviour and with finer critical judgements; an illusion of cerebral stimulation is thus precipitated. Chronic alcoholism, however, almost inevitably leads to physical and social degeneration, inability to retain employment, disruption of the family and the like, followed by generalized cerebral deterioration. Dependence is often of extreme degree and the high cost of alcoholic drinks has two major effects – firstly, increasingly cheap and, concurrently, toxic forms of alcohol are consumed and, secondly, there is often a lapse into petty criminality designed to obtain and conserve supplies. The criminal alcoholic who develops has to be distinguished from the intoxicated criminal – that is, the person with criminal inclinations which are potentiated by consumption of alcohol.

While the distinction between the sporadic and the compulsive drinker is emphasized in this section, alcoholism as a disease state will be discussed in detail in Chapter 28; the present concern is, in the main, to discuss the association of acute alcoholism with injury and sudden death and the resulting legal consequences.

PHYSIOLOGY OF ALCOHOL

Alcohol is absorbed rapidly from the stomach and especially by the upper intestine – if the stomach empties unduly fast, as in persons who have had certain surgical operations, absorption is likely to be more rapid and the effects more obvious; conversely, the commonly observed 'sobering' effect of a full stomach is probably due to delayed emptying. Once absorbed, the alcohol is dissolved in the body water and distributed according to the water content of the tissues – thus, the blood, in which there is much solid material, contains less alcohol, volume for volume, than does, say, the cerebrospinal fluid. The amount of alcohol in the body is expressed in the United Kingdom in terms of milligrams of alcohol per 100 millilitres of blood.[1]

The greater part of the ingested alcohol is destroyed by the liver. Approximately 10 per cent is excreted in the urine, sweat and breath. The combined effect of destruction and elimination is to reduce the blood alcohol by a variable amount which approximates to 15 mg/100 ml blood/hour.

Since alcohol diffuses uniformly in the body fluids, it will be present in the urine which is formed in the kidneys. But as urine contains very little solid material, there will be more alcohol per 100 ml of urine than per 100 ml of blood and, in order to compare the two fluids, a ratio of 1·3 : 1·0 is usually accepted. This, however, assumes that the urine and blood are in equilibrium, and this cannot be so in practice because urine is isolated and stored in the bladder. The nearest one can get to equivalence of blood and urine is to empty the bladder and test the smallest amount which can next be voided naturally – a matter of some 20 minutes' excretion by the kidneys. Direct comparison of urine and blood has been found to be so inaccurate that few forensic medical experts would nowadays be prepared to make the attempt – results are given either as urine alcohol or as blood alcohol. Breath, however, is another matter, as the alveolar air is in immediate contact with the blood in the capillaries; theoretically, a constant breath/blood ratio should be achieved and this is accepted as approximately 1 : 2000. Again, however, it is difficult to make a direct comparison in practice because an inconstant amount of a breath sample will be tidal air which has not been in contact with the blood – the proportion which is true alveolar air cannot be judged with certainty. The breath cannot, therefore, be used as a direct measure of the precise quantity of circulating alcohol in the body.[2] On the other hand, it is quite feasible to use it in an easily performed screening procedure on which to justify more accurate but more complicated tests.

It will be seen that the amount of alcohol present in the blood at any time is determined by many more factors than the simple measure of the quantity ingested. It depends on the method of dosing, on the rate of absorption, on the available water for distribution – which is reflected in the body weight and stature – and on the capacity of the liver to metab-

---

[1] In all the EEC countries, the expression is in grams per litre ('Promille'); the result is that the bald number quoted in the United Kingdom is 100 times that quoted for a similar concentration on the Continent.

[2] The recommendations in the *Report of the Departmental Committee on Drinking and Driving* (F. Blennerhassett, Chairman), London, HMSO, 1976, indicate that this view does not now hold. Breath analysers are now available which are of sufficient accuracy to replace the conventional blood test.

olize the dose. It is, therefore, surprising that the courts often require that an estimate of the amount of alcohol consumed be derived from the reported blood or urine level – only a very wide approximation can be given in the context of normal social drinking. As a consequence, it is common practice to assess only the *minimum* alcoholic intake likely to correspond to the analytic finding and, for this purpose, the tables prepared by the British Medical Association are generally acceptable to the courts.[3]

The expert witness will also be asked what was the likely practical effect of a given blood concentration of alcohol. Again, the answer to this can only be given in wide terms. Much depends on the conditions for drinking, the availability of food etc; there is also no doubt that habituation to alcohol occurs – the reason for this not being entirely clear – and the same blood concentration will have a lesser effect on the regular drinker than on the novice. However, the following table represents an acceptable average assessment:

10–100 mg/100 ml: Loss of self-control, an increase in self-confidence, talkativeness and alterations in judgement.

100–200 mg/100 ml: Distinct loss of skill, slurring of speech and commencing loss of coordination.

200–300 mg/100 ml: Loss of equilibrium, decrease in pain sense, marked disturbances in vision.

300–400 mg/100 ml: Increasing dissociation, stupor and probably coma.

400+ mg/100 ml: Coma (with its attendant hazards such as hypothermia) and possible death.

These are, however, subjective criteria. Objective measurements show that even low concentrations – of the order of 50 mg/100 ml – cause a lengthening of the reaction time in response to a complex situation and a decrease in visual function. If one adds to this the impulsive psychological effects, there is good reason to suppose that the most dangerous person on the roads with respect to alcoholism is the man who is only moderately intoxicated; while he is not able to react in an emergency in the normal way, he is, at the same time, unable to appreciate his deterioration in performance.

Such subtle changes are not disclosed by normal clinical tests – probably only those with a blood level of more than 150 mg/100 ml are detected as being unfit to drive by this means. Most countries have accordingly settled on holding it an offence to drive or to attempt to drive a motor vehicle when the proportion of alcohol in the blood exceeds x mg/100 ml; the figure x is variously defined – in Ireland it is 125 mg/100 ml; it is 80 mg/100 ml in Great Britain.

---

[3] *Relation of Alcohol to Road Accidents.* (1960) London, British Medical Association.

Alcohol is of medico-legal significance in relation to accident, suicide, homicide and natural death. The first of these, which includes the topic of road traffic legislation, is by far the most important.

AIRCRAFT ACCIDENTS AND ALCOHOL

A momentary digression to aircraft accidents is excusable in so far as they illustrate an important point in relation to alcoholism.

Table III. INTOXICATING LIQUOR AND THE GENERAL AVIATION
PILOT IN 1971

Fatal accidents studied for ethanol	256
Number positive (more than 15 mg/100 ml)	52 (20%)
15–49 mg/100 ml = 25%	
50–99 mg/100 ml = 12%	
100–149 mg/100 ml = 21%	
150 mg/100 ml+ = 42%	

The proportion of 'Ethanol Positives' has remained stable since 1968 and the proportion of accidents with ethanol 50 mg/100 ml or more is fairly stable. However, the proportion of accidents with ethanol 150 mg/100 ml or more is higher since the introduction in 1970 of an 8-hour abstinence period before flying.

It is not generally appreciated that, just as in the case of cars, a proportion of light aircraft accidents are alcohol-associated. The figures shown in *Table III* are extracted from a survey of such accidents ending fatally in the USA.[4] The fact that 13 per cent showed alcohol concentrations which would be significant in any circumstances is, in itself, interesting. However, the authors of the study noted that since the Federal Aviation Authority had introduced a regulation forbidding private flying within 8 hours of alcoholic intake, the proportion of fatal accidents associated with a *very high* blood alcohol had, in fact, risen. Only one conclusion is possible – that there is one cadre of drinkers who are amenable to reason and regulation – that is, the social drinkers; at the other end of the scale lie the hardened alcoholics who are indifferent to moral or punitive measures. The same thing probably occurs in motorists[5] and it is difficult not to infer that, if there are two classes of offender, there should, on general criminological grounds, be two types

---

[4] Ryan L. C. and Mohler S. R. (1972) Intoxicating liquor and the general aviation pilot in 1971. *Aerospace Med.* 43, 1024.

[5] Witness the study by McCarroll J. R. and Haddon W. (1962) A controlled study of fatal automobile accidents in New York City, *J. Chron. Dis.* 15, 811, in which 4 per cent of a controlled accident group had a blood alcohol in excess of 250 mg/100 ml, which must indicate a flagrant disregard of consequences.

of penalty.[6]

It is an offence to fly anywhere any aircraft registered in the United Kingdom or any other aircraft within the United Kingdom while under the influence of drink or drugs so as to impair the capacity of the crew member to do so.[7] Surprisingly, there is no authority to test the biological fluids of living pilots for alcohol content comparable to that which exists in regard to drivers of automobiles.

MOTOR VEHICLE ACCIDENTS AND ALCOHOL

There is abundant evidence that alcohol is a potent source of automobile accidents. The results of four well-controlled surveys are summarized in *Table IV*; although the figures differ in degree, the association of accidents with rising alcohol concentrations is clearly reproducible. Some minor interest attaches to the consistent finding that very small amounts of alcohol actually reduce the accident rate. It is submitted that this does not represent a beneficial effect of alcohol but rather that persons who know they may be at risk are at particular pains not to be discovered.

The current United Kingdom (excluding Northern Ireland) legislation on drinking and driving is contained in the Road Traffic Act 1972 which repeals the whole of the Road Safety Act 1967. Section 5 prescribes the offence of driving or attempting to drive a motor vehicle on a road or other public place when unfit to drive through the action of drink or drugs; Section 6 makes it an offence to drive or attempt to drive 'having consumed alcohol in such a quantity that the proportion thereof in the blood . . . exceeds the prescribed limit at the time the specimen is provided.[8] Refusal to provide a specimen when charged under Section 5 may, unless reasonable cause is shown, be treated as supporting any evidence given on behalf of the prosecution (s. 7), but the conditions defining refusal are very clearly laid down and allow for the provision either of blood or of two specimens of urine, the first of which is disregarded for the reasons discussed above. The procedure for screening by a breath test is detailed in s. 8 but a person whose ability to drive properly is for the time being impaired may be arrested without a breath test (s. 5(5)).

All specimens must be divided into two portions, one of which is

---

[6] Indeed, the Blennerhassett Committee (*see above*) acknowledges this. Much of the subsequent section may be irrelevant if the recommendations of this Committee are put into force.

[7] Air Navigation Order 1974, Article 45(2).

[8] The current prescribed limit means 80 mg/100 ml of blood; 107 mg/100 ml urine is regarded as equivalent (s. 12(1) and (4)).

given to the accused (s. 10(5)), and all analyses must be carried out by an 'authorized analyst' as defined in s. 10(7). Although there seems some

Table IV. ALCOHOL AND TRAFFIC ACCIDENTS

Approximate band of alcohol concentration (mg%)	Ratio of accident/non-accident drivers			
	I	II	III	IV
0–50	0·7	0·8	0·3	0·9
50–100	3·3	1·3	2·4	1·5
100–150	8·7	2·1	10·2	4·0
Over 150	33·1	8·1	41·8	18·0

The figures have been modified from the following reports: *I.* Holcomb R. L. (1938) *J. Am. Med. Assoc.* **111**, 1076. *II.* Lucas G. W. H. et al. (1955) *2nd. Int. Conf. Alcohol & Road Traffic, Toronto,* p. 139. *III.* Vamosi M. (1961) *Traff. Saf. Res. Rev.* 4.8. *IV.* Borkenstein F. et al. (1964) *The Role of the Drinking Driver in Traffic Accidents.* Indiana University Department of Police Administration.

doubt as to the absolute need for the use of a particular analytical apparatus, the amount of blood which must be provided is correlated with the amount needed for gas chromatographic analysis (*see* Chapter 26). The doctrine of *de minimis* – that something is too small to be taken notice of – is specifically nonapplicable to the Road Traffic Act; it follows that great responsibility rests on the analyst when dealing with blood or urine concentrations which are only slightly above the prescribed limits. Using the gas chromatograph, a skilled analyst should provide results which show a standard deviation of no more than 2 per cent from the actual concentration. To be absolutely safe, a possible scatter of three standard deviations is accepted. Thus, whenever a result is 100 mg/100 ml or less, an amount of 6 mg/100 ml is automatically deducted; above 100 mg/100 ml, the deduction is 6 per cent of the actual figure. The result is then expressed as 'not less than [the corrected figure]'[9]

The use of a motor car is almost essential for the discharge of many professions and the obligatory disqualification for driving consequent upon conviction for driving or attempting to drive with a blood alcohol concentration in excess of the prescribed limit can be draconian in its effects – it is not surprising, therefore, that a mass of case law has been

[9] For a simple exposition of accuracy in analysis, *see* Walls H. J. and Brownlie A. R. (1970) *Drink, Drugs and Driving*, London, Sweet & Maxwell, Ch. 7.

built up on the basis of all conceivable methods of outwitting the statute – so much so that textbooks have been devoted to the subject;[10] it would be invidious to attempt to select illustrative instances for inclusion here.

One aspect – that of what constitutes reasonable excuse to provide a specimen – is, however, of sufficient interest to both the medical and legal professions to merit comment. The Act (s. 7(2) and s. 9(5)) lays down the ground rules – for a person to be said to have refused a specimen there must be refusal to provide a blood specimen; there must then be refusal to provide the proper urine samples; and, finally, a second invitation to a blood test must be rejected. It is not, however, necessary for the police officer to specify the precise conditions.[11] The criteria for 'reasonable excuse' would seem to be very strict – 'no excuse can be adjudged reasonable unless the person from whom the specimen was required was physically or mentally unable to provide it or the provision of the specimen would entail a substantial risk to his health';[12] this last condition will be most obviously fulfilled when the person concerned is in hospital and his doctor objects that the provision of the specimen would be prejudicial to the proper care or treatment of the patient (s. 9(2)). If the conditions for reasonable excuse are not met the question can, as a matter of law, be withdrawn from the jury; otherwise, it is a matter of fact for decision. One can imagine certain conditions – for example, a severe skin disease or a horror of injections – which might constitute good reason for not wishing a needle prick; but there is always the possibility of providing a urine specimen, the legal importance of which is considerable. It has been held that failure to provide a urine specimen even after three unsuccessful attempts had been made by the police surgeon to obtain blood – a thoroughly unpleasant experience – still did not qualify as a reasonable excuse.[13] Insistence upon giving a blood specimen from part of the body other than that specified by the police surgeon would be regarded as refusal to provide a specimen.[14] Moreover, one cannot consent to the removal of the specimen by a doctor of one's own choice yet refuse the offices of the police surgeon.[14] But once a specimen has been provided, it is perfectly proper for the accused to refuse to give a second one; neither the police nor the police surgeon can retrieve a technical error made by them.

Charges under the 1972 Act can still be made without the use of a blood or urine test (s. 5) and this will always apply when there is a possibility of driving under the influence of drugs. In this case, a medical

[10] Strachan B. (1973) *The Drinking Driver and the Law*, London, Shaw & Sons, is indispensable reading in this context.

[11] R. v. Pursehouse [1970] R.T.R. 494, C.A.

[12] R. v. Lennard [1973] R.T.R. 252.

[13] R. v. Harling [1970] 3 All E.R. 902, C.A.

[14] Rushton v. Higgins [1972] R.T.R. 456, D.C.; R. v. Godden [1971] R.T.R. 462, C.A.

examination must be undertaken and the results of this are certainly open to the court as matters of fact; police surgeons do have, as a point of policy, a standardized form of examination and reporting which eliminates much argument. Fortunately, these cases are now very rare.

Perhaps the function of the clinical examination which has the greatest medico-legal significance is not so much the detection of alcoholism as the exclusion of other causes of abnormal behaviour – head injury or disorders of carbohydrate metabolism spring immediately to mind. The distinction is even more important when the subject is being detained in custody on account of apparent drunkenness for reasons unconnected with motoring offences; death of a person in detention dictates a Coroner's Inquiry with jury in England and Wales and will precipitate a Public Inquiry in Scotland (Fatal Accidents and Sudden Deaths Inquiry (Scotland) Act 1976, s. 1(1)(a)(ii)).

Studies of pedestrians killed in road traffic accidents indicate a very similar pattern of alcohol association to that shown by drivers. *All* persons killed in traffic accidents should be examined post-mortem for evidence of alcoholic intoxication; the fact that a killed pedestrian was drunk to the state of muscular incoordination should be available to the defence of a driver.

ACCIDENTAL DEATH OF OTHER TYPES ASSOCIATED WITH ALCOHOL

Consumption of sufficient alcohol to remove the constraints of normal care is very often associated with accidental firearm injuries.[15] Theoretically, the level of blood alcohol might be expected to be of diagnostic significance in this connection. Reported results are, however, equivocal, some authors having noted that a high proportion of suicidal gunshot wounds are alcohol-associated, and there is no reason why a drunken argument should not end in a shooting. The finding of alcohol in a victim of a gunshot incident is but one piece of evidence to be assessed in conjunction with the findings discussed in Chapter 9.

Other accidental deaths associated with alcohol are directly related to the more severe physiological effects. At a level of about 200 mg alcohol/100 ml blood, a loss of equilibrium will be superimposed on inhibition of the critical faculties. Falls from heights, particularly out of windows, are likely to be precipitated and it may be extremely difficult to establish the total innocence of the death in conditions of group alcoholism; very little force will be required to overbalance an intoxicated person and any minor marks sustained in a mêlée might be obscured by,

---

[15] Before issuing a Firearms Certificate, the Chief Constable must be assured that the applicant is not of intemperate habits (*see* Chapter 9).

and would certainly be difficult to differentiate from, the effects of terminal impact. Similarly, drowning is associated with alcohol particularly in docks or canals beside which the less uninhibited would be wary of walking and where the high sides make escape from the water very difficult. The author has, however, been impressed by the high incidence of artefactually-raised blood alcohol levels (*see* p. 332) in cases of drowning and this possibility should be excluded before a firm association is accepted in individual cases.

Stupor is likely at higher blood levels and this is a very common underlying cause of death from burning, a cigarette dropped from the hand setting light to the bedclothes; many such deaths are due to the synergistic effects of alcohol and carbon monoxide poisoning. Other forms of carbon monoxide/alcohol deaths include the situation in which the subject 'passes out' in front of a carboniferous source of heat which burns with decreasing efficiency. Overlaying of small children while in alcoholic stupor is fortunately uncommon now that adequate housing is more widely available; it is an offence both in England and Wales and in Scotland for a responsible person to be drunk while in bed with a small child (*see* p. 250). At comatose levels, hypothermia constitutes a major hazard, the physiological protection provided against the cold by constriction of the peripheral blood vessels being countered by the pharmacological action of alcohol; the man who lies down in a field on a cold night on the way home after a drinking bout is at great risk. At even higher levels of intoxication, accidental death may be due to no more than the action of the alcohol itself; this may well be the tragic ending to the 'dare' or race to drink an entire bottle of spirits which, if done rapidly, can elevate the blood alcohol level to an order of 600 mg/100 ml.

The problem of asphyxia due to inhalation of aspirated stomach contents has been discussed in Chapter 13; while many experts are sceptical, the author believes massive inhalation of vomit to be a genuine cause of death which is particularly associated with intoxication by drugs or alcohol.

SUICIDAL ALCOHOLISM

Deliberate suicide through the use of spirits which are ordinarily consumed must be extremely rare though it has been reported. There are, however, two other aspects which are relevant. Firstly, suicide may well be effected by the consumption of toxic alcohols of which ethylene glycol, available mainly as antifreeze, is the most probable. Secondly, ethanol is most commonly associated with suicide when both alcohol and drugs, particularly barbiturates, have been taken together. There is no doubt that an additive effect occurs – indeed, the action of very many drugs is enhanced by alcohol – and many apparent suicides may be accidents which are due to sheer ignorance of the possible consequences. Others have suggested that these deaths are accidental in that the subject, who is accustomed to taking a hypnotic as a routine, fails, in a state of alcoholic confusion, to distinguish the number of capsules he or she is taking; this seems unlikely. Many such deaths are undoubtedly suicidal but, even then, it is doubtful if the alcohol component is taken with deliberate self-destructive intent; it is more probable that a state of alcoholic depression contributes to the suicidal frame of mind. These distinctions have become of less importance since the passing of the Suicide Act 1961.

One form of alcoholic suicide, which probably occurs more often than is recognized, is the deliberate contrivance of a vehicular crash while under the influence of alcohol. In a case investigated by the author, a man with flying experience and of unstable personality had a series of altercations with his family and, on being left alone, went to an airfield where he borrowed a light aircraft; he crashed after 60 minutes flying which was observed to be of progressively more dangerous character. A broken half-bottle of spirits was discovered in the wreckage and the post-mortem blood alcohol level was 313 mg/100 ml. Similar cases have been reported by others both in aircraft and in motor vehicles. The function of the alcohol in these tragedies is probably of two types. Either it is consumed in the certainty that it will ultimately precipitate an accident – a type of subconscious guilt transference; or the alcohol consumed merely serves, deliberately or otherwise, to inhibit a normally dominant moral rejection of self-destruction.

ALCOHOL AND SERIOUS ASSAULTS

The most obvious association of alcohol with serious assaults is the typical 'pub brawl', so liable to end in a fatal stabbing. Such cases raise the question of diminished responsibility due to acute alcoholism. The major decision on the point has held that drunkenness cannot excuse or mitigate homicide except when the accused was so drunk as to be incapable of forming an intention to kill or do serious injury; if the latter condition holds, the case is one of manslaughter or of culpable homicide.[16] These conditions were fulfilled in *R. v. Donoghue* in which a drunken man stabbed his friend thinking him to be a dummy; he was

---

[16] D.P.P. v. Beard [1920] A.C. 479. Gordon states that the decision in this case has been adopted in Scotland (*The Criminal Law of Scotland, p. 359*). A very recent report, however, indicates that this may not be so (*The Scotsman,* 4 June, 1977, pp. 1, 6). The press account suggests that the offence in Scotland would be one of involuntary murder.

convicted of manslaughter.[17] The law is, however, strict; it has been said that the Homicide Act 1957, in introducing to England the concept of diminished responsibility due to abnormality of the mind (s. 2), was neither intended to be, nor was it, a charter for drunkards.[18]

The interpretations of the relationships between alcohol and the specific assault of rape which are made in England and Wales and in Scotland are discussed in detail in Chapter 21. Such considerations apply both to the state of the victim and of the rapist.

Rape is an example of a crime which may involve the type of injury likely to cause death from vagal inhibition of the heart. As discussed elsewhere (p. 152), an association has been noted between such deaths and a state of alcoholism, generally of moderate degree only, in the victim. There is little doubt that the finding of a level of, say, 150–200 mg alcohol/100 ml blood in a fatality resulting from an assault – particularly one involving the neck – could be taken as supporting a claim by the assailant that the death was unexpected.

Excessive alcoholic intake is positively associated with the currently widespread assaults of baby- and wife-battering. In criminal proceedings, the general principles derived from *Beard's* case would almost certainly apply and alcoholic intoxication would have to be recognizable as insanity if it was to be used as a successful special defence – the insanity could be either temporary or permanent by reason of alcoholic brain disease; otherwise, any mental or pathological condition short of insanity is relevant only to the question of mitigating circumstances and sentence.[19] The same thinking would apply both in England and in Scotland. As to civil litigation – e.g. in divorce proceedings based on cruelty – it is doubtful if even true alcoholism would provide a defence for a husband accused of inflicting cruelty upon a wife in a divorce action.[20]

ALCOHOLS OTHER THAN ETHANOL

Alcoholic addiction is not confined to ethanol intended especially for human consumption; unusual preparations containing alcohol – such as cheap eau-de-Cologne – are often used, while hand lotions and rubbing alcohols can be ingested; the alcohol involved is isopropyl alcohol which is more toxic than is ethanol.

The main alcohols other than ethanol which are of medico-legal significance are methanol (methyl alcohol) and ethylene glycol. The latter

---

[17] Simpson K. (1954). *Police J.* **27,** 110.

[18] Donovan J. in R. v. Dowdall, *The Times,* 22 January, 1960.

[19] Clyde L. J.-G. in H.M.Adv. v. Cunningham 1963 J.C.80.

[20] *See* Simpson K. (ed.) (1965) *Taylor's Principles and Practice of Medical Jurisprudence,* 12th ed., Vol. 1., p. 465.

requires only a brief mention – it is the basic ingredient of many anti-freezes and produces much the same effects as does ethanol but in far more exaggerated form. There is severe involvement of the central nervous system and death in coma is to be expected when more than 100 ml is drunk. There may be severe damage to the kidneys in the event of survival from the immediate effects.

Methyl alcohol is absorbed in the same way as is ethyl alcohol but it is metabolized far more slowly by the liver. As a result there is a cumulative effect in addition to its inherent toxicity. Methanol is used in industry and is a constituent of some antifreezes but it is most generally available as 'methylated spirits'. Industrial methylated spirits, consisting of ethanol with 5 per cent methanol added, is widely used in medicine and can be obtained from pharmacists on a written order by medical practitioners, laboratories and the like; not more than one pint can be dispensed to a patient at any one time and the container must be marked 'for external use only'. The ordinary household equivalent is known as mineralized methylated spirits which is 9 per cent methanol in ethanol with added disgustants and colouring matter.

A blood level of 80 mg methanol/100 ml is dangerous, the toxic action being twofold – the body is rendered severely acidotic and there is depression of the central nervous system. Methanol almost specifically affects the eyes and, even if a generally toxic dose is survived, visual impairment of permanent or temporary nature, or even complete blindness, may persist. Very occasionally, methanol poisoning is caused by the use of lotions containing the substance but, in general, it results from either involuntary or voluntary ingestion. Involuntary ingestion is associated with drinking ordinary commercial spirits which have been deliberately or accidentally contaminated. The writer was once confronted in the Second World War by a body of foreign combatants who had visited a 'strip club' the night before – all were suffering from temporary methanol-induced loss of vision. Voluntary 'meths' drinking – often in association with a cheap source of palatable ethanol – is a resort of many impoverished alcoholics; there is no doubt that some habituation to methanol, similar to that seen in ethanol drinkers, must occur. The sale of methylated spirits is controlled in Scotland where it can be retailed only by authorized sellers under similar regulations as apply to Part II poisons.[21]

ALCOHOL AND DISEASE

Alcoholism is associated with disease both directly and indirectly.
Direct association is represented by disease of the mind – alcoholic

---

[21] Methylated Spirits (Sale by Retail) (Scotland) Act 1937.

dementia – and by conditions which are primarily centred on the gastro-intestinal system.

Alcoholic dementia – of which the most prominent examples are Korsakov's psychosis and delirium tremens – is of little direct medico-legal importance other than as to testamentary capacity. It is sufficient only to emphasize that crime committed while suffering from such conditions is clearly committed within the legal concept of insanity. In addition to causing mental disturbance, alcohol also has a direct toxic effect on the peripheral nerves (alcoholic peripheral neuritis).

Alcohol associated gastro-intestinal disease may be of relatively minor character, such as the so-called alcoholic gastritis which is a degenerative process in the stomach lining rather than a true inflammation. This condition may lead to malabsorption of essential foodstuffs; an unsatisfactory diet may compound a deficiency of protein and of vitamins. Coincidentally, there is degeneration of the liver of fatty type with, ultimately, fibrous destruction of the liver tissue; the condition of alcoholic cirrhosis is established and this may well be fatal.

Indirect association of disease with alcohol is of little medico-legal significance. Most examples stem from the inhibition of higher critical faculties; thus, sexually-transmitted disease is often mediated alcoholically while unwanted pregnancies contracted under the influence of alcohol may pose problems in relation to legal abortion.

There is a distinction in the medico-legal disposition of alcohol-associated deaths in England and Wales on the one hand and in Scotland on the other. In the former, the mere mention of alcohol in the death certificate – e.g. liver failure due to chronic alcoholism – would dictate reference of the case to the Coroner by the Registrar. There would appear to be no such obligation on the Procurator Fiscal in Scotland unless the death was sudden and unexpected – as, for instance, an accidental death associated with acute alcoholism.

ALCOHOL AND THE DOCTOR

Alcoholism represents a main reason for disciplinary action against doctors and dentists by the General Medical and Dental Councils.

The subject is discussed in greater detail in Chapter 30. Any court conviction of a medical or dental practitioner will be reported to their respective disciplinary bodies. Proven motoring offences are reportable and convictions under the Road Traffic Act relating to alcoholism will certainly result in warning letters if not more serious reaction. Less commonly, but certainly more seriously, professional negligence resulting from alcoholism virtually 'speaks for itself' and will inevitably result in a complaint to the GMC or GDC. In the extreme case, alcohol may be the factor which precipitates a prosecution for criminal negligence. A doctor, above all persons, should be able to appreciate the likely effect of alcohol on his clinical judgement and expertise; in the case of a medical practitioner convicted of delivering an obstetric patient while under the influence of a drug (chloral hydrate), the judge, in passing sentence of 3 months' imprisonment, indicated that a much more severe sentence would have been passed had alcohol been proved to be the cause of the prisoner's condition.[22]

---

[22] R. v. Wight, quoted in Rentoul E. and Smith H. (1973) *Glaister's Medical Jurisprudence and Toxicology*, 13th ed., p. 13.

Chapter 26

Methods and Limitations of the Toxicology Laboratory*

THE role of the toxicology laboratory is to provide information about the nature and amount of any poisons which may be present in the body during life or after death. The word poison here is taken as meaning any noxious substance as well as including an excess of what is generally regarded as a 'normal' substance in the body, e.g. insulin.

For the detection of poisoning, the clinician or pathologist provides the toxicologist with biological specimens the nature of which is determined by the circumstances. In life, it is generally possible only to obtain specimens of blood, urine, vomit and faeces. The pathologist who performs the post-mortem examination can, in addition, provide organs and other body fluids, the most useful of which are liver, bile, kidneys, brain and lungs; the intestinal contents can also be fractionated. Each of these samples is placed in a separate and suitably-labelled container. The best containers are glass, screw-capped jars but, for economic reasons, plastic bags are now commonly used for all samples except blood and urine. Proper labelling is important to ensure continuity of identification. In respect of blood (and sometimes urine) two samples should be provided for the toxicology laboratory. One contains a 'preservative', the other has 'no preservative'. The reason for this is that some poisons, e.g. alcohols, may either be produced in blood which has been exposed to yeast spores in the air or they may be destroyed during decomposition after death. The 'preservative' used in the case of blood is usually sodium fluoride; phenyl mercuric nitrate is used for urine. The sample without preservative is taken in case the added preservative may interfere with other parts of the analyses. It is important that the samples be sent to the laboratory without delay to avoid possible loss of volatile poisons such as cyanide. It is to be noted that any material inside the alimentary tract should be regarded as being 'outside' the body and that, although a large amount of a poison may be detected in, say, the stomach contents, it does not necessarily mean that sufficient of the poison has been absorbed into the body to have caused death. For proof of this, the poison must be shown to be present in

---

* By H. V. Street, DSc, PhD, FRIC, FRCPath.

321

lethal amounts in one or more of the body organs or 'internal' fluids.

Requests for analysis of samples may be made in three different ways depending on the amount of relevant information available in the case being investigated. The first is where the evidence points to a particular drug (or drugs) having been ingested. An example of this type would be where the toxicologist is asked to examine the specimens for the presence of barbiturates and alcohol, and to estimate the amount of these drugs if they were found to be present. Note that a distinction is made here between qualitative analysis, which deals with identification of the poison, and quantitative analysis, which is concerned with estimating how much of the poison is present.

The second type of request asks that a particular group (or groups) of drugs be searched for in the analysis. It is here that the difference between pharmacological and chemical analytical classifications of drugs must be emphasized. *Table V* gives a list of some substances arranged in both ways. The pharmacologist and the medical practitioner classify drugs according to the effect they will have on the body. The analytical chemical toxicologist, however, lists drugs according to the chemical functional group(s) which each may possess. These two types of classification are by no means the same. For example, a request may be made to the toxicologist to search for the presence of tranquillizers. Now, although the drugs which come into this category have a similar pharmacological effect, they may have widely different chemical properties. Chlorpromazine and meprobamate are both tranquillizers but they bear no resemblance to each other from the viewpoint of analytical chemistry. It will be seen, therefore, that a request for a particular pharmacological group of drugs usually involves a search for a wider variety of chemical types than is apparent from the simple demand.

The third type of request is where no information at all about the nature of any poisons present is available. This is the toxicologist's 'general unknown' or 'drug scan' which obviously requires considerably more analytical time than do the first two groups. The narrower the field covered by the request, the more rapid can be the answer. Much unnecessary effort and frustration can be avoided if there has been close cooperation to this end between police, pathologist and toxicologist. The experience of the pathologist is also important not only as to limiting the number of poisons to be sought but also in determining the need for any toxicological investigation. In some countries, lack of such expertise leads to large numbers of nonspecific requests for analyses with consequent accumulation in the laboratory of specimens awaiting analysis. In some places, the backlog is anything up to three years! Proper training and close cooperation are, therefore, essential.

Before discussing methods of analysis, it may be of value to lawyers to

refer to Appendices M and P which explain some of the nomenclature of
weight, capacity, wavelength, etc. used by the toxicologist. The analysis

Table V. CLASSIFICATIONS OF DRUGS

Pharmacological	Chemical
Tranquillizers	(Necessary for systematic analysis)
Narcotics	Acids
Hypnotics	Bases
Anticonvulsants	'Neutrals'
CNS Stimulants	Amphoterics
Antihistamines, etc.	Phenols
	Phenothiazines
	Carbamates, etc.

The pharmacological properties of two drugs may be similar but their chemical constitution is different (*see text*).

itself may be seen as involving four separate stages. These are isolation,
purification, identification and quantitative assay. In some procedures
there may be an overlap between one or more of these stages. The main
purpose of this section is not so much to teach toxicology as to explain
to the lawyer the meaning of some of the terms which may be used in
reports.

ISOLATION

The analysis is started by separating the drug or poison from the tissue.
It may be extracted by an organic solvent or it may be distilled; in either
case the tissue protein may be first removed by precipitation. This is a
crude separation since substances other than drugs, e.g. natural body
constituents, may be co-extracted. The main point of this stage is to remove the protein–fat complex of the tissue. The particular procedure
used will depend on the nature of the drug being sought. In the 'general
unknown' type of analysis, it may be necessary to use several isolation
procedures.

As was seen in *Table V*, the toxicologist classifies the drugs according
to the presence or otherwise of chemical functional groupings. Broadly
speaking, these are of four types: acidic, neutral, basic and amphoteric.
The acidic drugs are further classified into 'weak' and 'strong' acids.
Neutral drugs display neither acidic nor basic properties. Basic drugs

include the natural alkaloids, a very large number of synthetic drugs such as the amphetamines and most of the tranquillizers. Amphoteric drugs, such as morphine, possess both an acidic and a basic group. By making the tissue sample acidic or basic (by adding an acid or an alkali) the analyst can control which drugs will be extracted into the organic solvent. This explains one of the difficulties encountered in the analysis of morphine in tissues. Because the drug behaves both as an acid and as a base, precise control of the balance between acidity and basicity is essential if extraction is to be successful.

PURIFICATION

This is really an isolation procedure. But whereas isolation usually refers to the separation of drug and other materials from the protein matrix of the tissue, purification generally means separation of the drug from other materials of a similar nature. The whole idea behind the analysis is to obtain the drug in as pure a form as possible so that impurities will not interfere with the tests carried out. In modern toxicological analysis, the purification step is usually carried out by some form of chromatography.

Separation of a mixture by chromatography depends on the fact that, if substances are encouraged to move over a 'stationary phase', the extent of their movement in the 'mobile phase' will differ according to their composition; the slower movers can then be separated from the faster. Reference may be made in reports to four types of chromatography: liquid, paper, thin layer and gas chromatography. The lawyer will not require to know the procedures involved in the majority of these but, briefly, liquid chromatography involves pouring a liquid containing the supposed drug through a powdered solid medium, a process which can be hastened by the use of high pressure; in paper chromatography, an organic solvent is allowed to flow over filter paper impregnated with water or vice versa; and in thin layer chromatography, the filter paper is replaced by a layer of an adsorbent such as alumina or silica gel. Provided the test conditions are standard, each dissolved drug will move a constant distance in relation to the substrate in which it is dissolved. This is known as its R_f value. The toxicologist can obtain a guide as to the identity of the unknown drug by comparison with tables of R_f values which have been prepared for the great majority of drugs. He will then repeat his experiment using an authentic sample of the suspected drug for comparison. Although all forms of chromatography have their particular uses, none is more valuable in the drug field than gas chromatography; it deserves fuller description.

Gas chromatography is the most useful of all forms of chromatography in current use, although high-pressure liquid chromatography may prove to be more valuable in the future. But each has its own particular merits and, ideally, the toxicology laboratory should possess equipment to carry out both types of chromatography. The high-pressure equipment is, unfortunately, currently very expensive.

The basic difference between gas chromatography (GC) and other forms of chromatography lies in the use of a gas to carry the test substance. The stationary phase may be either a solid (gas-solid-chromatography) or a liquid (gas-liquid-chromatography, GLC). The apparatus used in GLC is shown in diagrammatic form in *Fig.* 19. Carrier gas (usually nitrogen) is passed through a metal or glass tube (called the column) containing the liquid phase which has been deposited (prior to packing the column) on to a suitable, powdered solid. The column is kept in an oven, the temperature of which can be controlled. Nitrogen emerging from the column passes through a detector, the electrical signal from which is amplified and fed into a recorder. The pattern appearing on the recorder is called a (gas) chromatogram. The mixture to be separated is introduced (usually by syringe) into the gas stream just prior to the gas entering the column and is swept on to the column where the components of the mixture are separated. The

Fig. 19. Schematic diagram of gas chromatography.

signals representing these separated components are presented on the recorder chart paper as a series of peaks, as shown in *Fig.* 20. The time interval from the point of injection to the top of a peak is called the retention time (t_r) which, under standard conditions, is a constant and allows tentative identification by reference to standard tables. The term relative retention time (Rt_r) is sometimes used and refers to the t_r of a particular substance related to the tr of a 'standard' substance. Rt_r has no dimension and enables t_r values to be compared under less standard conditions, e.g. on a GC apparatus in another laboratory. The factors which affect the results obtained by GC are more controllable than those of other forms of chromatography and, hence, these results are more reproducible and reliable. Gas chromatography has a greater discriminating power not only between compounds of widely different size and physico-chemical properties but also between closely related chemical species; it is the most sensitive of chromatographic techniques currently available.

IDENTIFICATION

When the drugs have been separated from the biological matrix and from each other, it then is necessary to identify them. As seen above, chromatography may provide one parameter of identity through the R_f or t_r value. But to be 'reasonably' certain of identifying the drug correctly, at least two criteria are required. In some cases it is possible chemically to manipulate the isolated drug to form a new compound (derivative) which may have different R_f and t_r values. Or, use may be made of other physico-chemical properties of the drug. Techniques used in this connection include Ultraviolet (UV) Spectrophotometry, Infra-red (IR) Spectrophotometry, Mass Spectrometry (MS) and many others. The commonest of these, mainly because it is the cheapest, is UV Spectrophotometry, which makes use of the fact that when UV light is passed through a solution of certain drugs, the drug molecules absorb more light at certain wavelengths than at others. The UV spectrophotometer is a device which records on a moving paper chart how much radiation these drug molecules absorb at different wavelengths. This record is called the 'ultraviolet spectrum' of the drug. It is often loosely termed the 'absorption curve' or simply the 'UV curve'. The wavelength range for these instruments is usually from about 210 nm to 400 nm. *Fig.* 21 shows a typical UV spectrum for amylobarbitone in a solution of dilute aqueous ammonia. The wavelength at which the curve exhibits a maximum value is characteristic of certain groupings of atoms (functional groups) within the drug molecule and, again, can be compared with standard tracings for identification purposes. It is to be noted that the

UV absorption curve is not unique for the drug molecule as a whole but only for the functional groups which the molecule may possess. For example, the UV curve for amylobarbitone is the same as that for pentobarbitone because both drugs have a common functional group. The drugs differ in that they contain other (different) chemical groups which do not materially affect the UV absorption spectrum which alone does not distinguish amylobarbitone from pentobarbitone. UV spectrophotometry is very useful for assaying the amount of drug present (as will be seen later) and, at the same time, suggesting the presence of a particular type of barbiturate.

Infra-red spectrophotometry is similar to UV spectrophotometry except that, as the name implies, the radiation used is in the infra-red region of the electromagnetic spectrum (about 2500 nm to about 50 000 nm). The IR absorption spectrum is more characteristic of an

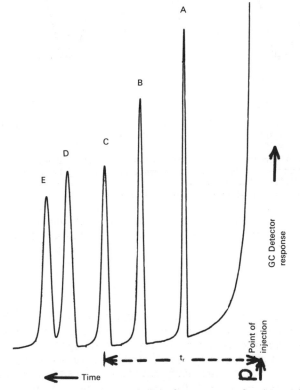

Fig. 20 Gas chromatogram showing resolution of components of a mixture of substances A, B, C, D and E. P = point of injection into the apparatus; t_r = retention time of substance C.

individual compound than is its UV spectrum and, for this reason, it is often used to identify a particular drug by providing a 'finger-print' spectrum.

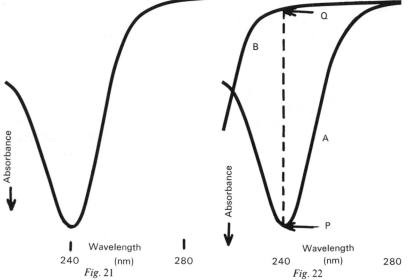

Fig. 21. Ultraviolet absorption curve of amylobarbitone in dilute ammonia solution. Note that the maximum absorption occurs at 240nm.

Fig. 22. Ultraviolet absorption curve of amylobarbitone in (A) dilute ammonia solution and (B) in acid solution. Note that the absorption maximum in (A) disappears when the solution is acidified. The difference in absorption in these two solutions at 240nm (i.e. PQ) is proportional to the amount of barbiturate present.

For details of other techniques used in identification of isolated drugs, the reader is referred to standard textbooks of toxicological analysis.

QUANTITATIVE ASSAY

Once the drug has been identified, the next stage is to find out how much drug is present. In this connection, some of the techniques used for identification purposes may be used quantitatively. Two such examples will be given. Firstly, UV spectrophotometry may be used to assay some drugs, e.g. the barbiturates. Reference to *Fig.* 22 shows that curve A is the UV curve given in *Fig.* 21 for amylobarbitone, in ammonia solution. Curve B is the absorption spectrum obtained when this same amylobarbitone solution is acidified with sulphuric acid. It will be seen that the peak, which occurs at 240 nm in ammonia, disappears in acid solution; the difference PQ in the amount of absorption at 240 nm in the two solutions is proportional to the amount of barbiturate present. Secondly, gas chromatography can also be used to estimate the amount of a drug present in a particular solution. In this case, it is usual to add a known amount of a standard substance to the sample at the start of an analysis. Such a substance is called an internal standard and is usually closely related chemically, but distinguishable from, the drug being investigated. This internal standard is taken through the whole analytical procedure. Comparison is thus made internally, as distinct from externally as is the case when reference is made to a standard result obtained on some previous occasion. At the present time, one of the most widely used methods for the analysis of alcohol in blood or urine employs gas-liquid chromatography with an internal standard of another alcohol, namely propyl alcohol (known to the chemist as n-propanol). The amount of alcohol injected into the gas chromatograph is proportional to the area under the curve displayed on the recorder chart. This area is usually measured electronically by means of an integrator[1] attached to the recorder, which prints out the area as an arbitrary number. The amount of alcohol in the original sample can be calculated by comparison with standard alcohol solutions.

Ideally, in the processes of isolation and purification, the whole of the drug present in the original tissue sample should be recovered. This state of affairs never occurs in practice. It is necessary, therefore, to perform experiments with drugs added to tissue samples to determine how much drug is 'lost' in the analytical process. These are often called recovery experiments. It is important to distinguish between apparent recovery and absolute recovery. If an internal standard is added at the start of the analysis and the amount of drug found is related to the amount of internal standard recovered, then this is termed apparent recovery of the drug. If for example, the extraction process recovered only half the amount of drug present and only half the amount of internal standard, the recovery would appear to be 100 per cent. But the absolute recovery of the drug was only 50 per cent because half was lost.

In quantitative work, there are two terms which require to be clearly defined. These are 'accuracy' and 'precision'. The accuracy of a determination is the concordance between it and the true or most probable value. The true value of a quantity cannot be determined experimentally, so that the result obtained must always be compared with the most probable value. Precision may be defined as the concordance of the results of a series of analyses of the same substance whether the re-

---

[1] When an integrator is not available, it may be permissible to use the height of the peak (in place of the area) which, provided the curves are 'reasonably' symmetrical, is also proportional to the amount of alcohol injected.

sults are accurate or not. Note that precision always accompanies accuracy but that a high degree of precision does not imply that the results are accurate.

OTHER ANALYTICAL METHODS

The above description of the analytical steps leaves out several important procedures which have to be used for poisons which do not fit into the general scheme for drugs. Some of the 'heavy metals' – arsenic, antimony, bismuth, mercury and silver – can be detected quite simply by immersing a clean piece of copper wire or foil in the acidified (with hydrochloric acid) sample and heating the mixture at 100° C. The foil is inspected after half an hour and 1 hour. A black deposit on the copper may indicate the presence of one or other of the above metals. This is the Reinsch test. A more sophisticated way of detecting (and estimating) a large number of toxic metals makes use of the expensive apparatus known as an Atomic Absorption Spectrometer, which utilizes the property of elements in a gaseous state to absorb energy at characteristic wavelengths. This type of spectrometry is very useful in assaying metals present in trace amounts in the presence of large quantities of other elements. It is thus of particular value in pollution and other environmental problems.

Toxic inorganic anions, such as chlorate (present in some weedkiller preparations), oxalate, fluoroacetate, fluoride, nitrite, etc. have first to be isolated from the sample by dialysis through a cellophane bag suspended (and often rotated) in de-ionized water.

Other poisons which do not fit neatly into the analytical scheme are:

i. Gases and vapours of highly volatile liquids which may be detected by gas chromatography using special columns.
ii. Carbon monoxide which combines with the haemoglobin of red blood cells to form carboxyhaemoglobin and which can be detected by spectroscopy. Carbon monoxide may also be separated and detected by gas chromatography but for quantitative work this requires, in addition, a separate determination of the haemoglobin content of the blood.
iii. Glycosides – such as digitoxin and digoxin, which are used as cardiac stimulants. These compounds are difficult to assay by 'ordinary' methods, but the recently-developed technique of Radio-Immuno-Assay is proving to be of great value in this respect. This method depends on the availability of radioactive forms of the substance being sought.

DIFFICULTIES IN THE LABORATORY

Most of the analytical problems in toxicology are really problems of extraction and stem from the fact that the poison being sought is hidden in a mass of tissue sample. In many cases, the toxicologist is searching for a few micrograms of drug in several grams of tissue, i.e. the ratio of weight of drug to the weight of tissue may be of the order of 1 to 1 000 000. Some of the newer drugs, such as phenothiazine derivatives, are bound so firmly to the protein-lipid matrix that 'ordinary' procedures fail to extract them in measurable amount. Recourse then has to be had to techniques which will release the protein-bound drug and which may destroy some of the drug itself.

Another problem is concerned with the presence of metabolites. The majority of drugs are altered in the body to varying degrees to form new chemical substances. These transformation compounds are called metabolites and represent the result of the body's efforts to make the drug less harmful. Metabolites are usually more water-soluble than the parent drug and are thus excreted more readily by the kidneys. The analytical problem here is that the metabolite may not be extracted with the parent drug and, as some metabolites are more pharmacologically active than the parent drug, difficulties in interpreting quantitative results may arise.

INTERPRETATION OF RESULTS

Some poisons, such as alcohol, are distributed fairly evenly throughout the body water. Having estimated the alcohol content of, say, a post-mortem blood sample, it is reasonably safe to assume that the same concentration will hold for the total body water (between 30 and 40 litres) thus enabling an assessment to be made of the minimum amount of alcoholic beverage consumed which would give rise to such a concentration. Other substances, e.g. imipramine (one of the so-called tricyclic antidepressant drugs), are found post-mortem to be distributed very unevenly throughout the body. Following a fatal overdose of such a drug, the liver may contain 30–40 mg of the drug per 100 g, whereas only 0·2–0·5 mg per 100 ml may be found in the blood. Such uneven distribution may lead to erroneous results when attempting to determine how much of the drug was probably consumed.

When the quantitative analytical results are finally obtained it then becomes necessary to decide whether such results indicate ingestion of

(a) a therapeutic amount of drug; or
(b) a fatal overdose of drug.

In order to make this decision, the results must be compared with figures obtained in fatal overdose cases either in the published literature or from the laboratory's own records. Difficulties arise here, firstly, from the fact that the analytical procedures in the published work may differ – and hence the accuracy may be different – from those used by the toxicologist himself and, secondly, because with newer drugs there is insufficient information available concerning fatal cases to enable comparisons to be made. If the toxicologist finds a level of a new drug which is higher than he would have expected from a therapeutic dose then, if no figures are available and no other cause of death has been found, it is reasonable to assume that the level found was a lethal concentration. The dilemma can only be solved on the bases of the circumstantial evidence and of consultation between pathologist and toxicologist.

PARTICULAR PROBLEMS OF POST-MORTEM BLOOD ALCOHOL ANALYSES

Many reviews involving post-mortem determinations of ethanol draw attention to the occurrence of certain artefacts.[2] Although the literature is confused, there is fairly widespread evidence that certain bacteria and yeasts can produce alcohol as part of their normal metabolism and that, prominent among these, are bacteria responsible for post-mortem putrefaction. Vehicular, and especially aircraft, accidents produce severe open injuries in which micro-organisms can flourish. Post-mortem enzymatic activity may also convert sugar to alcohol. There is, therefore, a potential for falsely raised blood alcohol values to be obtained using post-mortem specimens, and this applies particularly to those derived from accident cases; the possibility of artefact has to be taken into consideration when responsibility for the accident is being considered.

Experience has shown that a urine sample taken post mortem may be a more reliable qualitative index of antemortem intoxication than is blood but many courts are reluctant to accept quantitative urine evaluations. It has been recommended that, if a post-mortem blood analysis is to be interpreted with certainty, blood specimens should be obtained from three different sites in the body and that these should be tested by two gas chromatographic techniques; but it is doubtful if many laboratories abide by such counsels of perfection. These considerations apply only to putrefying blood specimens; in-vivo specimens taken from motorists are placed immediately in bactericidal containers and are extremely unlikely to show artefacts due to contamination.

---

[2] See, for example: 'Post-mortem alcohol', Lancet (1975) 1, 229.

THE TIME TAKEN TO PROVIDE A TOXICOLOGICAL REPORT

The requirement for a diagnosis is urgent in many cases of poisoning and it is important that those concerned with enforcement of the law should appreciate why this demand cannot always be met. Unless the poison sought is in a routine category, time may be needed to set up the apparatus and to prepare the necessary standards. The greatest cause for delay, however, rests in the often unavoidable indefiniteness of the request for analysis; the more specific the demand, the more prompt can be the answer.

The toxicology laboratory is also subject to logistical difficulties. The more trained staff available, the greater the case load which can be accepted. But adequate staff is dependent upon the availability of equipment of which even the most standard items are now very expensive. Much modern sophisticated apparatus, such as mass spectrometers, while being extremely useful for providing rapid and unequivocal results along with increased sensitivity, is beyond the economic potential of small laboratories. There is a strong case for concentrating analytical resources and manpower into major groups related to the demand for advanced technology. But in any event, an instant result is unobtainable and some delay must be accepted in the provision of analytical reports.

Chapter 27

Radiology in Forensic Medicine

RADIOLOGICAL techniques have many applications in forensic science. Amongst these may be included the examination of finger-prints and of documents. There is, however, no intention to discuss the purely scientific field in this section which is concerned to deal only with forensic medicine.

Forensic medical radiology falls into two functional categories – those investigations concerned with identification and those directed to diagnosis.

RADIOLOGY AND IDENTIFICATION

As described in Chapter 3, methods used for the identification of dead bodies may be, firstly, of a deductive nature. These are designed to indicate the type of person who should be sought in the missing-persons files; this approach is dictated when there is no clue as to identity. But once there is reason to suppose a personal identification, this is proved largely by means of comparative methods. Radiological assistance is invaluable in the former circumstance and has a very special place in the latter; only a few of those benefiting from a National Health Service have not been X-rayed at some time during their lives. It is noted, however, that current United Kingdom regulations require the retention of X-rays for five years only and there is no provision for microfilming.

Deductive Identification Methods

The age of a cadaver at death is particularly well estimated radiologically. In infancy and early childhood, the presence of centres of ossification can be demonstrated with accuracy and ease; the union of these centres can be observed in childhood and adolescence up to approximately 25 years of age; in later life, degenerative changes may give some indication of maturity, but this is only over a wide range – the chief value of X-rays of adult persons is to distinguish between two or three bodies who are known as a group but are of unknown individual identity. The main ossification details are given in Appendices F and G.

The sex of a mutilated or charred body can also be established with some certainty and without the need for extensive cleaning processes if

334

suitable bones are available for X-ray. The pelvis is by far the most useful bone in this respect (see p. 49).

Comparative Identification

Provided X-rays taken in life are available, any similar radiograph taken after death can be used for comparison. Identification can be based on similarities in either normal or abnormal structures; the value of the latter in positive identification is proportional to the rarity of the abnormality.

Of the normal structures routinely used for comparison, perhaps the skull sinuses – the frontal sinus in particular – are the most satisfactory; the number of variations in shape and size which are potentially available is so diverse as almost to make a radiographic outline unique to the individual; the problem is mainly one of obtaining an identical view in the cadaver to that available in life. If an adequate frontal view is not available, the general outline of the skull, including the shape of the pituitary fossa, may provide almost equally good evidence (Plate 19).

One particular form of comparison of the normal which should be mentioned is the process whereby a post-mortem X-ray is superimposed on a photograph of the living person. Again, the technical difficulties of obtaining a precisely similar scale and orientation are formidable but the method has been used with success in several classic cases of investigation of homicide.[1]

Abnormalities which may be of value are so numerous that only a few illustrations can be given. Congenital abnormalities such as absence of bones, displacement or malformation may be so rare as to be virtually diagnostic of identity. Others, such as fusion of the ribs, are not uncommon and should only be regarded as confirmatory of other circumstantial evidence. Pre-existing disease – in the form of changes in bone density, arthritic deformities and the like – may provide unequivocal evidence of identity of dead persons from whom films taken in life are available for comparison. Such opportunities are not confined to bone; unusual calcification – of tuberculous origin in the lungs or lymph nodes or due to degenerative changes in the uterus and many other organs – may show a pattern as individual as is that of a finger-print. The presence of healing fractures in sites known to have been broken in life would obviously provide strong confirmatory evidence of identification but, even more useful, is the presence of surgical prostheses or of supportive implants such as plates, pins or orthopaedic screws – not only can the X-rays be compared but the appliance can be removed

---

[1] R. v. Ruxton, 1936, Manchester March Assizes; see Glaister's Medical Jurisprudence and Toxicology, 13th ed., 1973. Edinburgh, Churchill Livingstone, p. 90.
R. v. Dobkin, 1942, C.C.C.; see Simpson K. (1974) Forensic Medicine, 7th ed., London, Edward Arnold, p. 34.

from the cadaver and superimposed. Surgical implants are of very great use in identification in the mass disaster situation; if, for example, one man is known to have a bone plated, it is simplicity itself to screen radiologically that bone in all unidentified bodies.

The importance of dental identification in both the single unknown body and in the mass has already been stressed. Dental radiography very greatly enhances the contribution of the odontologist. The mere presence of a single or double restoration in one or two commonly filled teeth would often be insufficient to prove a positive identification as opposed to an exclusion of identification. The precise shape of the fillings is, however, likely to be unique and it would not be impossible to make a reasonably certain identification from a comparison of post- and antemortem radiographs of a single filling. Dental radiography may also show up significant root shapes, socket outlines or abnormalities of tooth eruption, development or decay; it is the policy in the Scandinavian countries, among others, to record the dentition of their commercial aircrew radiographically as a routine.

Another useful adjunct provided by radiology in identification in the mass lies in the occasional localization of significant possessions which have been embedded in charred tissues; generally, this represents no more than a 'fringe benefit' of radiographic examination for other purposes – such as a search for injuries due to explosives – but it is, nonetheless, often of great value.

DIAGNOSTIC RADIOLOGY

Diagnostic radiological techniques are of value both in accidental and in criminal deaths.

Accidental Deaths
Accidental death is a major epidemic of modern times and is attracting increasing interest throughout the medical world; forensic pathology has a great part to play in satisfying this interest since all such deaths are investigated through the medico-legal system. It is doubtful if a busy forensic pathologist can be expected to demonstrate individually all fractures present following a fatal accident, despite the fact that some of these may be of research significance; routine X-ray coverage of accident cases simplifies the whole procedure. Moreover, some fractures – notably those of the spine – are difficult to demonstrate satisfactorily by post-mortem dissection. The prevention of spinal fracture in vehicular accidents is one of the main objectives of the bio-engineers; in some unusual procedures – such as escape by ejection from high speed aircraft – it is, perhaps, the main limiting factor to added safety. Ideally, the com-

plete autopsy in vehicular accidental death should include adequate radiography of, at least, the spine. X-rays may be of great assistance in distinguishing ante- from post-mortem fracture, an observation which may have profound significance in the reconstruction of both accidental and homicidal deaths. Finally, X-ray diagnosis is not confined to the study of bones; very useful information in relation to soft tissue changes can also be obtained.

Homicidal Death
The most obvious use of X-rays in potentially homicidal death lies in the demonstration within the body of bullets and other missiles (*see* Chapter 9). The technical difference between searching for a single bullet in a cadaver with and without the assistance of radiographic localization needs no emphasis; moreover, fragments of bullets or of bomb casings or contents can easily be missed in an unaided dissection; much important information might, thereby, be lost to the ballistics expert.

Hijacking of aircraft is a particular modern use of firearms. The diagnosis of sabotage has been discussed in p. 112; the possibility of demonstrating hijacking as a cause of a fatal accident would depend, to a large extent, on the finding of bullets in the crew members, a task which would be physically impossible to discharge with assurance in the absence of X-ray facilities. This particular aspect also highlights the importance of radiography in distinguishing a true shooting from artefact. *Plate* 20 shows bullets in the arm of a fatality from an aircraft which was carrying an important person and which was believed to have been shot down; the radiographic demonstration of percussion caps and fragments of cartridge case clearly shows that this appearance resulted not from criminal activity but from the explosion, during the post-crash fire, of bullets carried on the person of the V.I.P.'s bodyguard.[2]

The importance, both to the reconstruction of events and to the subsequent investigation, of localization of shot from smooth-bore weapons and of fragments of explosives has been discussed in Chapter 9. Any radiographs which have been taken for the purpose of investigation can be retained as permanent records and, if necessary, used as productions.

Other forms of homicide are also well illustrated in the form of X-rays. Particularly noteworthy is the radiography of the larynx in cases of strangulation; fractures of the thyroid cartilage or hyoid bone are generally well shown (*see Plate* 10).

Perhaps, however, radiography and radiology reach their apogee in the examination of suspicious infant deaths. X-ray examination in the non-accidental injury syndrome (discussed in detail in Chapter 20) does more than merely demonstrate the presence of fractures. Its particular

[2] Stevens P. J. (1970) *Fatal Civil Aircraft Accidents.* Bristol, Wright, p. 44.

value is to prove' the infliction of injury at various times – evidence which is essential to the concept of 'battering'. The X-ray picture can clearly demonstrate the difference between healing and fresh fractures and can often differentiate different periods of repair in the former. Attention has also been drawn to the possibility of indicating parental inattention to fractures sustained. Fractures unite by the elaboration of primitive bone known as 'callus'. The deposition of callus is particularly marked when the fracture has not been properly treated by immobilization.

Additionally, the radiologist may be able to demonstrate that a fracture has been caused in an unusual way – as, for example, by severe twisting. Such evidence strongly negates a defence, say, of an accidental fall.

X-RAY EXAMINATION OF THE LIVING

Industrial Diseases

The importance of X-rays in the assessment of dust diseases is discussed in Chapter 15. The diagnosis and assessment of disability due to coal miners' pneumoconiosis, being based on the distribution and size of pulmonary nodules, are virtually in the hands of the radiologist (*see* *Plate* 13b).

Angiography

Angiography or arteriography – the study of the arteries by means of X-rays – is performed by injecting radio-opaque material into a blood vessel and observing its subsequent movement and distribution. There are two major medico-legal applications of the technique.

Firstly, angiography of the cerebral vessels may be used as a test of brain death. It can be taken that a situation exists which is incompatible with function or revival of the brain if serial observations show the intracranial circulation to have been absent for 15 minutes; the permanence of the films provides lasting evidence of the fact of death and this method of establishing death is increasingly used in Continental Europe in relation to transplantation (*see* Chapter 12).

Secondly, angiography of the coronary arteries is achieving some prominence in relation to the diagnosis of disease of the coronary arteries in persons in whom sudden collapse poses a particular risk to public safety – the most obvious example is the commercial pilot. Although there have been no case decisions at the time of writing, there is the possibility that failure to diagnose arterial inadequacy prior to an accident attributed to such disease might result in a successful negligence suit and the diagnosis of coronary artery disease – as opposed to frank disease of the heart muscle – is impossible to make with certainty using current standard electrocardiographic techniques. Recourse to more specialized tests is sometimes indicated and the current position of coronary angiography in this situation seems to be as follows. Firstly, while the examination may show the presence of the disease, there is no certainty that the disease will prove fatal – in a recent series of observations, only 60 per cent of persons with 80 per cent narrowing of all three main vessels and, presumably, symptoms at the time of examination, had died from coronary heart disease 6 years after the test; the 6-year mortality for persons with obstruction of only one artery was 20 per cent. It follows that the test might unnecessarily prevent a competent person being properly employed; the risk would have to be balanced against the many other factors involved.[3] Secondly, the test is not without danger and has some mortality in its own right;[4] it follows that it would be quite unreasonable to suggest its use on a routine basis. In the writer's opinion, coronary angiography has presently no place in the *selection* of persons in high-risk occupations. It might well be useful in the evaluation of cases in which there was doubt of fitness on other criteria; but, if the doubt was sufficient to justify the investigation, common prudence would already have impressed the need for suspension from duty. When the test has been used along these lines, the specificity of results has been found disappointing.[5]

Routine X-ray Examinations and Negligence
Finally, it is noted that failure to make an X-ray examination in a case of head injury or in any other situation in which fracture might reasonably be anticipated might, in the circumstances of modern hospital practice, be difficult to justify no matter how full the clinical examination may have been.[6] The development of disability due to a fracture being undiagnosed for this reason would almost certainly result in an action for negligence; many cases would be indefensible. The same might well be so were the presence of a foreign body to remain undiagnosed. The

---

[3] It might, for example, be difficult to find an experienced airline pilot without some degree of coronary narrowing; the results of reducing the overall experience of airline pilots might well be worse than the risks involved in well-organized 'double-crewing' by older men.

[4] The overall incidence of complications is in the region of 8 per cent and the mortality lies somewhere between 0·3 per cent and 1·0 per cent. This applies to investigations performed on persons with symptoms; certainly, the risk in 'normals' would be expected to be less.

[5] Froelicher V. F. et al. (1973) The correlation of coronary angiography and the electrocardiographic response to maximal treadmill testing in 76 asymptomatic men. *Circulation* **48,** 587.

[6] *See* Nathan H. L. (1957) *Medical Negligence*, London, Butterworth, p. 45.

presumption of negligence is, however, by no means certain. Denning M. R.[7] is reported as stating, 'In some of the earlier cases the doctor had been criticized for not having taken X-rays with the result that they had sometimes been taken unnecessarily. This case showed that the Courts did not always find that there had been negligence because a patient had not had an X-ray; it depended upon the circumstances of each case'. There is no doubt that the increasing number of radiographic examinations must make a significant contribution to the total dose of radiation delivered to the population and, in general, there should be a genuine medical need to justify such an examination.[8]

THE HAZARDS OF RADIATION

The dose of X-rays given to an individual during a single diagnostic procedure is well controlled and the earlier complications, such as radiation skin burns, are now unlikely to be seen. Nevertheless, radiation used outside the field of clinical medicine may affect the genetic structures or the blood-forming tissues and represents a hazard which is growing in importance. Radiation injury of all types falls within the ambit of forensic medicine and has potential, even if not current, medico-legal importance.

Radiation is of two types – non-ionizing, which includes infra-red and ultraviolet light, and ionizing, amongst which are X-rays, gamma rays and cosmic rays together with particulate radiation due to alpha and beta particles. Non-ionizing radiations are not without danger. Extreme exposure to ultraviolet light undoubtedly predisposes to cancer of the skin (of basal cell or 'rodent ulcer' type). In the industrial field, long exposure to microwaves may result in cataract (or opacity of the lens of the eye) while laser workers may develop burns of the retina; such cases are rare but may multiply as the devices become increasingly used. Ionizing radiations are more important and owe their biological effects to an ability to alter the chemical properties of 'ionized' cells. The unit of X-rays is the röntgen but, from the point of view of their effects, all ionizing radiations are measured in terms of rad, 1 rad being the energy absorbed when 1 röntgen is received by 1 gram of tissue. In order to allow for variations in response, the biological effect on man is measured in rem (rem being the röntgen equivalent for man); for practical

---

[7] In Braisher v. Harefield and Northwood Hospital Management Group Management Committee, C.A. July 13, 1966. This case is quoted by Jellie H. (1966) *Lancet* **2**, 235; the author cannot discover the definitive reference. See also an older case – Sabapathi v. Huntley [1938] 1 WWR 817, where a similar view was held.

[8] The medico-legal dilemma is ably discussed by Jennett B. (1976) Some medico-legal aspects of the management of acute head injury, *Br. Med. J.* **1**, 1383.

purposes, a rad can be accepted as being the same as a rem.[9] For ease of description it can be taken that rapidly growing and multiplying cells are the most sensitive to ionizing radiation. The organs within the body most easily damaged are the bone marrow, the epithelium of the bowel, the testes or ovaries and the lymphatic glands. Similarly, children, because they are growing faster than adults, are generally more sensitive to radiation. External sources of radiation, other than those of natural origin, act in a relatively transient fashion. But a source of radiation which is bound to the tissues will exert a continuous influence until it decays. Such foci of radiation can come, firstly, from radioactive substances deliberately introduced into the body, almost invariably for medical diagnostic purposes. It is imperative that such substances decay rapidly, the rate being dependent upon the 'half life' of the radioactive element; the half life is defined as the time taken for half the available radioactive atoms to disintegrate. An alternative source of internal radiation is food which has itself been contaminated by external sources of abnormal radioactivity. The half life of such radioactive elements may be long and in certain cases, notably strontium 90 (which is chemically similar to calcium), the element is actually stored in the body; this type of radiation therefore constitutes a serious health hazard.

The effects of radiation will vary from person to person but, in general, it can be said that high doses, of the order of 500–1000 rem and above, will kill within a matter of weeks; medium doses may cause malignant disease, particularly of the blood, several years after exposure; and low doses may cause genetic damage to future generations. It is small wonder that radiation hazards are strongly controlled by legislation.[10] In particular, the amount of radiation sustained by workers in occupations associated with the hazard is monitored by sensitive devices such as film badges or thermoluminescent dosimeters; the maximum permissible dose for such workers is set by international regulation at 5·0 rem per year.[11] The corresponding permissible dose for the public at large is 0·5 rem per year, the difference being accepted as a safe compromise which allows for the use of radiation in an advantageous way. Both limits exclude exposure for the purposes of medical diagnosis or treatment.

As indicated above, the ill-effects of radiation are of two types. First-

---

[9] The main exception being in alpha particle radiation for which 1 rem ≡ 10 rad. It should be noted that the rad is soon to be replaced by the gray (≡ 100 rad).

[10] Apart from international agreements, British legislation is contained in the Radioactive Substances Act 1960, the Sealed and Unsealed Source Regulations (made under the Factories Act 1961) and in the Health and Safety at Work etc. Act 1974. The Radiological Protection Act 1970 established a National Radiological Protection Board.

[11] Standard set by the International Commission on Radiological Protection.

ly, there is the production of disease which may result either from the destructive effect of ionizing radiations or from their capacity to stimulate cells into abnormal activity and, thus, predispose to cancer. The tissue most commonly destroyed is the bone marrow, a process which leads to very severe anaemia; the lymphoid tissue is also sensitive to radiation and its destruction results in an increased susceptibility to infection. Manifest acute damage of this type is limited to the levels of exposure sustained in an atomic bomb explosion or in the treatment of cancer; nonetheless, increasing exposure to radiation carries with it an increased statistical risk of disease of those systems which are most sensitive. Cancer may be provoked in many sites by radiation – particularly in the blood (leukaemia), lungs and thyroid gland. Symptoms of the disease may be delayed for many years after exposure, a fact which may be of very great medico-legal importance in establishing a cause-and-effect relationship.

Classic industrial examples include cancer of the lung occurring in miners in radioactive mines, particularly in Central Europe, and the malignancies induced in painters of luminous dials. Blood dyscrasia – which would include leukaemia – due to ionizing radiation is a prescribed disease when related to exposure to electromagnetic radiations other than radiant heat or to ionizing particles; since anaemia virtually always accompanies leukaemia, the latter could also be held to be notifiable as a form of 'toxic anaemia' (Appendix K).

The second group of adverse effects results from genetic damage; alteration of the chromosomes in the gonads may be caused by direct ionizing damage or by an increase in the rate at which spontaneous changes occur – the process of mutation. The dose of radiation required to produce genetic change is certainly less than that needed to provoke cancer and, for all that is known at present, it may be very small. The effects of abnormal gene changes are also problematical. As discussed in Chapter 18, most harmful genes are eliminated and are certainly recessive. But should there be a sudden widespread increase in altered genes there would follow an increase in homozygous, clinically abnormal persons – the elimination of the harmful genes might then be difficult; it is encouraging that there has been no obvious increase in genetically controlled abnormalities in the cities of Hiroshima and Nagasaki since 1945.

Although there is no certainty that even small doses of radiation are completely harmless, any estimate of the hazard induced by man himself must be measured against a natural radiation of approximately 0·5 rad per year, a value which far exceeds any effects from artificial sources. The bulk of this stems from the ground itself and therefore differs in magnitude geographically. About one-quarter of the natural dose results from cosmic radiation which, arising in space, is filtered by the atmosphere. Its effect is, therefore, greatly dependent upon altitude and dictates specific shielding for astronauts; perhaps of more general concern, some form of premonitoring is needed in supersonic transport aircraft, although the risk of significant exposure of crew or passengers is negligible save during the cyclical spasms of solar hyperactivity. Internal radiation constitutes the third most important form of natural exposure and is due to the presence of infinitesimally small amounts of radioactive potassium which are present as a proportion of the total amount of that element in the body.

Of the artificial sources of radiation, the most dramatic is that derived from the detonation above ground of nuclear bombs or test devices. The explosion of a nucleur bomb results in a central zone of massive destruction surrounded by a wide area of lethal heat; beyond this is a circle of radiation which falls off in intensity from an original area in which a rapidly fatal dose is sustained. Additionally, radioactivity is displaced into the upper atmosphere, returning to earth with rainfall over a prolonged period; it is this type of radiation fall-out which gives rise to a persistent hazard as the radioactive elements, being taken up by plant life, become a source of internal radiation to animals and humans – the particular importance of strontium 90, which is stored in bone, has been mentioned.

The possibility of dangerous leaks of radioactivity from nuclear power stations has recently been receiving much publicity. Fortunately, there have been very few actual accidents and, in these, a significant dose was sustained only by those working close to the plant. The risk from nuclear power plants can, therefore, be looked at in two ways. Either it may be seen as providing a potential disaster situation, or one could compare the total adverse effect of even occasional accidents with the amount of disease and suffering resulting from the production of other sources of power, especially coal. Perhaps a far more worrying aspect of nuclear power is the ultimate effect on world-wide natural radiation of the disposal of waste products in increasing quantities – a problem which is more one of economics than of technology.

In practice, however, the most significant source of man-made radiation stems from its use in medicine as a diagnostic aid and as a form of treatment. The hazard to the population is proportional to the sophistication of its medical services and, while there is no real danger from this source provided reasonable precautions have been taken, all radiologists are deeply conscious of their responsibilities in this connection. In Britain, the radiation dose to the population resulting from the use of X-rays in medicine approximates to one-fifth of the natural background exposure.

Exposure to a diagnostic X-ray constitutes very little hazard to the individual patient – particularly when this is balanced against the advantages derived. Nevertheless, there are certain circumstances in which a decision to make such an examination would be taken only after careful consideration, the absence of which might well constitute negligence. These mainly concern pregnant women and the possible effect on the fetus; diagnostic pelvic X-rays are seldom taken in pregnancy and, during this time, the internal use of radioactive substances for the diagnosis of disease in the mother is contra-indicated. Only in emergencies should a radiological examination be made below the waist of a woman more than 10 days after her last menstrual period.[12] Nonessential X-rays of all types are always to be deprecated, perhaps not so much for their possible effect on the patient as for their contribution to the total population exposure.

The hazards of ionizing radiation used for medical purposes are, however, well understood and are controllable; it is the nonmedical sources of exposure which are likely to have an increasing medico-legal significance.

---

[12] *See* The ten day rule, *Br. Med. J.* (1975) 4, 543.

Chapter 28

An Introduction to Forensic Psychiatry*

THIS chapter is not, in the main, concerned with the origins of mental disorder or with details of treatment;[1] rather it seeks to show the way in which people may offend because they are mentally disordered and how they may be most humanely cared for and rehabilitated. It is based on the generally accepted medical model of mental disorder; the legal framework within which the psychiatrist has to operate is also outlined.

Within that framework, the psychiatrist engaged in forensic work has a number of tasks. His first is to identify those who offend because of mental disorder; his second is to advise the Court on the most appropriate disposal; and his third is to treat and rehabilitate the offenders. The treatment and rehabilitation setting may be penal, in hospital, in the community or a combination of all three.

Identification of the mentally disordered offender, particularly the adolescent, can be very difficult. Adolescents are typically rebellious and ranged against authority, questioning the standards and philosophy of their elders. This is normal and healthy. The activities to which this attitude can lead them may depend on their environment. Fifty per cent of all crime is committed by youngsters under the age of 21. Their characteristics are well known. They tend to come from large families, from broken homes, are intellectually under-average, have under-achieved at school and live in a criminogenic area where their only chance of acceptance by their peers – and adolescents are rigid conformists within their own group – is to join them and emulate them in their usually petty criminal activities. These conformist youth groups tend to form themselves into gangs and the end result may be more sinister than is petty crime. Most violent crime is committed by the 17–21 age group, closely followed by the 14–17 age group.

It would be absurd to see all of these youngsters as psychiatric cases in need of treatment. Disturbed, wayward and antisocial they may be, but the solution to their problems and the prevention of repetitious behaviour lies less in the province of psychiatry than in socio-political action to counter the effects of ghetto areas (including high-rise flats and

---

* By A. K. M. Macrae, MB, FRCPE, FRCPsych.

[1] An authoritative exposition of psychiatry written in popular terms is to be found in Stafford-Clark D. (1971) *Psychiatry Today*, London, Penguin.

housing schemes with no amenities), of labelling and of our present meritocratic society.

It would seem reasonable to regard as abnormal only those who do not have this background and yet offend, together with those who show an escalation in the type of crime they commit.

Clearly this is a 'grey' area and there are many others. Since an individual's personality and his reaction to the strains and stresses to which he is subject arise from a combination of his heredity, innate intelligence, parental attitudes and environmental influences, there must be situations where one or other of these factors assumes a dominant role. Most people have flaws in their personality due to failure at some stage in its development during their formative years. Where such failure to adapt has been serious, the resultant personality may be clearly abnormal. Such abnormal personalities include the dependent (always leaning on Mum, demanding attention and unable to come to any independent decision), anxious (seeking reassurance and prone to hypochondriasis), obsessional (parsimonious, punctual, pernickety, pedantic, always double-checking, rigid, methodical and meticulous, obstinate and stubborn), assertive (hectoring and domineering with considerable drive but without consideration for the feelings of others), or hysterical (extroverted, histrionic, manipulative, suggestible and emotionally shallow).

The psychopath, who represents the most extreme example of abnormal personality, deserves further consideration. It has long been recognized that there is a type of person who displays no sign of disorder of thinking, of mood or of intellectual deficit and yet whose actions are inexplicable in ordinary terms. Such people have been termed 'psychopaths' and this term is incorporated in the Mental Health Act 1959. Unfortunately, the term has been used so loosely in the last 50 years that it has lost any precise meaning and has been dropped from the International Classification of Diseases to be replaced by the term 'Personality Disorder'. Yet, provided fairly rigid criteria are used, a group of people is fairly easily identifiable as being, by any reckoning, abnormal and who are some of the most disturbed, disturbing and dangerous members of our society. Let us still call them psychopaths.

Basically, although they have reached adult stature and adult intelligence, they have not progressed beyond childhood in their emotional development. They are still child-like in their impulsive demand for the immediate gratification of their wishes – no matter the cost. They will tolerate no frustration and will meet any with aggression. They have no capacity to love or be loved and no conscience.

They are, consequently, totally egocentric, they cannot relate to others, they have no remorse or guilt for whatever they do, they act on impulse with no regard for the consequences and they are unable to learn from experience. They will lie, cheat, swindle or defraud, embezzle or thieve to gratify their immediate desires or, if frustrated, they will assault or kill. They can be superficially charming – 'flowers without perfume' – but are emotionally cold with no feeling for anyone. Their treatment and rehabilitation has been a recurring disappointment to the extent that the *Report of the Committee on Mentally Abnormal Offenders*[2] has finally come out with the statement that 'the psychopath is, in general, untreatable, at least in medical terms'.

They are a small group, yet among the most destructive and dangerous members of our society. They remain a major challenge in criminology and forensic work.

In times of stress, neurotic disorders such as hysterical conversion, anxiety and phobic and obsessional states arise from abnormal personalities. Although they are widespread and disabling illnesses, neuroses have few criminal effects. The commonest anxiety states do not lead to criminal actions; neither do obsessional states, although it is not unusual for a defence to claim that some criminal action – e.g. fire-raising, shoplifting, indecent exposure – has arisen because of an obsessive compulsion and to enhance this with a pseudoclassical term such as pyromania or kleptomania. The true obsessional often has fears of committing some criminal act but rarely does so. Those offenders who claim an irresistible compulsion are usually acting either for material gain or for a generally superficial emotional satisfaction.

MENTAL HANDICAP

This is the most severe form of developmental defect and combines defect of intellectual development with social maldevelopment. It has a number of synonyms – mental retardation, mental subnormality (as in the Mental Health Act 1959) and mental defect (as in the Mental Health (Scotland) Act 1960). Basically people thus handicapped, because of a failure of brain development from whatever cause, are unable to learn at the same rate as their fellows and, indeed, may not be able to learn at all. The most severely affected have a multiplicity of developmental defects, physical as well as mental, and do not survive long, even with expert nursing and medical care.

Our concern is with those whose deficiency is of a more limited nature. Most defectives are genial, law-abiding citizens who are protected by their families and their community; those with an emotionally or socially unstable background are most at risk. It is a hard life being a

---

[2] Butler, Lord (Chairman) *Report of the Committee on Mentally Abnormal Offenders* (1975) (Cmnd. 6244.) London, HMSO.

defective in such circumstances. Even those who can read, write and count money – and many cannot do these basic essentials – have a very limited comprehension of what society expects of them and of fundamental concepts of right and wrong. Their inability to learn means that they tend to repeat their wrongdoings. They are gullible and are used by their more intelligent companions as the 'fall guys'. The common crimes committed by defectives are shoplifting, theft and housebreaking. Two more serious crimes are often, but not exclusively, committed by defectives – fire-raising and sexual crimes.

The frustrated defective may set fires for vengeful reasons – and repeat the act. He may also do so for the excitement that a fire arouses. A mentally defective fire-raiser is constantly in danger of doing so again.

Sexual crimes committed by defectives are more complex. Their limited comprehension of moral values is fundamental – and this applies to both sexes. Female defectives are often superficially attractive and have no difficulty in satisfying their sexual drives. They become promiscuous and are only criminal when they engage in prostitution. Male defectives, on the other hand, are generally unattractive to the opposite sex and, even if they are physically acceptable, their lack of understanding causes them to be rejected by girls of their own age. Baulked of a normal sexual outlet they turn to children. If the children resent or resist their advances they may panic and kill them. In any circumstances, a defective may kill because of frustration or a lack of appreciation of what he is doing, particularly when alcohol, to which he is unduly susceptible, is involved.

One way of identifying the defective is to measure his Intelligence Quotient (I.Q.) – that is, to measure his performance in various tests against that which would normally be expected from a person of his age. If he performs up to the standard of his own chronological age, then his I.Q. score is 100; his I.Q. is above or below 100 to the extent that he falls below or exceeds that standard. It would be generally accepted that anyone with an I.Q. of 75 or lower would be regarded as defective, although some would put it as high as 80 and others as low as 70. However, this is only one measure of how the individual copes with his social surroundings; many other factors come into account and a measurement of intellectual ability alone cannot be decisive.

MENTAL ILLNESS

So far, we have been considering only those whose disability is the result of developmental failure. We now come to consider those whose development is relatively normal but who are overtaken by an illness. We are entering the sphere of the major psychoses, the serious mental affections where contact with reality is lost. We shall encounter some 'grey areas' here too, but the main syndromes are clear cut. They divide into two groups – those called *organic*, where there is some clearly demonstrable structural or biochemical damage, usually in the brain, and the *functional* where such damage, although suspected, has not yet been conclusively demonstrated.

Organic Psychosis

The key disturbance in the organic psychoses is a degree of confusion and clouding of consciousness, either transient (acute) or permanent (chronic). The patient does not know the time or place and misidentifies people (disorientation). His memory, short-term or long-term, is defective. Such a confusional state may arise from damage to the brain itself (by trauma, tumour, toxins, infection or vascular accident) or from systemic disease in other parts of the body which affects either the quantitative or qualitative supply of blood to the brain (e.g. congestive cardiac failure, hypoglycaemia, liver disease, vitamin or hormone deficiency).

The damage to the brain may be small and discrete and clinically interesting but, criminologically, it is only occasionally important. A lesion in the frontal lobes may totally change the individual's personality, making him asocial, tactless, fond of silly jokes and uncaring for the feelings of others; a lesion in the temporal lobe can produce not only epilepsy but also all the characteristics of the 'epileptic personality' (*see below*); other lesions in the region known as the hippocampus may produce an aggressive, assaultive individual.

These, however, are rare; the most common brain defects are due to diffuse processes occurring in old age including arterial disease, general degeneration or, more rarely, infection and trauma. These are, moreover, of most legal significance.

The normal process of ageing, whether or not complicated by minor arterial accidents (or strokes) leads to changes in the person's ability to grasp new ideas, in his memory (most commonly his recent memory) and in his personality. Personality characteristics tend to be exaggerated so that a person with a lifelong suspicious nature believes that objects he cannot find, because he cannot remember where he put them, have been stolen by some malevolent neighbour; he becomes a persistent nuisance to the police to whom he is always complaining. A person in such a senile paranoid state can be a source of embarrassment to his family, neighbours and local police. Another source of discomfiture is the process of disinhibition which accompanies the ageing process; the elderly man may rediscover an uninhibited sexual drive which may be directed towards children or expressed in exhibitionism.

Two areas where the individual's failing may have legal significance are shoplifting and testamentary capacity. An elderly person may take something from a shop without realizing that he has not paid for it. Only an expert examination may reveal a disturbance of memory which explains his action. As to testamentary capacity, it is important that the testator knows not only the extent of his property but also those who ought to have a claim on his bounty. Unfortunately these are questions that tend to be asked after the testator is dead; in such circumstances one inclines to the view that such clinical retrospection is not a medical function.

Acute brain damage, either from infection (encephalitis), trauma or deficiency of hormones or vitamins is unlikely to lead to any criminological problem. Long-term effects of infection such as that due to syphilis (general paresis) used to be important but are now very rare.

More important, nowadays, are the effects of trauma. Road traffic accidents, if not fatal, can lead to a range of disability from the totally disabled to the minimally brain-damaged. We are not concerned here with those who have a clearly demonstrable neurological deficit from actual brain injury but rather with those who have no such deficit and yet show a change of personality which may be attributable to their head injury. First, there are those who complain of the effects of the head injury upon themselves and, secondly, there are those whose behaviour after the accident gives rise to complaints by others.

The first group are variously described as suffering from postconcussional or postcontusional states or from compensation neuroses; they have certain characteristics in common. They have suffered a change from stable, outgoing personalities into nervous, apprehensive individuals, prone to severe headaches, intolerant of noise, emotionally labile and unable to follow their previous occupation. They have suffered a head injury in circumstances in which someone else or some corporation is to blame and they expect compensation. This is a 'grey area' between hysteria and malingering. There is no doubt that their symptoms are genuine and unconscious and, yet, the longer the compensation is delayed, the longer the symptoms will last; moreover, the symptoms will clear up after adequate compensation is paid. Recovery is not immediate as it would be in malingering and may take some years.

In the second group the patient has no complaints and yet those who know him well describe a change in personality. A previously mild and stable person has become unusually aggressive, irritable and liable to be assaultive especially after taking small amounts of alcohol which he could previously tolerate well. Such people can be very dangerous.

The final group of brain-damaged people are the epileptics. The vast majority are perfectly normal people but they do suffer from social disadvantages in that they are barred from certain occupations and certain pastimes. This may not matter if they are socially accepted but, if they are not, they may react in an antisocial way. Prior to the 1939–45 War, it was thought that there was a definite 'epileptic personality'. Affected persons were thought to be impulsively assaultive, ingratiating, religiose and untrustworthy. It was then realized that the epileptic personalities described were those of seriously disturbed epileptics who were in mental hospitals; the picture was not that seen in the epileptic living in the ordinary community, who was no more assaultive or criminal than was the rest of the population. Recent research has, however, shown that epileptics have a higher expectancy of criminal conviction than have the rest of the population but this, curiously enough, is not for violent crime. It seems likely that, while the majority of epileptics do not differ from the rest of the population, those who are rejected and socially disadvantaged react by committing crime. Those who are impulsively assaultive are very quickly steered into the hospital – and particularly the Special Hospital (*see below*) – system rather than into the penal system, and they remain there for a long time.

Functional Psychoses
These are called 'functional', as opposed to the organic, because although the basis of their abnormality is suspected to be genetic, biochemical or metabolic there is, as yet, no clear evidence that this is so; indeed, many of them appear to be explicable on a psychological basis.

As with the organic psychoses the gross abnormality appears to be determined by a break with reality caused either by pathological variations of mood or by catastrophic disorders of thinking. The two broad groups concerned therefore are the *affective psychoses*, where the disorder is primarily in the sphere of mood, and the *schizophrenic psychoses*, where the disorder is primarily in the thought processes of the individual.

Affective Psychoses
We are all subject to changes of mood ranging from deep despair to wild elation. Such changes are usually reality-based and depend upon external events; sometimes they appear to arise *sui generis*. Whatever the cause, external pressures and our own resilience usually ensure that we return to an even keel within a short time. In the affective, or manic–depressive, psychosis, however, the change of mood, in either direction, may not appear to have an adequate precipitant or, if it has, its intensity and duration may be quite out of keeping with that precipitant. A bereavement, for example, is a saddening affair which normally lightens as time goes on; but in an affective psychosis the depression deepens and intensifies until all contact with reality is lost.

This loss of contact with reality is demonstrated by the appearance of delusions and hallucinations. A *delusion* is a mistaken belief which is out of character with the individual's background and is unshakeable by reasoned argument. A *hallucination* is a sensory experience without any real sensory stimulus. In this it differs from an *illusion* which is a mis-interpretation of a sensory stimulus.

Manic–depressive psychosis derives its name from the fact that sufferers are, at different times in their lives, either profoundly depressed or unduly elated. They tend to come from families whose members show the same tendencies; they incline to a certain body build (short, thick-necked, barrel-chested and prone to vascular disease); and they have cyclothymic personalities – they are subject to unpredictable swings of mood. In the extreme example of this syndrome there are swings from deep depression to exalted elation with only brief spells of normality. It has become fashionable to emphasize that the depressive swing is much the more common and to talk of unipolar and bipolar depression depending on whether or not a manic phase has appeared.

In the manic phase the patient is elated, has considerable pressure of talk and of ideas, is convinced of his own ability to carry out new schemes and of his financial wizardry. He is therefore at risk of being charged with assault and breaches of the peace (due to his intolerance of the fools around him), of road traffic offences (his judgement being impaired) and of fraud or embezzlement because he has used money which is not yet there.

In the depressed phase he is despondent to the point of despair. It seems that there is no future for him or for his family; not only is he doomed, but everyone connected with him is equally damned. Suicide is, of course, the major risk but when a depressive includes his family in his delusional system there is the danger that he may decide to 'save' them at the same time as himself and thus perpetrate a ghastly family tragedy. One-third of all murder suspects in England and Wales commit suicide; only about 5 per cent do so in Scotland and North America.

The other crime characteristic of the depressive is shoplifting. The person concerned may not necessarily be of the classical manic–depressive, or 'endogenous', depressive type but may be one of those who are overwhelmed by external circumstances and who have a depressive and anxious personality. Typically, the culprit is a middle-aged woman of hitherto impeccable character and with a full purse who shoplifts in a state of confusion as a 'cry for help' and as an indication of her depressed state of mind. The shoplifter who does so because she is depressed may be in need of urgent help, and a significant percentage of women in the age group 40–60 years who are caught shoplifting are suf-fering from some degree of depression. Most shoplifters are psycho-logically normal and a small percentage are professionals.

Schizophrenia

Schizophrenia is probably a group of conditions which have certain characteristics in common and which may arise in a number of different ways. They key factor is a disorder of thinking; the component from which it derives its name, a split between the affect and the content of thought, is a secondary factor. In essence, schizophrenia can be seen as a disorder of perception; the world the schizophrenic sees around him is one which is distorted by hallucinations, illusions and delusions. Because of his perceptual distortions, the schizophrenic lives in an environment of fantasy. This may so beguile him that he lacks all drive and ambition – the once-promising pupil fails to fulfil his early promise (schizophrenia simplex). On the other hand, he may be so beset by his fantasies and delusions that his whole thinking becomes too distorted for clear expression; he talks in a confused 'word salad' with numerous *neologisms* (hebephrenic schizophrenia). Thirdly, his perceptual distortion may lead him to a total withdrawal (stupor) or to a wild and impulsive attack on those around him (catatonic schizophrenia). Finally, he may translate his distorted view of the world around him into an aggrieved sense of a hostile environment and, while retaining much of his original personality, he will interpret any action or spoken word in the belief that everyone is against him (paranoid schizophrenia). There is a withdrawal from the real world and a lack of emotional response in all the varieties of schizophrenia. There is also a lack of appropriateness between the thoughts expressed and the emotion accompanying these thoughts, e.g. the expression of a belief that a person is about to be disembowelled may be accompanied by a fatuous smile.

The schizophrenic's delusional ideas are so bizarre and the personality dilapidation is so marked that there is no difficulty in seeing him as insane; he is none the less potentially dangerous. His auditory hallucinations may command him to attack an innocent bystander. Most dangerous of all is the well-preserved paranoid schizophrenic who, convinced of the evil intentions of certain people who are plotting against him, retains enough grasp on reality to counter such plots with deliberate action.

Schizophrenics may commit any sort of crime but, in practice, their crimes are mainly petty. Their lack of drive and persistence leads many of them into a vagrant existence and they steal in order to live. This leads to a well-known vicious circle in which they steal and are apprehended; they are admitted, either informally or through the courts, to a mental hospital where they are treated with psychotropic drugs; they are discharged, discharge themselves or, most commonly, abscond; they stop taking their medication, they relapse into schizophrenia and, with no job, stable background or support, they steal in order to live.

Occasionally, a series of petty crimes by a previously blameless individual may be the prodromal phase of schizophrenia. More dramatically, the first sign may be a sudden unprovoked homicidal attack on a member of the family, an acquaintance or a stranger, often prompted by hallucinatory voices. A careful history will, however, usually reveal that the young person concerned (schizophrenia most usually begins in the late teens or early twenties) had recently been rather strange and withdrawn and had been falling off in his performance at work, all of which had been abscribed to an 'adolescent phase'.

While a schizophrenic may kill anyone, the very rare crime of matricide is characteristic of the condition and, in general, the more bizarre and unusual a crime, the more likely it is that it was committed by someone mentally disordered.

The very dangerous state of morbid jealousy, sometimes referred to as the 'Othello syndrome', is allied to paranoid schizophrenia but generally occurs without the characteristic thought disorder of true schizophrenia. In the 'Othello syndrome', the person, usually male, has delusions of infidelity about his wife or mistress. The man is usually in his 40s, has been married or associated for 10 or more years and has held his delusional ideas for 4 or 5 years during which time he has frequently upbraided or physically assaulted his partner. The end result may be murder or attempted murder. In such a situation, divorce is probably the only safe course for the spouse.

FORENSIC PSYCHIATRY IN PRACTICE

The major categories of mental disorder have now been all reviewed but clinical cases are seldom as clear cut as are the syndromes that have been described. Many are more complex and there are gradations between one form of illness and another. For example, one may encounter an elderly woman, accused of some crime, who is clearly depressed. Further examination may reveal that she has been subject to episodes of depression throughout her life, that her forebears were similarly affected, that she has always been a dependent personality, that her adult life has been beset with serious problems and that she is now showing signs of early intellectual deterioration. In such a case it is neither easy nor helpful to arrive at a single diagnosis; it is more profitable to state a formulation of her present mental state and relate that to the crime she is accused of committing.

Serious forms of mental disorder are found in a small proportion (1–3 per cent) of offenders but psychological factors may be found in many cases. Reference has already been made to crime in adolescents. Very few of these youngsters have a serious mental disorder other than some degree of personality disorder but many thieve – the commonest form of delinquency – because of psychological factors which range from simple bravado in an attempt to prove themselves to themselves or to their peers, through complex unconscious desires to hurt their parents to a desire to be punished due to a sense of guilt.

Psychological mechanisms also enter into the use and abuse of alcohol, which is an important factor in many crimes. Alcohol is a central nervous system depressant and its apparent stimulant effect is due to its disinhibiting action which releases tendencies which might otherwise be resisted. This effect is so well known that it is common for offenders to plead that they were acting under the influence of alcohol. It is, therefore, difficult to estimate the true part played by alcohol in the commission of crime but it is probable that its influence is related to the extent to which the abuse of alcohol is tolerated in the community. Its role is particularly important in assaultive crime and research has shown that, in such instances, intoxication in the victim is almost as important as it is in the assailant.

Persistent excessive drinking can lead to the disease of alcoholism. Alcoholics are those excessive drinkers who become so psychologically dependant on alcohol that it interferes with their health, social functioning and interpersonal relationships. The development of alcoholism follows a familiar pattern. It begins by the person choosing his social activities according to the amount of alcohol to be expected, then 'doubling up' on his drinks, surreptitious drinking from an ensured supply, increasing tolerance of alcohol, amnesic episodes with no more than the normal amount of alcohol and the experience of general tremulousness and irritability every morning. The tremulousness may lead on to 'the shakes' and eventually to delirium tremens (D.T.'s) with vivid and terrifying hallucinations. The psychological dependence on alcohol may take the form of an inability to abstain (a need for a constant blood level of alcohol) or an inability to stop (continued drinking until all resources are expended). This progressive dependence may be spread over a number of years during which jobs, driving licence and marriage are lost. The stereotype picture of the skid-row alcoholic, living on meths on a bomb-site or in a model lodging house on social security is, in reality, less common than is the business executive gradually slipping down the socio-economic scale.

The need for alcohol – and the occurrence of withdrawal symptoms show it to be a physiological as well as a psychological need – may involve alcoholics in many crimes such as breach of the peace, road traffic offences and dishonesty. Depending on the social level of the alcoholic, offences of dishonesty may take the form of fraud and embezzlement or breaking and entering – in each case in order to acquire money for further drinking. It is only rarely that an alcoholic is involved in major crime such as murder, although alcohol is a potent factor in murder. One must learn to distinguish between those who commit crime after normal drinking and alcohol dependants who commit crime because of their dependance.

Sexual offences are also influenced by psychological abnormality. A distinction must be made between those crimes in which the direction of the sex drive is normal (indecent assault, rape and attempted rape) and those where it is abnormal (homosexuality, paedophilia, incest, bestiality). In the former, there may be either an unconscious resentment of women, stemming from a poor mother–child relationship, or an immature inability to make proper heterosexual contacts; but the majority stem from a combination of strong normal sexual drive in a compromising situation, lubricated by alcohol and with an aggressive component. There is an aggressive factor in most rapes and it is interesting that, while convictions for abnormal sexual crimes have remained steady, those for rape have tended to rise, *pari passu*, with the increasing occurrence of crimes of violence.

Abnormal sexual drives result from developmental failure or from immaturity. The offences arising are best understood as an attempt to achieve sexual expression in one who has not attained full sexuality. Many homosexuals enrich our lives in cultural and artistic fields while others spell misery for themselves and others. The majority of sex offenders are pathetic people trying to find their own solution and most offend only once. Those whose offences escalate are very dangerous. Child sex murders are very rare and usually the result of panic in the offender.

THE ELECTROENCEPHALOGRAM

We have already talked of those who are brain-damaged in various ways. Some of these – particularly the epileptics – may be identified by the use of the electroencephalogram (EEG).

An EEG abnormality is not pathognomic of brain damage since nonspecific abnormalities occur in about 12 per cent of the adult population and in a much higher proportion of adolescents in whom the brain takes a variable time to mature. It is significant that there is a very high incidence of abnormal EEGs in those who are recidivist criminals and particularly in those who are repeatedly convicted of assaultive crime. It would seem that a considerable number of these individuals have some form of nonspecific brain damage.

CRIMINAL RESPONSIBILITY

It has long been accepted in all civilized countries that children and those who are seriously mentally disordered are not responsible in law for any crime that they may commit. This is enshrined in the old doctrine of '*Reum non facit nisi mens rea*' which means that there cannot be a criminal act without criminal intent.

The difficulty has always been in determining what degree of mental disorder is necessary to absolve the person from responsibility. Until relatively recent times, the test applied was whether his or her powers of reasoning were impaired and, indeed, this was the basis of the McNaghten Rules. Daniel McNaghten was a paranoid schizophrenic who held the delusional belief that he was being persecuted and that this could only be stopped by shooting the Prime Minister of the day – Sir Robert Peel. He attempted to do so but, by mistake, shot and killed the Prime Minister's Private Secretary – Mr William Drummond. He was acquitted on grounds of insanity but his aquittal raised such public concern that the House of Lords put a series of questions to the Judges. The Judges' answers are contained in what are known as the McNaghten Rules, the most relevant portion of which reads:

'The Jurors ought to be told in all cases that every man is to be presumed to be sane and to possess a sufficient degree of reason to be responsible for his crimes until the contrary be proved to their satisfaction; and that to establish a defence on the ground of insanity it must be clearly proved that at the time of the committing of the act the party accused was labouring under such a defect of reason from disease of the mind as not to know the nature and quality of the act he was doing or, if he did know it, that he did not know he was doing wrong.'

The Rules would have very limited application if they were strictly interpreted and they have been criticized ever since their introduction in 1843. Nevertheless, they have been followed in most English-speaking countries although their application has been, generally, liberal.

The main criticisms of the Rules stem from their emphasis on reason as the main factor in determining an individual's behaviour while ignoring the potent effects of emotion, delusional beliefs and hallucinations.

Several attempts have been made to find an alternative, particularly in the United States. The first of these was the New Hampshire formula in 1865:

'So far as a person acts under the influence of mental disease, he is not accountable.'

The second was the so-called Durham formula of 1954:

'The accused is not criminally responsible if his unlawful act was the product of mental disease or mental defect.'

The most recent is the proposal in the American Law Institute's model penal code of 1959 that:

'The question be whether the defendant as a result of mental disease or defect lacked substantial capacity either to appreciate the

criminality of his conduct or to conform his conduct to the requirements of law.'

The difficulties of these formulae lie in the fact that mental disease or
defect is not defined in any of them and, in giving evidence, psychiatrists
are apt to be drawn into stating a conclusion about the nature of the
accused's mental disorder and its relationship to his responsibility
rather than concentrating on the facts indicating mental disorder and
leaving the question of responsibility to the jury.

In the United Kingdom, the first attempt to modify the McNaghten
Rules was in the Scottish case of *Dingwall* in 1867[3] where Lord Deas
first proposed the doctrine of 'diminished responsibility'. This doctrine
has been developed over the years and has for a long time been a well-
established part of Scottish law. It recognizes that there are differing
degrees of mental disorder and, in general, a defence of diminished responsibility requires evidence of 'a state of mind bordering upon but not
amounting to insanity'. This would cover certain organic states, de-
pressions, obsessional states and some paranoid states.

This doctrine of diminished responsibility, limited in its application
to cases of murder, was incorporated in English law in the Homicide
Act 1957, s. 2(1) which provides that: where a person kills or is party to
the killing of another he shall not be convicted of murder if he was suffering from such abnormality of mind (whether arising from a condition
of arrested or retarded development of mind or any inherent causes or
induced by disease or injury) as substantially impaired his mental responsibility for his acts and omissions in doing or being a party to the
killing'. The effect of a successful plea of diminished responsibility is to
reduce the charge from one of murder to one of culpable homicide in
Scotland or manslaughter in England. This reduction of the charge
gives a wide discretion to the Court in disposing of the offender and includes the use of the provisions of Part V of the Mental Health Act 1959
and its Scottish equivalent (*see below*) to provide a hospital disposal if
the condition of the accused so warrants. Originally, psychopaths were
not regarded as falling into the category of those whose responsibility
was diminished but, in recent years, particularly since the 1957 Act,
severely abnormal psychopaths have been dealt with in this way.

Just as it has been accepted that it is inhuman to punish someone who
is not responsible for his actions, so it has been accepted that it is inhuman to subject to trial someone who by reason of mental disorder is unable properly to defend himself; such a person is judged to be unfit to
plead. The generally accepted criteria for fitness to plead are that the
accused should be able to:

---

[3] Alex. Dingwall (1867) 5 Irv. 466.

a. Understand the nature of the charge and the possible consequences to himself;
b. follow the proceedings in court;
c. challenge the jurors; and
d. properly instruct his defence.

If the accused is unable to fulfil these requirements and is found to be unfit to plead, the trial does not proceed and he is committed on a Hospital Order. In serious cases, this Hospital Order will be to a Special Hospital with a restriction order without limit of time. It is possible for the prosecution to reopen the case if the accused recovers quickly from his mental disorder and thereby becomes fit to plead, but this seldom happens since the degree of disorder leading to unfitness to plead is usually of a very serious nature. The disposal may seem an unsatisfactory one from the point of view of the accused since he sees himself as being confined to and restricted in hospital by reason of a crime which has never been proved against him. Because of this it is important that unfitness to plead should be used only very sparingly and, indeed, there are some authorities, particularly in the United States, who would abolish the concept and insist that everyone be tried no matter what his mental state.

The Butler Committee[4] considered the questions of fitness to plead and of insanity at the time of the crime in considerable detail. They recommended that the term 'Unfit to plead' should be replaced by the phrase 'Under disability in relation to the trial' which could be shortened colloquially to 'Under disability'. They also recommended the introduction of an 'Interim Hospital Order' which would have the effect of postponing the trial until such time as hospital treatment might enable the accused to become fit to stand trial. This Order would have a limit of six months. Such an Interim Hospital Order would also be useful where the defendant required medical care during a custodial remand and where a period in hospital was required to determine whether a Hospital Order was appropriate. The Interim Hospital Order would have the effect of ensuring that only those who were likely to be permanently unfit to plead would be denied the opportunity of defending themselves.

In relation to insanity at the time, the Butler Committee recommend a new formulation of the Special Verdict, namely 'not guilty on evidence of mental disorder', the grounds for which should comprise two elements, (*a*) a *mens rea* element approximating to the first limb of the McNaghten Rules (Did he know what he was doing?) and (*b*) specific exemption from conviction for defendants suffering from severe mental

[4] Butler, Lord (Chairman) *Report of the Committee on Mentally Abnormal Offenders* (1975), (Cmnd. 6244). London, HMSO. The recommendations of the Committee were concerned with England and Wales only.

illness or severe subnormality at the time of the act or omission charged.
They propose a definition of severe mental illness which details the clinical features which would have to be present in order to justify such a
finding. The clinical features are those which would only be present in
someone who is seriously psychotic. It would be for the examining psychiatrist to show clearly that they were present in the accused and for the
jury then to determine whether the defendant was 'not guilty on evidence of mental disorder'.

THE LEGAL FRAMEWORK

The vast majority of people suffering from mental disorder are treated
informally, i.e. without any legal compulsion on either an out-patient or
in-patient basis. Even about 90 per cent of those admitted to mental
hospitals are admitted informally. The prosecution will sometimes drop
minor charges in the case of a mentally abnormal offender if he or she
agrees to enter hospital for treatment as an informal patient. One quasi-
informal disposal available to the courts is a probation order with a condition of treatment, either as an out-patient or in-patient. In such a case,
the patient is free to discontinue treatment at any time but in doing so
runs the risk of being held in breach of his probation order. Such orders
have only a limited usefulness.

The provisions of Part IV of the Mental Health Act 1959 or the
Mental Health (Scotland) Act 1960 may be invoked in those few
instances in which a mentally disordered person does not recognize that
his mental state may constitute a danger to the health or safety or himself or others. Sections 29, 25 and 26 of the 1959 Act and Sections 31 and
24 of the 1960 Act provide that a mentally disordered person may be
compulsorily detained for 3 days (s. 29 of the 1959 Act) or for 7 days
(s. 31 of the 1960 Act) as an emergency on the certificate of one doctor.
He may be detained for 28 days (s. 25 of the 1959 Act) or for up to a year
(s. 26 of the 1959 Act and s. 24 of the 1960 Act – subject to review at 28
days) on the agreed recommendations of two doctors – preferably the
one who knows him best (his family doctor) and the one who knows
most about his condition (the hospital consultant). In all of these cases,
the test is that he must be in such a state of mental disorder that either
his own health or safety or that of others is at risk.

In recent years it has been argued that to take compulsory powers
over someone whose own health or safety only is at risk is paternalistic
and an infringement of the individual's liberty to dispose of his own life
as he thinks fit; such compulsory powers should only operate where the
health and safety of others are compromised. This argument might have
some force were it always possible to separate the two hazards but, as we

have seen with the depressive and schizophrenic murderers, it may be a matter of chance whether the afflicted person kills himself or others or both. Furthermore, the argument rests on the assumption that the individual is making a rational choice, whereas the people catered for in the Acts are those whose actions are determined by totally irrational forces.

Two classes of mental disorder are excluded from the operation of Part IV of the Acts – those over age 21 who are suffering from psychopathic disorder or from subnormality as defined in the 1959 Act. Under age 21 they may be admitted and detained compulsorily, if necessary up to the age of 25, but they may not be admitted for the first time if they are over 21.

Special provision is made in Part V of the Acts for those mentally disordered individuals who have committed crimes. Under s. 60 of the 1959 Act,[5] where someone has committed a crime normally punishable with imprisonment and where the court is satisfied, on the evidence of two doctors, one of whom must be approved for the purpose, that the offender is suffering from mental disorder, the court may impose a hospital order instead of a penal disposal. The effect of such a hospital order is virtually the same as a committal under Part IV of the Acts. There are two differences – the one statutory, the other practical. Under s. 60, the 21-year-old limit no longer applies; that is to say that a psychopath or subnormal person who has been convicted of a crime may be committed to hospital even if he is over 21. The practical difference is that the responsible medical officer may be more chary of discharging someone who has committed a crime than one who has not.

An extension of this caution in discharging those who have committed crimes is exemplified in s. 65 of the 1959 Act which empowers the court, having regard to the seriousness of the crime and the likelihood of its repetition because of mental disorder in the offender if he were prematurely discharged, to impose a restriction order on his discharge. Such restriction orders mean that the patient cannot have parole, be transferred from one hospital to another or be liberated either conditionally or unconditionally without the express and personal consent of the Secretary of State. It is increasingly the custom to make such orders without limit of time; this not only means that a person who does not recover can be held indefinitely but also allows for someone who makes a rapid recovery to be disposed of more readily than if he were subject to a fixed term of restriction. It is thus more flexible. Furthermore, a fixed term implies a prognostic skill that neither the judge nor his psychiatric advisers are likely to possess.

The whole question of compulsory committal is at present controversial. There are those who would argue that the mentally disordered

[5] The corresponding sections in the 1960 Act have recently been incorporated in the Criminal Procedure (Scotland) Act 1975.

commit no more crimes than do their fellow citizens. This is statistically true but it ignores the fact that most of those who are mentally disordered and likely to commit crimes are safely tucked away in hospital. In recent years the liberalization of mental hospitals has led to the presence in the community of many more patients than before and recent research has suggested that, under this policy, more crimes are committed by the mentally disordered. Emphasis is placed on the common-sense view that a mentally disordered individual who is prone to antisocial acts should be prevented from perpetrating them by being contained.

Mental hospitals currently adopt a very liberal policy with open doors and a minimum of compulsion and supervision; this has greatly increased the dignity of the individual patient and the therapeutic relationship between patient and staff at the expense of making it more difficult to control those few who may be disruptive, destructive and dangerous. Modern methods of management in mental hospitals have been a great advantage to the majority of patients but have posed dangers to the public because of the unrealistic actions of the few really dangerous patients. In consequence, an increasing burden has been thrust on the Special Hospitals set up by the Government for the treatment of those patients with violent and dangerous propensities who require treatment under conditions of special security. These hospitals – Broadmoor, Rampton, Moss Side, Carstairs and, now, Park Lane – were originally established to care for those patients who could not be dealt with by the ordinary locked mental hospital and, in the main, took their cases from the courts where the individual had been convicted of a serious crime and had been found to be mentally disordered. They must now deal, as well, with those who are unmanageable within the open-door policies of ordinary mental hospitals.

Because they have special skills in the management of these patients, they are also expected to have special skills in the prediction of the future behaviour of those patients they discharge. They tend to be over-cautious because the safety of the public may seem to be more important than is individual liberty. Hence, their problems are compounded by overcrowding. It was because of this that the Butler Committee recommended the setting up of regional secure units to deal with the lesser degrees of dangerousness. The Butler Committee recognized that too great a gap existed between the open units dealing with non-dangerous persons within their own area and the Special Hospitals dealing with the dangerously mentally disordered on a country-wide basis.

It is difficult to strike a balance between the right of the individual to lead – and end – his own life and the right of the community to be protected from the irrational acts of those whose perceptions of the world about them are distorted by mental disorder. On the whole, our Mental Health Acts are fair. They put no obstacle in the way of those who wish treatment for their distress on an informal basis and yet provide that persons without insight who might be a danger to themselves or to others can be contained and treated. At the same time, they ensure that the latter are safeguarded not only by the knowledge and qualifications of those who commit and treat them but by the number of people – their doctor, the Mental Health Review Tribunals in England and Wales, the Sheriff and the Mental Welfare Commission in Scotland and the nearest relative and managers of the hospital – who can demand their discharge.

MENTAL DISORDER AND CIVIL ACTIONS

Aside from criminal acts, the mentally disordered person is at risk in civil actions. In making a contract, for example, one who is mentally defective or mentally ill may be held to be incompetent. While this is generally true, the law recognizes that such a person may have a lucid interval and, if his medical attendant is prepared to certify that at the relevant time the patient was capable of understanding what he was doing in making the contract, that contract may be valid.

Marriage is a special form of contract which was previously considered separately under the Matrimonial Causes Act whereby it was possible for a person to petition for divorce on the grounds that the spouse had been continuously under care and treatment for five years and was incurably insane. Under the new divorce laws, however, these provisions will hardly ever be used since it will be easier to prove an irretrievable breakdown of the marriage, even where such breakdown has resulted from mental illness.

Reference has already been made to testamentary capacity in which the testator needs to know not only the extent of his estate but also those who would normally be expected to benefit from his bounty. His will may be invalid if his dispositions are distorted by delusions. Mentally disordered persons may make invalid wills either because their knowledge is wrong – by organic mental disorder – or because their dispositions are unfair – by paranoid ideation, of schizophrenic or depressive type, or by hypomanic overevaluation.

Similarly, a mentally disordered person may be incapable of managing his affairs either because he is mentally defective or because he is mentally ill. In such a case it may be necessary to appoint someone else to manage his affairs, either through the Court of Protection in England and Wales or by the appointment of a Curator Bonis in Scotland.

Chapter 29

Forensic Odontology

HUMAN dentition is of two types – the deciduous of infancy and the permanent; the former consists of 20 and the latter of 32 teeth. The permanent dentition comprises 4 symmetrical quadrants each containing 2 incisors, 1 canine, 2 pre-molar and 3 molar teeth. Although the differentiation of individual molars, pre-molars and lower incisors presents some complications, it is generally not difficult for a dental practitioner to identify an individual tooth on the basis of its size and shape; for court purposes, however, the opinion of a specialist dental anatomist may well be sought.

Several systems for recording the dentition are current but that attributed to Zsigmondy and used in the National Health Service can be regarded as the standard method in Great Britain. In this, the teeth in each quadrant are numbered consecutively from the midline in the front; the second molar tooth in the right lower jaw thus becomes lower right 7 or, in common dental notation, 7⌋. The 5 deciduous teeth are annotated A–E in a similar fashion. An alternative system, which is being lobbied at an international level, substitutes the prefix 1 for right upper, 2 for left upper, 3 for left lower and 4 for right lower quadrants; using this notation the second molar in the right lower jaw would be designated 47.[1] The deciduous teeth are prefixed 5–8 according to quadrant. This is known as Viohl's Two Digit System.

If one considers a tooth for descriptive purposes as a cube projecting from the jaw, it has five surfaces. The surface which is opposed to its fellow in the other jaw is called the occlusal surface (O in shorthand); except in unusual circumstances, such as the loss of rear teeth, there is no occlusal surface on the incisor and canine teeth which are sharp. The surface nearest the anterior midline is called the mesial surface (M), and that furthest away the distal (D). The surface contacting the cheek is called buccal (B), and the inner surface is designated palatal (P) in the upper and lingual (L) in the lower jaw. Thus, the common massive

---

[1] The commonest notation in the USA numbers the upper right third (back) molar tooth as 1. Each tooth is then numbered consecutively, the upper back molar on the left side being 16. The lower left back molar is then numbered 17 and the process continued to 32 which represents the lower right back molar.

filling which involves the biting surface and the mesial and distal walls of a tooth would be noted as MOD.

Any tooth may be unerupted, it may be normal, it may contain a cavity caused by caries or a lost filling or a cavity may have been restored. The restoration may be by synthetic porcelain or epoxy resin complexes, by a silver/tin amalgam or by gold; the tooth may have been capped or crowned. A tooth may have been extracted and, if so, been replaced by a partial denture, or bridge, or there may be a complete denture; the dentures may be made of a plastic or of metal, they may be deliberately coloured, marked or even numbered and national practices lead to characteristic designs. Add to all these variables the possibilities of removable or fixed mechanical devices to straighten the teeth (orthodontic appliances) or of obvious deformities together with characteristics associated with race or with occupation, not forgetting changes due to age, and it will be appreciated that the potential variations in the mouth are so great in number that the dentition may provide as personal a method of identification as can finger-prints.

A brief comparison of odontology with dactylography as a means of personal identification is not out of place at this point. Odontology scores in two main areas. Firstly, in a country provided with a National Health Service, it is at least probable that a record of the dentition of a missing person will be available somewhere – either in the files of a practitioner or at the Dental Estimates Boards where records of treatment are maintained for up to 4 years. By contrast, permanent records of finger-prints are maintained in the United Kingdom only rarely (*see* p. 53); there is no way of tracing a *completely* unknown body through its finger-prints although, given some clue to identity, a match may be made with impressions obtained from selected personal possessions. It should be noted, however, that these considerations would not apply in the United States where filed finger-prints are a commonplace throughout the population. Secondly, the teeth are very resistant to fire. Odontology therefore becomes the method of choice for identification of that major group of bodies which is unsuitable for visual recognition.

On the other hand, although developmental differences between two persons are almost always demonstrable by X-rays etc, the dentition can only become 'personalized' if abnormalities have arisen or have been induced. The fewer the deviations from the normal, the less precise can be the identification and it is difficult to identify with certainty from the mouth someone who has had no treatment or dental investigations; it may be hard even to distinguish between two persons of similar age and race with such an unblemished dental history. Finger-prints, on the other hand, are personalized from birth and remain so until death. It follows that odontological identification finds its greatest use either in confirming or denying an identification suspected in an individual on other grounds or in discriminating the bodies of a large number of known but individually unrecognizable persons.

ESTIMATION OF AGE FROM THE TEETH

Four observations can be made on the teeth with relative ease. In chronological order of appearance these are: mineralization, formation of the crown, eruption of the tooth and completion of the root of the tooth.[2] These are applicable to both the deciduous and permanent dentition and observations may be made on two or more changes at the same time; one can, for example, estimate the eruption of the deciduous teeth and their degree of root development at the same time as assessing the state of completion of the crowns of the following permanent teeth embedded in the jaw.

These variables are shown in diagrammatic form in *Fig.* 23. It is seen that there is considerable variation in the appearance of each characteristic. For example, the range of eruption of the first lower deciduous incisor is from 4 to 10 months and, although the remaining deciduous teeth behave more regularly than this, the 'scatter' in the permanent teeth is far greater; in addition, the teeth generally develop rather earlier in girls than in boys. The more characteristics that are examined and taken into consideration, the more accurate will be the final assessment of age. In brief, the dental practitioner will utilize X-ray or microscopic evidence of early tooth development in the fetus or neonate; up to the age of 1 year the eruption of the deciduous teeth combined with an evaluation of the oncoming permanent teeth will give a most useful assessment of age. Following this – up to the age of about $2\frac{1}{2}$ years – age can be estimated from the state of tooth eruption, always accepting the proviso in each case of a 'bracket of probability'. Eruption of the permanent teeth generally begins between 6 and 7 years. Eruption proceeds in a fairly standard order in each individual but the range among different persons may be up to $\pm$ 2 years; it is of some interest that Gustafson's *average* ages for eruption are, in many cases, rather higher than those given in standard works on forensic medicine – much depends on the phase of eruption intended. The development of the third molar or wisdom tooth is not shown in *Fig.* 23; its eruption is variable but its roots are important in the young adult – if its roots are incompletely formed it can at least be said that the body is aged less than 25 years.

After eruption of the permanent teeth there are still characteristics which may lead to a reasonably accurate estimate of age. These are attrition, or wearing down of the teeth; paradentosis, or loosening of the

---

[2] For full discussion of estimating age from the teeth, *see* Gustafson G. (1966) *Forensic Odontology*, London, Staples Press.

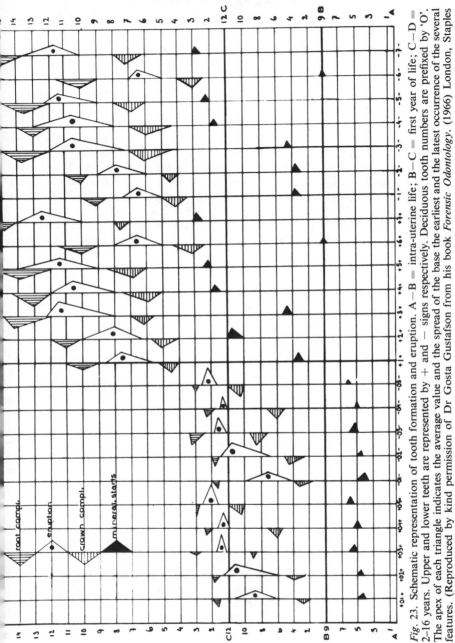

Fig. 23. Schematic representation of tooth formation and eruption. A — B = intra-uterine life; B — C = first year of life; C — D = 2–16 years. Upper and lower teeth are represented by + and − signs respectively. Deciduous tooth numbers are prefixed by 'O'. The apex of each triangle indicates the average value and the spread of the base the earliest and the latest occurrence of the several features. (**Reproduced by kind permission of Dr Gosta Gustafson from his book** *Forensic Odontology.* (1966) London, Staples Press.)

teeth; infilling of the normal root cavity (secondary dentine formation); increase in the tissue holding the root in place (cementum apposition); resorption of the root; and transparency of the root. All but the first two of these six changes need careful laboratory preparation of the material and their assessment is certainly a process requiring previous experience. Gustafson has evolved a mathematical formula which attempts to arrive at a nominal age on the basis of all six characteristics and this gives promising results in *specialized hands*; the current order of accuracy, using computer techniques, is about ± 5 years. It is the author's experience that a dental practitioner interested in the subject can give a very fair estimate of age – in the region of a decade – from a simple estimate of attrition, paradontosis, mouth hygiene and the like; certainly the odontologist's assessment tends to be more accurate than that of the pathologist in the face of burning or severe mutilation.

Perhaps it is fair to say that odontology as an aid to ageing is most valuable in the comparative context, a further reflection of the importance of the dentist at the major disaster.

RACIAL AND OCCUPATIONAL CHARACTERISTICS

The assessment of race or occupation may be of help in the identification of the single unknown body. A few traits approach diagnostic value but most are, again, of greatest use in a comparative role; racial characteristics may be very useful in a preliminary sorting of multiple casualties from, say, an air accident. Except in such a circumstance, when the tentative isolation of a *known* group of negroids from a *known* group of caucasoids may be relatively easy, the problem is essentially one for the specialist anthropologist and little will be said here save to draw attention to the evidence which he might obtain. Three lines of observation might be followed – the size and shape of the teeth themselves, the extent and nature of any restorations and the quality of prostheses (bridges or dentures).

The size of the teeth, which are said to be larger in primitive peoples, is so variable as to be virtually useless save at extremes of the scale. Mention may be made of the high incidence of so-called shovel-shaped upper incisors in mongoloid and eskimo races. Subtle differences in the pre-molar and molar teeth are also to be found in these groups. The arch of the jaw is wide in negroid persons and the teeth are usually in good alignment and occlusion; this is in general contrast to the European caucasoid in whom a narrow arch predisposes to crowding and misplacement of teeth – the wisdom teeth are very commonly unerupted or are extracted.

As to the recognition of restorations and prostheses, it has been

pointed out that it is far easier to say that a given piece of work was unlikely to have been done in a certain place rather than to identify the
area in which it was performed; moreover, the place of treatment is not
necessarily the same as the homeland of the person treated. There are,
nevertheless, some interesting geographical variations in dental restoration. Certain nationals, in particular Africans, have remarkably good
teeth requiring virtually no restorative treatment; they are therefore
very difficult to identify individually from their dentition. The use of
gold is far less common in the United Kingdom than elsewhere; it is particularly prevalent in southern Europe and in the mongoloid races.
Silver alloys for fashioning false tooth crowns are said to be common in
eastern Europe and, while silica and epoxy resin is generally used in
Great Britain for restoring front teeth, porcelain is rather more likely to
be used in the United States.

Such findings are, however, no more than guides to identification and
the same is true of bridges and dentures. Certain types of work may be
more common in one country than another but to make an 'exclusion'
type of identification solely on this basis would be a hazardous undertaking.

Occupational stigmata can arise from mechanical or chemical injury.
Classical mechanical injuries are said to be found in the form of notches
in the incisors of those who grasp the nails or twine in the mouth – shoe-
makers, upholsterers and seamstresses. Gustafson has also described
changes in the front teeth of musicians, those working in dusty environments and in miners; most of these changes can now be relegated to historical interest. Chemical stains are most frequently due to the use of
tobacco which, in pipe smokers, may also produce highly personalized
mechanical injury, but chemical injury due to occupation is most frequent in those whose work involves the use of strong acids. Such observations must, however, be of forensic interest only very rarely.

IDENTIFICATION

Dental identification of the dead at the personal rather than exclusion
level depends upon the availability of antemortem records. *Fig.* 24
shows how this operates in practice. It follows that nothing can be done
in the absence of a retrieval service for these records and it is this which
so severely limits the value of the method in the case of the wholly unknown body. It is certainly true that in cases of major importance, a description of a cadaver's teeth can be sent to every practising dentist and
hospital but the process is time-consuming and expensive. An identification service has been set up in Scotland under the aegis of the Home
and Health Department utilizing the Regional Dental Officers through

Fig. 24. Dental identification in practice. The lower chart shows the teeth as recorded in the cadaver; the upper is prepared from previous dental records. Note that the lower 6 is charted as missing at post-mortem examination with a drift of lower 7 and 8 on each side to close the spaces; the lower 8 on each side is charted as missing in the dental records. The cavity recorded in the dental records in the lower right 5 was found to have been filled at post-mortem. A new cavity, not previously recorded, was found in the lower left 5 at post-mortem. Such inconsistencies are all compatible with a positive identification which can be made despite the loss of much of the anterior jaw during the process of the accident. (The example has been kindly contributed by Wing Commander Keith Ashley, R.A.F.)

whom dental charts, with X-rays when available, are distributed on a scale commensurate with the information available; but success generally attends only when there is *some* indication as to identity. Dental charts are seldom absolutely correct even when they are available. Some dentists record only the work which they have done, others are not so thorough as perfection would demand, while a large number of persons undergo emergency treatment which may not appear in their records until noted at a later date. For all these reasons combined, dental identification is at its most useful in a comparative or exclusive role and has been most used in the mass disaster, in particular the aircraft accident in which an especially good indication of the group identity of the dead is available through the list of passengers.

The essence of rapid dental identification lies in the speed of retrieval of the records of the missing person – the conventional methods of the International Police Organization are generally too slow to satisfy public demand for rapid restitution of the dead. British airlines are given service by a firm of funeral directors who maintain a control room for this purpose and whose facilities are at the disposal of the police wherever the accident occurs; the use of the telex system is an essential element in the rapid provision of information.

Dental identification then depends mainly upon comparison between the records of the missing persons and the findings in the bodies in relation to:

a. *Restorative work*: Teeth may require treatment, have been filled, have been extracted or replaced by prostheses.

b. *Unusual features*: Important features may include absence, persistence, malformation or discoloration of teeth; malocclusion of the jaws; abnormalities of the mouth or lips.

c. *X-rays*: If antemortem X-rays are available, matching radiographs taken post mortem may provide unequivocal evidence of identification.

Comparison in any form may be affected by trauma – the possibility of fillings having been dislodged, and the like, must always be considered. A comparison of restorations may result in inconsistencies which can be either compatible or incompatible with a positive identification.

In general, a compatible consistency is one which can be explained either by the failure of the dental practitioner to record what he has done or by the treatment having been given subsequent to the last recording. Thus, a filling discovered in a tooth of a cadaver which is not shown in the chart of a missing person need not necessarily exclude a match. An incompatible inconsistency is one which involves negation of a recorded treatment. Thus, the discovery of a single filling in a tooth said to have had three treatments would normally exclude identification. Even so, very occasionally an identification is so certain on other grounds that it must be accepted despite the presence of an incompatible inconsistency. Usually such a situation is attributed to clerical error or slipshod record keeping. It is, however, possible that the phenomenon of tooth migration, which occurs particularly in the molar region, may pose real problems both for the recorder and observer. Identifications allowing for such anomalies must, however, be accepted only after careful analyses by competent authorities of all the relevant factors.

Strong confirmatory evidence of identification can also be provided by dentures. As discussed previously, many of these may have national characteristics. Different colours are used and the majority of laboratories incorporate some mark by which they can identify their work. Such observations are particularly useful, say, in separating the last three bodies from a large number of casualties. There is also a growing habit of incorporating a number in the denture; once the laboratory performing the work for the deceased has been identified, this number may be as certain evidence of identification as is the use of identification discs.

ACCIDENT RECONSTRUCTION

A large proportion of persons killed in automobile or aircraft accidents sustain maxillofacial injuries. The precise distribution of these when correlated with the crash environment and the safety harness in use may give invaluable information as to the direction and strength of the deceleration forces involved; the observations made may also have a profound influence on the design of equipment, instrument panels and the like.

This aspect of forensic odontology has not received the attention it deserves.

BITE MARKS

Animals may bite humans either in life or after death. However, such injuries are not the concern of this chapter,[3] which will deal solely with human/human bites and bites in food.

The value of bite mark evidence lies predominantly in two fields of examination:

 a. Of the skin of a person assaulted, a prime objective being to identify or exclude the assailant.

---

[3] The general medico-legal associations of vaccine therapy which might arise in the prevention of rabies are discussed in Chapter 6.

b. Of food and other inanimate objects in an attempt to prove the presence of someone at the locus at some time.

In either case, the evidence must be of a comparative nature – the dentition of a person must be examined and compared with the mark before he or she can be identified or excluded as a suspect.

Human/human bites are most commonly associated with sexually motivated assault with or without rape and with nonaccidental injury inflicted on children. The examinations may, therefore, be required in both the living and the dead and, while the majority of evidence is likely to be derived from an examination of the victim, the reverse might hold if biting has formed part of a defence reaction to assault.

The comparison of records falls into two phases. The first, recording the bite mark, is a matter of urgency in the living person as the mark may alter in intensity and definition with time; indeed, such alterations may also occur in the dead body even before the process of putrefaction intervenes.

In instances of recent biting, say within 5 hours, the first stage of the examination should be to swab the mark for saliva; previous physical examination, or interference by other investigators or mortuary technicians, may remove a large proportion of the saliva available and may contaminate the area with the examiner's own secretions. Approximately 76 per cent of people secrete readily recognizable amounts of either A, B or O ('H') antigens in their saliva and these antigens correspond to the blood group (*see* Chapter 18). The typing of saliva, which is obtained by swabbing the area with damp cigarette papers,[4] may, therefore, positively exclude a suspect as having inflicted a bite – always provided the group of the suspect is known. Alternatively, a match of antigens may add further to the evidence giving rise to suspicion. Failure to identify antigens may be due to the absence of saliva, to the saliva coming from a 'non-secretor' or to poor collection technique.

Following this, the bite is photographed both in black and white and in colour. Both sets of prints must incorporate a suitable linear scale following the natural curves of the part bitten, and the latter should also show a colour comparison chart; this has special importance in that repetitive colour photography is useful to follow the changes in the appearance of a bite mark and it is important to ensure a standard colour balance. The photographs should be supported by a sketch or tracing showing the actual measurements between landmarks. Useful landmarks are variable but would normally include such items as the distance between the canine teeth and the width of any clear individual

---

[4] The subject's own sweat may contain her or his own water-soluble antigens. Control specimens taken from elsewhere (ideally from the same area on the opposite side of the body) are, therefore, essential. For the same reason, the examiner's hands should be gloved.

tooth mark. Obvious abnormalities of size or position will be of major importance. Removal of post-mortem specimens *in toto* may be found useful but it must be remembered that tissues shrink in preserving fluids even if pinned on a board.

Recognizable marks on the skin may not be due only to direct pressure by the teeth. Scrape marks may provide valuable information in demonstrating characteristic contours of the cutting surface of the front teeth. The combination of suction and pressure by the tongue may result in bruises derived from parts of the mouth other than the teeth or from the surfaces of the teeth in contact with the tongue. It is probably true that no two persons have *exactly* the same tooth characteristics when these are expressed as a bite impression; in fact, it is difficult to reproduce perfectly a bite mark made under experimental conditions by the same participant. Nevertheless, it is a general rule that the more unusual is an abnormality, the more useful it is as evidence of positive identification.

Consideration should be given during this part of the investigation to the possibility of self-infliction. If there is any doubt, evidence which might be needed – i.e. models of the victim's teeth – should be made available.

The second phase of comparison requires the recording of, and obtaining impressions from, the teeth of a suspect and it is here that important considerations as to the legal admissibility of bite mark evidence arise. The police have clear power to finger-print, to have physically examined, to take rubbings from the hand and even from the orifices of an arrested person and it would be a logical extension to suppose they also have authority to examine the mouth of an accused in order to establish whether there is evidence which bears on his/her guilt or innocence. So far as is known, the law of England has never been tested in this respect but it is certainly possible that the dental officer who attempted to take impressions from the teeth of a person under arrest without his written permission – and after full explanation of the purpose of the examination – might be held guilty of an assault.[5] The position in Scotland is almost as uncertain because, once a person is no more than under suspicion, he is protected by traditional rights based on the principle that he should not be placed in the position of self-incrimination. Certainly an examination should not be made after arrest without the consent of the accused and, ideally, this should be backed by advice from his legal adviser. On the other hand, it is noticeable that the Scottish courts, in balancing the interests of the State

<hr>

[5] *See* discussion on Simpson K. (1951) Dental evidence in the reconstruction of crime, *Br. Dent. J.* **41,** 229. In R. v. Gorringe, Maidstone Ass., 1948, the taking of dental impressions from the suspect was not subsequently opposed by the defence: the man concerned had given his consent after the purpose had been explained.

against the rights of the accused, are tending to give rather more weight to the former in disclosing evidence with a view to securing conviction than to the interests of the latter in preventing disclosure so as to avoid conviction.[6] In these days, evidence derived from findings of a transient nature might well be accepted in serious cases even if it was obtained in the face of an arguable technical irregularity. This tendency was particularly expressed in relation to forensic odontology in the greatly publicized case of *H.M.Adv. v. Hay*,[7] where a warrant obtained to make impressions from the mouth of a close suspect, who happened to be detained in an approved school, was held to be valid or, at least, granted in accordance with the overriding public interest.

Having obtained impressions of a suspect's dentition, the next step is that of comparison with the bite mark and, if a match be obtained, the presentation of the case in an acceptable fashion. There is no 'minimum number of points of conformity' required to prove the identity of a biter – it is simply a matter of the skill of the advocate and of the credibility and weight to be attached to the evidence of the expert witness. This is primarily because, in contrast to finger-printing, the possible configurations in bite marks are less systematized. Similarly, there is no standard system of notation or presentation of the results, various experts having their own chosen methods. Certainly, photography must play an important part and the author's preference is for superimposition techniques involving the use of transparencies. The criteria to be met are that the deductive processes should be easily demonstrable to and understandable by a jury and, perhaps more importantly, that the method should be free from attack on the grounds of unwitting distortion of the evidence.

Compared with those in flesh, bite marks in food are stable evidence and, while it is possible to take impressions from marks in the former, they are not nearly so satisfactory as those which can be obtained from apples, cheese and the like. Nevertheless, all foodstuffs lose moisture and become deformed as they decay and this process must involve any tooth marks present. From the evidential aspect, therefore, impressions must either be taken with a reasonable sense of urgency or it must be established that the specimen was preserved in a solution known to preserve the original size and shape of the material. Within these limitations there is no doubt that models made from foodstuffs can provide positive comparisons with those made from the teeth, which are easily understood by juries. What seems less credible is the likelihood of criminals leaving such evidence at the locus in any but extraordinary cir-

---

[6] *See*, for example, the opinions of Lord Cameron in Brown v. H.M.Adv. 1966 S.L.T. 105, and Lord Wheatley in Miln v. Cullen 1967 J.C. 21.

[7] 1968 J.C. 40. The case is very fully reported from the odontological aspect in *J. Forensic Sci. Soc.* (1968) **8**, 156–217.

cumstances – but it does seem to occur.

It is apparent that the science of bite mark investigation is still in the developmental stage,[8] largely because practical research presents obvious difficulties. Few dentists can claim to be experts and, as a result, it may be difficult for the police to obtain the essential expertise at short notice. It seems, in fact, that opinion is hardening towards the view that bite mark evidence is of firmer value in excluding suspects when there are several rather than in confirming the identity of an assailant.

---

[8] A further extension of forensic odontology – identification by lip prints – has also been introduced recently, particularly in Japan. It has interesting theoretical possibilities but must, for the present, be regarded as mainly an experimental procedure.

Chapter 30

Legal Aspects of Medical Practice

A REGISTERED medical practitioner is one who is registered with the General Medical Council. While anyone may practise his 'healing art', it is an offence to pretend in so doing to be properly registered. A person who has passed the necessary examination and who has received the relevant diploma (Appendix N) may be duly qualified but, without registration, he is denied certain privileges and protection and he is disqualified from holding medical office under the Crown, from holding medical appointments in the public services and from practising under the National Health Service Acts. An unregistered practitioner cannot prescribe or supply certain poisons (*see* Chapter 23), he cannot treat venereal disease, he cannot attend a maternity case without supervision except in emergency[1] and he cannot sign valid medical certificates required under many statutes.

This supervision is based on the various Medical Acts of which the first was passed in 1858 and the most recent is dated 1969. The principal cumulative effect of these has been to establish the General Medical Council[2] with the following major functions:

a. To maintain the official register of medical practitioners.

b. To supervise the standard of qualification for registration.

c. To exercise discipline over the medical profession.

The lawyer should have some knowledge of all these duties.

The Official Register

The register, which contains the names of all fully and provisionally registered practitioners on 1 January of the year in question, is divided

---

[1] Venereal Disease Act 1917, s. 1; Midwives Act 1951, s. 9.

[2] The present General Council consists of 18 representatives appointed by universities in Great Britain and Ireland, 9 appointed by the Medical Corporations, 8 by the Privy Council (including a compulsory 3 laymen) and 11 elected by the medical profession. There are Branch Councils for England and Wales, which is now inactive, and for Scotland and for Ireland; the Branch Councils have no major formal powers but the General Council can delegate matters to them. The *Report of the Committee of Inquiry into the Regulation of the Medical Profession* (A. W. Merrison, Chairman), 1975, London, HMSO, Cmnd. 6018, has recommended changes in this constitution; a Bill or Bills are likely to be laid before Parliament in 1977–8. The dental profession is controlled under the Dentists Act 1957.

377

into a register of medical practitioners and a register of temporary medical practitioners. The main register consists of a Principal List and an Overseas List, the latter including registered practitioners who are not practising in Great Britain. Entries in the main Register for those practitioners undergoing a compulsory year of postgraduate training are marked by an asterisk; during this time their practice is limited to their appointment.

An annual retention fee of £8 is currently levied and it is within the powers of the registrar to erase a practitioner's name by reason of non-payment of this fee; there is a £10 charge for reinstatement. Erasure may otherwise follow due to loss of contact with the practitioner or as a result of disciplinary action. Reinstatement involves a charge of £10 in the former case; in the latter, provision is made for suspension as an alternative to erasure.

Supervision of Educational Standards
This function has little immediate interest for the lawyer. It is sufficient to say that the Council can look into the courses given by, and the methods of examination practice of, the universities and other bodies empowered to grant qualification for registration; the Privy Council can take any appropriate action. The General Medical Council is responsible for deciding upon the reciprocal acceptability of qualifications which is agreed with most Commonwealth countries and is in the discussion phase in relation to the European Community.

The Disciplinary Function
Although the General Medical Council may itself instigate actions against doctors on information received, it most commonly acts only in the event of an allegation being made. The disciplinary charge which can be brought before the Council against the doctor is that he was guilty of 'serious professional misconduct', which is to say that his conduct was such 'as would reasonably be regarded as disgraceful or dishonourable by his professional brethren of good repute and competency'. Thus, to some extent, serious professional misconduct is judged on current public attitudes, although professional men are, perhaps, rather less liberal in their views than are the majority.

There are two main ways in which the General Medical Council may become aware of matters needing their attention in a disciplinary role:

a. On a doctor's conviction of a criminal offence by a court in Great Britain and Ireland (including Eire) or in the Isle of Man or the Channel Islands, the Clerk of the Court will inform the Council of the fact. This applies also to courts martial. Although such cases have greatly reduced since the enactment of the Divorce Reform Act 1969, a doctor justifiably cited as co-respondent in the Family Division of the High Court in a case involving a patient might also be reported.

   b. Complaints against a doctor's conduct may be made by members of the public, including other doctors acting in a private capacity or by such bodies as a Family Practitioner Committee of the NHS, a Hospital Authority or the relevant Department of Health.

   Information is first laid by the Registrar before the President of the Council who rejects complaints which are obviously insignificant and passes the remainder to the Penal Cases Committee who may invite the doctor to explain his conduct. Three options are then open: the case may be dismissed, the doctor may be sent a warning letter or the case is referred to the Disciplinary Committee consisting of the President and 18 members (6 of whom must be elected and 2 must be laymen) of whom half usually sit at one time.

   It is at this point that the lawyer becomes actively involved as the Committee is advised on questions of law by an Assessor and the hearings conform to the practices of a court of law. The respondent may be represented, usually through his protection or defence society, and there is provision in all parts of the United Kingdom for appeal to the Privy Council against suspension or erasure (*see below*). A similar right of appeal applies to a dentist appearing before the General Dental Council. Findings in a previous court are accepted as factual and may not be argued.[3] The hearings are public, and this is one of the main complaints against the system levied by those seeking its reform – no matter what his innocence in relation to professional conduct, a doctor's standing in a community can seldom be unaffected by sensational reportage of his private life.[4] The Disciplinary Committee has only two courses open to it – to dismiss the complaint or to find the allegations proved and amounting to serious professional misconduct.

   There is no delimiting definition of serious professional misconduct but, in general, the Committee is likely to regard as most serious any misconduct which implies that the doctor has taken advantage of his privileges and of his special training and position as a professional man. Thus, false certification and the improper prescription of – or self-indulgence in – drugs are bound to be censured; in the latter case, further action may be taken by the Secretary of State under the Misuse of Drugs Act 1971 (*see* Chapter 23).

   Use of his training to procure an illegal abortion will certainly not go unpunished and such cases still occur despite the wide compass of the Abortion Act 1967. The most widely publicized abuse of the doctor's

<hr>

   [3] There is some doubt as to whether the findings in a Coroner's Court would be so accepted and the doctor may dispute the facts on which his conviction was based in an overseas Court.

   [4] An interesting discussion of the disciplinary function of the GMC is given by O'Donnell M. (1973) Yesterday's gentlemen, *World Med.* 9(3),15.

professional position relates to adultery with a person with whom he or she is in a professional relationship. Such accusations may often be made in a spirit of revenge and much of the case may depend upon the definition of a professional relationship; recent cases indicate that the Disciplinary Committee's interpretation is generally strict. Other manifest abuses of position, such as indecent assault or attempted rape, will usually reach the Disciplinary Committee by virtue of notification from a Criminal Court and are, therefore, irrebuttable.

Advertising is one aspect of professional misconduct which illustrates how the climate of public opinion may influence professional ethics. The age of 'instant television' and the widespread interest in medical matters have dictated a relaxation of the old rule of professional anonymity in public. The current view seems to be that, as long as a doctor is already a recognized authority in the field under discussion, the public have a reasonable right to know his name and its publication would not constitute an offence; such an attitude would probably not be held, however, were the doctor using a television interview to raise his professional reputation. A far more dangerous source of potential misconduct in the course of an interview lies in the unwitting criticism of a fellow practitioner.

Probably the most frequent cause for notification is conviction for the abuse of alcohol, particularly in association with the Road Traffic Acts. Most first offences are dealt with by warning letter, but repeated convictions not only bring the profession into disrepute but also indicate that the doctor may be a danger to his patients; more serious action is likely in the end.

Following a finding of proven 'serious professional misconduct', the Disciplinary Committee may postpone sentence, in which case the practitioner is, in effect, put on probation, or it may suspend the doctor's registration for a period not exceeding 12 months. The most severe penalty is that of erasure from the Register. In addition to the general right to appeal to the Privy Council, applications for restoration to the Register may, in this case, be made any time after 10 months have elapsed.

It will be seen that the disciplinary function of the General Medical Council is directed to misconduct. Except in unusual circumstances, it is not concerned with negligence. Professional negligence is a matter of civil litigation, as is any other tort or delict, and is discussed later in this chapter.

MEDICAL ETHICS

Much of the ethics of medical practice represents a purely intraprofessional code of conduct. The maintenance of good relations often devolves on the professional associations, for example the British Medical Association, and seldom involves the lawyer. Ethics in relation to the patient are, however, another matter and may well result in litigation. Since much of this is based on common or case law, complex arguments may arise. Little more will be attempted than to mention some of the typical problems which may occur.

The Medical Code

It is doubtful if any universities now require the recitation of the 'Hippocratic Oath' at graduation. Nonetheless, it is a reasonable assumption that the act of qualifying for registration implies acceptance of a code which has been fashioned over centuries of development and it is worth reiterating the main components of what is held to be the original work.[5]

The primary consideration is the welfare of the patient; not only is a general affirmation given to apply one's skills to his or her benefit but it is positively declared to be improper to do anything which might harm the patient. Euthanasia and abortion are specifically condemned and, by implication, so is exceeding one's skill in undertaking specialist treatment. Improper association with patients or their families is specifically mentioned and, finally, much importance is attached to what is now known as professional confidence.

These principles, together with those arising from the barbarities peculiar to the twentieth century, are restated in the Declaration of Geneva approved by the World Medical Association.[6]

Consent to Examination and Treatment

The examination or treatment of a patient without his consent may constitute assault unless an emergency situation exists. The form of consent is, however, not uniform, and special difficulties may arise in relation to medico-legal examinations which may be positively to the subject's detriment.

Consent may be taken as implied when the patient presents himself or herself for examination and treatment. Even so, the implication only pertains to what the patient would reasonably expect – a patient does not expect a vaginal examination if she complains of a cough, although a really dedicated physician might contend that a *full* examination of every patient is necessary for accurate diagnosis. In this case, he should obtain specific consent for unusual clinical methods and it is well to have such consent given in front of a witness. Examinations of the opposite sex, particularly of women patients by male doctors, should ideally always be chaperoned; unfortunately, the current shortage of nursing

---

[5] *See: Medical Ethics* (1974, London, British Medical Association) for this and other ethical definitions.

[6] Produced in 1947 and amended in 1968.

staff makes this a counsel of perfection which it is almost impossible to observe.

Minor invasive investigations – such as withdrawal of blood from a vein – which might cause pain and have a very small morbidity can, as a matter of practicality, be undertaken without specific consent; they are no more than part of the normal practice of patient care. The problems of consent to major surgical procedures are discussed in Chapter 31.

The legal age above which valid consent can be given is now 16 in England[7] and is probably the same in Scotland.[8] Any consent to examination or treatment of a person below that age must be obtained from a parent or guardian. The doctor is in a dilemma if this is not forthcoming, say on religious grounds, and each such case must be decided, firstly, on the doctor's assessment of the importance of the matter and, secondly, on the chance of mishap; any decision to override parental opposition must be made on the basis of adequate justification. Such situations can stem from parental resistance to blood transfusion. The legalistic escape of applying for transfer of the child to the care of the local authority[9] has been advocated but is seldom needed, or now recommended, in the present climate of public opinion.

Unconscious patients or those incapable of understanding for other reasons cannot give consent. In such cases, the consent of a relative should ideally be obtained but is not needed when treatment is immediately necessary to protect life or health. In dire circumstances, such as a road traffic accident, it may even be reasonable for a doctor to give treatment which he knows to be inadequate – for example, in the absence of sterile gauze, it would be quite proper to use unsterile material to stop lethal bleeding. Such treatment should, however, be confined to the actual emergency; any which could be postponed pending admission to hospital should be left aside. The problems of consent to procedures which bear upon others, especially a husband or wife, are considered elsewhere (Chapter 17).

Examinations for legal purposes, the results of which may be damaging to the patient, constitute a special category but, again, a general rule is that, with a few well-defined exceptions, consent is necessary to eliminate any suspicion of assault. The most obvious examples of such

[7] Family Law Reform Act 1969 (s. 8).

[8] The author is unable to find an authority for this generally accepted practice. It is recommended by the *Report of the Committee on the Age of Majority*, 1967 (Cmnd. 3342, London, HMSO), but the recommendation was not included in the Age of Majority (Scotland) Act 1969. There seems no absolute reason why a Scottish minor (a female over the age of 12 or a male over 14) should not give consent of this type, but prudence would dictate that, up to the age of 16 supplementary consent be obtained from a parent or guardian.

[9] Children and Young Persons Act 1969, s. 23; Social Work (Scotland) Act 1968, s. 16.

examinations are those requested by the police who have, themselves, no authority to compel anyone to undergo medical examination whether he be accused or victim. It would even appear that examinations directed to no more than identification might be improper especially if they extended beyond the normal. Thus, an accused person must submit a finger-print recording; a Magistrate's Order or a Sheriff's Warrant might well be needed to take a dental impression without consent. These problems are specifically argued elsewhere (p. 262).

Professional Secrecy

It is accepted as a principle that the patient, in confiding in the medical practitioner, can expect that confidence to be sustained. The moral obligation is clear and extends, save in certain circumstances, to include the rights of maturing children to secrecy in relation to their parents; it would be difficult today to claim that a person aged less than 16 was not protected from such disclosure and, in some sections of society, the critical age might even be placed lower. Decisions in such cases must rest with the individual doctor – aided by his protection society – but the results of any subsequent action based on a breach of professional secrecy will be decided largely on the qualification of the party to whom the information was given.

The legal basis for the doctrine of medical confidentiality is probable but less certain.[10]

The fact that some qualification of an apparently absolute dogma exists has been recognized for a long time, perhaps the classic reference being Lord Riddell[11] who, describing the necessity and importance of medical confidence, was of the opinion that 'We must recognize also that the rules regarding them exist for the welfare of the community. . . . We must recognize also that they must be modified to meet the inevitable changes that occur in the necessities of various generations'.

This adaptation to changing circumstances has gained momentum in recent years particularly in relation to the prevention of road traffic accidents. Thus, it now seems perfectly clear that a doctor who is aware that a driver is subject to epilepsy has a right, if not a duty, to report the case to a licensing authority.[12] Such an ethical duty certainly exists when

---

[10] Kitson v. Playfair (1896), *The Times*, March 28 is a doubtful authority. Smith S. and Fiddes F. S. (*Forensic Medicine*. (1955), 10th ed., London Churchill, p. 366) cite McCardie J. as referring, in 1927, to the medical profession's duty of keeping inviolate the secret knowledge that they might gain from treating their patients and as stating that a medical man who, without lawful excuse, broke the duty of confidence would be liable to a civil action for damages. A general, but certainly indirect, statement of the position rests in the judgment of Lord Denning M.R. in Att.Gen. v. Mulholland and Att.Gen. v. Foster [1963] 2 Q.B.477.

[11] *Medico Legal Problems*. (1929) London, Lewis.

[12] There is a statutory obligation to do so in Canada (Quebec Transport Act 1972).

the patient is in a position to damage large numbers of persons as, for example, in the case of a driver of public transport;[13] moreover 'it is not out of the question that a doctor who knew an unsafe patient of his was continuing to drive and yet did nothing about it might be liable in damages for negligence to anyone harmed by his patient on the roads.' [14] The important principles lie in the 'right to know' of the person informed and the degree of public risk; with road traffic accidents accounting for 7000 annual deaths in Great Britain, the public need is clear. It is equally obvious that, even in cases involving criminality, the doctor's actions should be tempered with discretion and with humanity. For example, self-induced abortion is a statutory offence in England and an offence at common law in Scotland. The clearly adverse medical reaction to disclosure of such cases is described in Chapter 19; but the doctor's decision may indeed be difficult to make if a third party is involved.[15]

In general, such difficulties arise only when the doctor is providing care for his patient. A person submitting to examination for, say, life in- surance purposes or for obtaining a pilot's licence is not 'in care' and consents to disclosure of the result of his examination to the appropriate body by virtue of his signature on the document. It would seem, how- ever, that, in default of such consent, insurance companies are not en- titled to medical information as of right; the results of a post-mortem examination, for example, would not necessarily be privileged without the consent of the next-of-kin. It is also doubtful whether such consent is implied when the examination is carried out at the request of an employer; if the doctor fails to persuade the person examined either to report an abnormality himself or to change his occupation, the need for breach of confidence must be carefully balanced against any public hazard.

Many such cases are covered by statutes, generally related to public health, e.g. the notification of infectious disease. The Notification of Addicts Order 1968 (now replaced by the Misuse of Drugs (Notification of and Supply to Addicts) Regulations 1973) extended this principle to conditions which, strictly speaking, do not necessarily involve others than the individual concerned; there is little doubt that legislation will continue to recognize the rights of the community as often transcending those of the individual. *Pari passu*, the important principle of the need for transmission of medical information only from doctor to *doctor* is gaining ground.

---

[13] Medical Defence Union, *Annual Report, 1969*.

[14] *Br. Med. J.* (1974) Doctors, drivers, and confidentiality. **1**, 399. The proposition seems very doubtful.

[15] At one time, a doctor who failed to report his knowledge of a crime would probably have been guilty of an offence (*See* Lord Goddard L.C.J. in Sykes v. D.P.P. [1962] A.C. 528). Misprision of felony has, however, now ceased to be unlawful (other than in relation to treason) by virtue of the Criminal Law Act 1967.

Of the other circumstances in which a doctor is certainly privileged to break his contract of confidence, major importance attaches to statements made in courts of law.

There is no doubt that, in English and Scots law, the doctor cannot refuse to give evidence in court simply because such evidence is based on information received in the course of a professional relationship.[16] The courts normally exercise great care in enforcing this doctrine and devices for satisfying the ends of justice and the doctor's conscience – such as passing information on paper – may be used; in the end, however, the implications of Lord Denning's opinion must apply – that judges have the power to direct a doctor to answer a question which is not only relevant but is also a proper and necessary question to be put in the course of justice.[17] Absolute immunity from allegations of breach of contract then follows and this applies also to statements made to lawyers during preparation of a case prior to hearings; Scottish precognitions are equally privileged. It is interesting that a doctor is not excluded when there is a statutory obligation for 'any other person' to disclose information to the police.[18]

The provision of confidential medical records is closely bound up with this problem and, again, only the order of a court can give absolute justification for their publication in advance of trial. This is now a statutory right under the Administration of Justice Act 1970, s. 31 and s. 32 and the Administration of Justice (Scotland) Act 1972, s. 1. A potential plaintiff or pursuer can now obtain medical records from a defendant at an early stage – even before proceedings have been started.[19] Furthermore, in cases in which a claim in respect of personal injuries is made, either party can demand a sight of a doctor's or hospital's records once proceedings have started; it is now, however, established that this disclosure of confidential medical documents should be made only to the medical advisors of the parties concerned.[20] Beyond this, while there is no doubt that some parties – for example, insurance companies – have a legitimate interest in medical records in certain circumstances, it seems that such records should not properly be disclosed without the specific consent of the patient or of his guardians or next-of-kin. Good sense must, however, prevail – consent unreasonably withheld can only provoke an adverse reaction and there are now clear

---

[16] See transcript of Nuttall v. Nuttall and Twyman (*Lancet* (1964) 2, 145).

[17] In Att.Gen. v. Mulholland and Att.Gen. v. Foster [1963] 2Q.B.477.

[18] Road Traffic Act 1972, s. 168; see Hunter v. Att.Gen., *The Times*, 9 February, 1974.

[19] Dunning v. Board of Governors of United Liverpool Hospitals, *Br. Med. J.* (1973) 1, 623.

[20] Davidson v. Lloyd Aircraft Services Ltd, *The Times*, 15 May, 1974. *See also* Lord Thomson in Connolly v. Edinburgh Northern Hospitals 1974 S.L.T. (Notes) 53.

indications that reports on medical examinations made for the purpose of litigation should be exchanged if so requested.[21]

The Doctor and the National Health Service

Up till the passing of the National Health Service (Scotland) Act 1972 and the National Health Service Reorganization Act 1973, doctors involved in the National Health Service were administratively divided. Those practising in hospitals did so through Regional Hospital Boards; those in general practice were contracted through Executive Councils.

The reorganization of all aspects of the service under Area Health Authorities or Boards has modified the administrative and disciplinary procedures within the service although the contrasting concepts of servants to the hospital and contractors in general practice have, if anything, sharpened. There is now no doubt that Hospital Authorities are liable for the actions of all their staff irrespective of their seniority and their consequent freedom to adopt working methods of their own choice. The liability of a master (i.e. the hospital) for the wrongful or negligent acts of his servants extends throughout the hospital hierarchy from nonmedical staff to senior consultants. This was clearly laid down by Lord Denning who stated 'when the doctor or surgeon, be he consultant or not, is employed and paid not by the patient but by the hospital authorities, I am of the opinion that hospital authorities are liable.'[22] Whether it be *post hoc* or *propter hoc*, all hospital medical staff in the National Health Service are now required to belong to a defence society.

The general practitioner is in no sense a servant of the Health Authority or Board, but, in providing his services, he accepts certain terms of contract which have been drawn up in the interests of the patients dependent upon the service. Breach of responsibility in relation to contracts may be the subject of complaint either by the administration itself or by the patient, or by the patient's spouse or (if the patient is deceased, ill or young) by any person; in this respect, the practitioner is liable for lapses by his nursing or secretarial staff and by any registered medical practitioner acting as his deputy, though he may, at the discretion of the Chairman of the Medical Service Committee, be released from the investigation if his deputy is a principal on the list of the same Family Practitioner Committee (Primary Care Committee in Scotland).

The terms of contract accepted by a practitioner in the Health Service include that he is obliged to take medical responsibility for patients on his list and for certain other relatively minor categories which include any person in need of emergency treatment. A patient may leave the list of a doctor immediately if he obtains that doctor's signature on his

[21] Civil Evidence Act 1972, s. 2(3) (not applicable in Scotland).
[22] In Gold v. Essex County Council [1942] 2 All E.R. 237.

medical card and another practitioner accepts him; without the doctor's signature, he must give notice to the Family Practitioner or Primary Care Committee and must wait fourteen days before he can register with another doctor; the practitioner can ask the relevant Committee to remove the name of a patient from his list and removal takes effect on the eighth day after the request is received or upon the patient's acceptance by another doctor – whichever is the earlier. If the doctor who wishes the patient to be removed from his list is treating him once a week or more often, he must so inform the Committee. Transfer can still take place immediately upon acceptance by another doctor but, in the absence of such acceptance, the doctor must inform the Committee when he ceases to treat the patient at intervals of seven days or less; removal takes effect eight days after the Committee has been so informed.

Inevitably, conflict must occasionally arise as to the interpretation of the terms of contract, the commonest source of complaint being from those patients who believe they have received inadequate consideration. A system of investigation of such complaints exists and has not been significantly affected by the implementation of the 1972 and 1973 Health Service Acts.

Discipline is vested in Service Committees consisting of 3 professionals – doctors, dentists, pharmacists, etc., as applicable – 3 lay members and an independent Chairman. Complaints are originally screened by the Chairman who, with or without consultation with the practitioner concerned, may decide that no hearing is necessary; he will then take it to the Service Committee, who may decide the issue without a hearing. Hearings are of little significance to the legal profession as they are private, and paid legal representatives may not address the Committee; only occasionally are solicitors present to advise. The Committee can make various recommendations to the Family Practitioner or Primary Care Committee, including one to take no further action. The Health Authority or Board can, should they so wish, modify the recommendations. In the event of a decision to withhold remuneration from the practitioner, there is provision for appeal to the appropriate Minister who, if he does not dismiss the appeal on documentary evidence, can call for an oral hearing by the Appeal Body. Evidence at this point is taken on oath and legal representation is permitted on both sides. If it is suggested that the inclusion of a practitioner's name in the appropriate List is prejudicial to the welfare of the Service, the Family Practitioner or Primary Care Committee may refer the matter for consideration by a statutory Tribunal. The practitioner may be represented before the Tribunal, against whose findings he has a further right of appeal.

There is, therefore, a remarkable contrast between the publicity afforded to hearings before the General Medical Council and the privacy of investigations under the National Health Service Acts. The latter process is, however, cumbersome and, while the new process has not yet been fully agreed, it would seem that some of the functions of investigation may be undertaken by the Health Service Commissioner.

The Health Service Commissioner will be specifically excluded from action in any case in which the complaint has a remedy through a court of law. Having assured himself that the body complained of has had a reasonable opportunity to investigate and reply on its own accord, the Health Commissioner can instigate further investigation by his department. Again, it is considered that, in view of the informal nature of the investigation, legal representation should not normally be necessary. Individuals under investigation may be accompanied by a friend, trades union representative or member of a staff association.[23]

Outwith the Health Service

Doctors working wholly in private practice clearly have no contract with the Health Service but nevertheless have similar duties to their patients which are based on medical ethics. However, in the event of treatment being considered to be of inadequate quality as, for example, by failure to make a home visit when asked, the patient would probably need to show that damage had resulted before legal action could be taken against the doctor; a complaint might, however, be laid before the General Medical Council. Such conditions must be rare in private practice, in which economic laws operate as effectively as do the statutory rules of the Health Service.

Employment in industry carries some ethical difficulties. If employed as a Health Officer, the doctor still must base his professional conduct on a doctor/patient relationship; the acceptance of a contract involving disclosure of confidential information to employers against the wishes of the persons in medical care would certainly lead to a charge of unethical conduct against which there would be no defence. It is generally advised that the employment advisory medical officer should firmly dissociate his function from that of an employee's regular medical attendant. Other problems in industry – for example, those associated with experimentation, advertising and the like – might arise and are dealt with below.

On the face of things, the position of Medical Officers in the armed forces is equivocal in that they are the regular medical practitioners of the service personnel and yet at the same time are paid by and clearly owe an allegiance to the Crown which also employs their patients. The

---

[23] There has recently been a marked increase in attention to what may be loosely termed 'patients' rights'. The interested reader is referred to (a) Davies M. (Chairman) (1973) *Report of the Committee on Hospital Complaints Procedure*, London, DHSS and Welsh Offices; (b) Elliott-Binns E.U.E. (Chairman) (1969) *Suggestions and Complaints in Hospital: Report of the Working Party*, Edinburgh, SHHD.

principle governing medical practice in relation to servicemen – but not their dependants – must be modified to some extent in favour of the need to benefit the specialized 'community' as a whole. Two main factors work to minimize difficulties which are often the subject of ill-informed exaggeration. In the first place, by accepting service in the armed forces, the patients have accepted – and appreciate that they have accepted – both the advantages and disadvantages of a corporate system while, secondly, the service authorities themselves are only too anxious to preserve a normal doctor/patient relationship in all matters which do not directly and adversely affect the efficiency of a fighting unit. The relevant Service Acts and Queen's Regulations will normally cover any situation in which a service doctor, or a service patient, is in a position of professional uncertainty.

Medical Experimentation

A discussion of the ethics of experiments in medicine need only be brief as the lawyer will seldom be involved.

Some form of human experimentation is essential if medical knowledge is to advance to the good of the community; much preliminary work can be done on animals, but, ultimately, it is the effect of the procedure upon human beings in controlled circumstances which will determine its use in practice.

Experiments can be intended as treatment in an experimental fashion, they may be designed to increase academic knowledge with little prospect of immediate practical application or they may be needed to test the efficacy of an accepted treatment or to study the spread of disease. The subjects may be the researchers themselves, healthy volunteers or sick patients.

Experimental treatments are ethical only provided that there is no recognized alternative or that the recognized treatments have failed and the patient is seriously ill; the situation should always be explained and consent obtained – certainly if the treatment is painful or possibly liable to shorten life still further; in this case, the additional consent of a spouse or a close relative would be desirable. In general, the principles defining medical negligence (*see below*) will obtain in these cases.

Experiments designed mainly for academic advancement of knowledge are inapplicable to patients and are the prerogative of dedicated research workers and their assistants; much heroic work of this type is undertaken by physiologists – it is doubtful, for example, if modern air travel would have been possible in its absence. Two points of medico-legal importance arise. Firstly, the head of department must ensure that the risks taken are calculated to eliminate so far as is possible any serious danger to health. Secondly, the problem of the use of students as volunteer subjects often arises; such students will be of adult status but, while 'paternalism' is currently deprecated, most teaching organizations are conscious of some responsibility *in loco parentis* and formulate very stringent rules.

Greatest interest centres around the use of disinterested groups who are easily controlled – prisoners, soldiers, etc. – and of patients themselves for observations on disease processes and on the value of new medicines. These experiments can only be justified provided that they do no significant harm to the subjects and that the results are likely to be generally beneficial. Harm to patients would, of course, include the withholding of a reasonable treatment in order to study the effects of an untried remedy, particularly by using placebo controls – the principles are clear but each experimental project needs individual consideration. Consent is, perhaps, the most important single factor governing the ethics of an experiment. It need only be emphasized here that valid consent must be informed – the exact nature of, and the discomfort associated with, the experiment must be explained; it must be freely given and not associated with unreasonable reward – it is at least arguable whether prisoners can ever meet these requirements; withdrawal must be possible at any time; and the subjects must be capable of consent – a matter of mental capability and of age. The use of children for medical experiments is a particularly emotive subject and one which has medico-legal implications in that it is doubtful if a parent or guardian has the right to consent to a technical assault on a child unless the procedure is of positive benefit to that individual child. It should be noted that, whereas minors above the age of 16 are empowered to consent to medical treatment or examination, they have no similar statutory authority in relation to research investigations.[24] Nevertheless, advances in paediatric medicine must be made despite the evident difficulties. On one occasion in the United States of America, the child inmates of a home for mental defectives were infected with the virus of infective hepatitis as part of a manifestly useful research study in preventive medicine. Although one may, on the bald facts, reasonably doubt the ethical basis of such a project, the action of the investigator was strongly upheld by his national medical association; it is clear that there can be no 'blanket' approach to a subject which is governed, in the end, by humane pragmatism.[25]

Medical Negligence
The lawyer may well become involved in cases of medical negligence, which is a subject so wide that it cannot possibly be covered fully. Only an outline of the principles involved will be attempted.

---

[24] Family Law Reform Act 1969, s. 8(3) (not applicable in Scotland).

[25] The various views on this case are admirably argued by Golman L. (1973) The Willowbrook debate, *World Med.* **9** (1), 79. This article summarizes previous publications on the subject.

Criminal negligence can be dismissed rapidly. It is virtually confined to situations in which the patient has died, and it then implies negligence involving such a degree of recklessness as to amount to culpable homicide or unlawful killing 'not amounting to murder'. The great majority of such cases are associated with drunkenness or with impaired efficiency due to the use of drugs by doctors. The museum of Forensic Pathology in Edinburgh contains a specimen of some 8 ft of small intestine removed by a drunken obstetrician in mistake for an umbilical cord. Such cases are scarcely defensible; as Simpson has said, since a professional man should be more able than most to appreciate his impairment of function due to alcoholism, the fact that he was drunk at the time of a negligent act merely aggravates the offence.[26]

The vast majority of actions for negligence are civil actions for tort or delict and certain well-known facts must be proved for the action to succeed.

Firstly, the doctor must have owed a duty of care to the complainer or plaintiff. This, as has been seen, may not always exist despite the fact that an examination has taken place as, for example, in relation to fitness for employment. On the other hand, no bilateral agreement is needed to establish a duty of care. The essential feature appears to be the intention of the doctor to treat or to heal; once the intent is established, the duty continues until the need for care is past or until alternative arrangements have been willingly made.

Secondly, it must be shown that the doctor failed in his duty of care. Failure is a relative term; its degree must be measured against the skill that might reasonably be expected of the individual doctor. Much will depend upon the diagnostic and therapeutic aids available at the time; a doctor would be expected to be more efficient in an intensive care unit than by the roadside. The acceptance of such common-sense principles in British law makes it unnecessary to pass 'Good Samaritan' protective legislation as has been required under many other jurisdictions. Provided he has executed reasonable skill and care, a doctor cannot be held negligent for a mistake in diagnosis or treatment. The classic authority for this is Lord Clyde who, when Lord President, stated, 'In the realm of diagnosis and treatment, there is ample scope for genuine difference of opinion, and one man clearly is not negligent merely because his conclusion differs from that of other professional men, nor because he has displayed less skill or knowledge than others would have shown'.[27] In the same judgement, Lord Clyde introduced the concept of 'accepted medical practice', giving his opinion that, having shown that there was an accepted practice and that the doctor failed to follow that practice, the

[26] In *Forensic Medicine*, 7th ed., p. 49.
[27] In Hunter v. Hanley 1955 S.L.T. 213 at p. 217.

plaintiff in an action for medical negligence must further show that the course the doctor adopted was one which no professional man of ordinary skill would have taken had he been acting with ordinary care. This proviso is vitally significant. Accepted practice may differ from hospital to hospital; the important point is whether an approach to diagnosis and therapy was or was not reasonable. Nonetheless, the fact that a doctor has been found negligent in his use of antibiotics despite the evidence of witnesses for the defence to the effect that the doctor's treatment was acceptable appears to have undermined this principle to some extent.[28]

Thirdly, the patient must have suffered damage. The definition of 'damage' is certainly widening, and, when extended to mental distress, is almost all-embracing. It is, however, a function of the court to measure the loss or damage in terms of money and it is this which must ultimately deter the frivolous action. Negligence resulting in death can be the subject of an action by surviving kin – including those illegitimate or adopted – on similar grounds to those which would have been available had the patient lived.[29]

In certain circumstances, negligence as defined above is self-evident. For example, there has clearly been negligence if a pair of forceps is left in the abdomen and the patient is thereby subjected to a second operation. The doctrine of *res ipsa loquitur* then operates and it is for the doctor to prove that he was not responsible or to demonstrate extenuating factors.

Such cases are commonly settled but, in the event of their being contested, it would seem that this plea is rarely accepted by the court and, almost invariably, it is for the complainer or plaintiff to prove the fact of negligence. The doctor, generally in concert with the hospital or other employing authority, may claim that no negligence existed in the true sense; he may defend himself on the grounds that his course of action carried well-known risks which were fully explained to the patient and which the patient accepted; or he may assert that the patient himself contributed to his own disability.[30] It is apparent that two patients can leave hospital each with a disability of comparable gravity and each deriving from the treatment received; yet one may receive substantial damages while the other is not compensated, depending on whether 'fault' was proved. There is much to be said for the introduction of a 'no-fault' scheme of compensation operated by some form of compulsory insurance. Unfortunately, there is a great deal of practical diffi-

---

[28] Hucks v. Cole (1968) 112 S.J. 483.

[29] Law Reform (Miscellaneous Provisions) Act 1934; Fatal Accidents Act 1976.

[30] The acceptance of contributory negligence would not affect the fact of negligence but only the damages awarded.

culty in the application of such a policy which is one of the subjects under review by the Pearson Committee currently considering civil liability and compensation for personal injury. The operation of the law in respect of medical negligence may change dramatically in the not too distant future.[31]

[31] The 'no-fault' compensation scheme operating in New Zealand (Accident Compensation Act 1972) may prove a valuable example.

Chapter 31

Deaths Associated with Surgery and Anaesthesia

MEDICO-LEGAL interest focuses on deaths occurring during or as a result of surgical operations for several reasons. Firstly, a thorough investigation of fatalities is one means by which surgical treatment can be improved and unsatisfactory techniques can be eliminated. Secondly, such deaths cause considerable concern among those indirectly affected, and actions for negligence may result. Related to both these considerations is the availability of major surgical procedures to patients in increasingly 'high-risk' categories; forensic medicine has a part to play in maintaining a balance in advances in treatment.

Deaths of this type are often loosely referred to as 'anaesthetic deaths'. This is a misnomer which, apart from its undeserved professional implications, may, by limiting the field of investigation, be positively detrimental to progress. The term should be confined to those deaths which, *after full investigation*, can properly be attributed to the anaesthetic; phrases which presuppose this conclusion should be avoided.

Notification of deaths associated with surgery varies between England and Scotland. In the latter, 'anaesthetic deaths'[1] are reportable as a statutory duty and a particular procedure is followed in their investigation. This involves, firstly, the completion of a standard questionnaire (Appendix O) which is signed by both the surgeon and the anaesthetist and is forwarded to the Fiscal.[2] The case is then referred to the Police Surgeon who may or may not advise the need for a postmortem dissection. The Fiscal will then report the facts to the Crown Office who will dispose of the case according to the findings. In England, the obligation upon the Coroner to inquire into such deaths is no more specific than that they come under the general heading of violent or unnatural deaths. However, the Registrar is required to report any

---

[1] Defined as deaths occurring during the administration of an anaesthetic or before recovery from the effects of an anaesthetic.

[2] The Association of Anaesthetists of Great Britain and Ireland clearly approved this practice in their evidence to the Brodrick Committee (*Report of the Committee on Death Certification and Coroners*, 1971, para. 17.12).

death appearing to have occurred during an operation or before recovery from the effects of an anaesthetic,[3] while many coroners, acting on a purely local basis, insist that deaths occurring within 24 hours of the administration of an anaesthetic should be reported by the hospital authority. The Brodrick Committee has deprecated the isolation of anaesthesia as a medical hazard attracting particular attention.[4] Certainly there are many medical procedures, some of a purely diagnostic nature, which carry comparable risks yet excite less official interest.

HAZARDS OF SURGICAL OPERATIONS

All surgical operations, whether accompanied by local or general anaesthesia, or when performed without anaesthesia, have some morbidity and mortality. Efficient surgical practice is based on accurate clinical judgment as to whether the risks outweigh the dangers or discomfort to the patient of withholding operation.

Proper consent to operation is mandatory. The patient should be fully apprised of the balance between probable success and probable failure in his or her particular case; this is of special importance when consent is being given on behalf of another – e.g. a minor or an unconscious relative – or when an operation attended by some risk, such as the examination of an organ by biopsy, is performed mainly or partly as a research procedure. Consent after full explanation implies acceptance of the risks and, provided the operation has been carried out in accordance with the principles of good practice (see p. 391), there can be no question of negligence.

The Decision to Operate

The correctness of the decision to operate has to be considered whenever a death occurs during or is obviously referable to an operation.

No one would question the validity of an operation of even heroic proportions undertaken to save a life which would otherwise undoubtedly be lost. Very few would dispute the need for an admittedly palliative procedure designed to alleviate the pain of a terminal illness. But what if the risks to life of operation can be assessed as greater than those of inaction? Or what if the disease underlying severe pain has a negligible mortality in relation to suppressive surgery?

Obviously, no general ruling can be given and each case must be assessed by the surgeon and the anaesthetist acting together. Balanced decisions must be based on full preoperative information and must take into account the availability of measures to counteract difficulties

---

[3] Registration of Births, Deaths and Marriages Regulations 1968, reg. 51.

[4] Report of the Committee on Death Certification and Coroners, Ch. 17.

which are reasonably foreseeable. It might, for example, be justifiable to perform an operation which would be expected to result in severe blood loss; it would be unjustifiable to do so without previously arranging for a readily available supply of replacement blood known to be compatible with the recipient (*see below*, p. 406).

The Choice of Patient

Recent advances in anaesthesia, particularly the introduction of muscle relaxants, allow for a level of narcosis in major surgery which is far less deep than was possible, say, twenty years ago. As a result, patients in an older age group and less physically fit can be anaesthetized with increasing confidence. But, although surgical techniques are continually improving, the physical damage resulting from a given surgical operation remains the same and must affect the old and infirm more adversely than the young and healthy. Paradoxically, therefore, the effect of improvements in anaesthesia may be to increase marginally the statistical mortality of a particular operation, but this merely reflects the widening availability of complex surgery. An implication of negligence based on the death of a patient in a suspect category might well have the effect of depriving elderly patients of a potentially fuller remaining life simply because of apprehension of the consequences of failure. There are, therefore, very good reasons for dispensing with public inquest in all cases in which there is no evidence of avoidable mishap.[5]

The problems facing the investigating pathologist are often formidable and are certainly greatest in relation to the hazards specific to anaesthetics. These must, therefore, be considered separately – but still without prejudice to the thesis that they are only one aspect of the whole spectrum of major surgery. It is convenient to discuss individually local, spinal and general anaesthesia.

Local Anaesthetics

These agents, which may be given by infiltration of the area or by blocking specific nerve bundles, act by paralysing the sensory nerves with which they come in contact. Thus, a localized area can be made pain-free without narcotizing the whole organism, an obvious advantage when only minor surgery is to be performed or when the subject is unfit for a general anaesthetic.

All these drugs are absorbed to some extent and a maximum therapeutic dose is established for each agent on the assumption that absorption and detoxication will be normal. The old and debilitated may

---

[5] While the Brodrick Committee could not agree with this entirely, there is a clear indication from their report that they favoured some form of selection in relation to the type of inquiry (*Report of the Committee on Death Certification and Coroners*, 1971, p. 57, p. 207). Such a situation does, of course, obtain in Scotland.

destroy the drug less efficiently but, young or old, the major hazard lies in rapid absorption through widely dilated vessels in the part injected. Absorption is notoriously rapid from some areas – e.g. the nose and throat – and these are well known to anaesthetists. In order to reduce the size of the available vessels, it is common practice to inject a vaso-constrictive agent such as adrenaline at the same time as the anaesthetic. The dilemma then raised is that adrenaline, of itself, may produce adverse reactions. Moreover, the possibility of accidental injection of the drug directly into a major vessel – which will result in the sudden absorption of the whole dose – still remains.

The hazards of local anaesthesia can, therefore, be summarized as:

a. Overdosage of either the anaesthetic or vasoconstrictive agent, the total quantity and concentration of which must be related to the age, stature and fitness of the patient.

b. Rapid absorption from highly absorptive areas or as a result of local vasodilatation.

c. Accidental injection of a vessel.

d. Hypersensitivity reactions which most authorities now regard as being, in fact, due to overdosage.

In the event of serious error, there may be a general effect on the central nervous system which is either excitory – in which case convulsions may occur – or depressive – when the danger to life is from respiratory paralysis. Far less commonly, the heart may be directly affected.

Very occasionally, there may be local residua which result in long-term damage to the patient. Thus, an abnormally high concentration injected directly into a nerve may lead to permanent loss of function. As with any injection, there is the possibility of needle breakage.

The incidence of severe reactions to local anaesthesia is very low – in the region of 0·05 per cent – but the risks certainly increase with infirmity – so much so that many anaesthetists may prefer to use a modern, relatively nontoxic general anaesthetic in 'high-risk' patients.

Spinal Anaesthesia

Whole areas of the body can be rendered insensitive if a local anaesthetic is applied to the spinal cord through the cerebrospinal fluid (CSF). Since the nerves which supply the life support functions are placed high in the cord, the dangers of spinal anaesthesia increase as the anaesthetic is allowed to rise in the CSF. Some diffusion is inevitable and spinal anaesthesia has a definite mortality which is probably slightly higher than that of even relatively primitive general anaesthetics, particularly when the risks of introducing infection are included. Accordingly, the more difficult technique of epidural anaesthesia, in which the nerve roots are involved but the agent is separated from the central nervous tissue by the thick dura mater, has been introduced; it achieves much the same result as injecting the anaesthetic into the CSF and is far safer.

The problems of the standard method of spinal anaesthesia can be summarized as:

    a. those due to unwanted action on the nerves;
    b. those due to alteration in the volume of fluid protecting the brain and spinal cord.

As to undesirable action on the nerves, the difficulty is that, in addition to paralysing the sensory nerves, there is an action on the sympathetic nerves which control the strength or tone of the blood vessels; a fall in blood pressure is the almost invariable result. A moderate fall in a healthy person is of little significance; but the effect may be very severe if it occurs in the elderly, in those with pre-existing heart disease or in association with haemorrhage. The results may be disastrous if some degree of respiratory hypoxia is added; true coronary insufficiency may be precipitated and there may be either cardiac or respiratory arrest due to the impossibility of maintaining the circulation. In addition, the vagus nerve is commonly left unaffected. Death may, therefore, occur suddenly and quite unexpectedly due to cardiac inhibition following an unnatural stimulation of the nerve.

The hazards related to the changes in the volume of cerebrospinal fluid are less dramatic but may cause appreciable disability.

Lumbar puncture headache occurs in about a quarter of those recovering from spinal anaesthesia. It is probably due to continuing leakage through the hole made by the needle, so much so that the incidence and severity of the condition is almost proportional to the size of needle used. In addition to headache, the patient may complain of vomiting, dizziness and abnormal hearing. The condition is usually transient but may on occasions last for months.

More significant is the occasional double vision which occurs as a marked complication once in some one thousand cases treated. The probable cause is movement of the brain following removal of protective fluid. Recovery within a month is usual but a few cases sustain permanent paralysis of the muscles of one eye.

Permanent nerve damage associated with the actual agent used may occur in a very small proportion – of the order of 1 : 10 000 – of spinal anaesthetics, while the possibility of haemorrhage following puncture of a vessel also exists. The introduction of sepsis into the spinal canal is a hazard peculiar to the method and one which must almost always result from some form of negligence.

General Anaesthesia
General anaesthetics may be given by inhalation or intravenously.

Anaesthetics entering the body by inhalation combine with the body tissues in order to produce a narcotic effect. By any definition, they are toxic substances and it is remarkable that pharmacological and medical skills have combined to limit to miniscule proportions the mortality from a deliberate interference with the patient's physiological balance.

Children and the very aged are rather more susceptible to general inhalation anaesthetics than are adults in the middle age range; there is some suggestion that negroes are more susceptible to their ill-effects, particularly those with sickle cell trait (*see* p. 11). The general mortality rate is probably in the order of 1 : 1500 and the causes can be summarized as being due to:

a. the technique of administration;

b. the actual anaesthetic agent;

c. hazards associated with unconsciousness;

d. external problems – e.g. explosion.

Death due to inadequate techniques are of two main kinds – vagal stimulatory and hypoxic. Cardiac inhibition due to vagal stimulation is a real threat because the autonomic system is relatively spared in the process of nervous suppression; the patient is susceptible to abnormal stimuli despite apparent unconsciousness. Thus, stimulation of the respiratory lining by a high concentration of irritant gas or the passing of a tube through an inadequately anaesthetized larynx may result in sudden arrest of the heart. Vagal inhibition of the heart is much more likely in the presence of oxygen deficit. Cardiac failure of a rather different type (ventricular fibrillation) can result from excessive secretion of adrenaline by patients who have been inadequately sedated; dental patients are particularly susceptible by reason of their generally ambulant treatment while the actual use of adrenaline during the induction of anaesthesia obviously increases the risk.

By far the greatest risk in relation to technique is the provocation of tissue hypoxia due to true oxygen deprivation. The skill of anaesthesia lies in reducing hypoxia to a minimum while achieving an unconscious patient; this is done by the addition of oxygen to the anaesthetic mixture supplemented, if necessary, by forced ventilation of the lungs. An inadequate oxygen supply may derive, firstly, from the apparatus itself. Murder mysteries have been written around mistaken colouring or filling of gas cylinders – and it can happen accidentally. Cylinders may run dry or taps may be inadvertently turned off – or may not turn on in an emergency. Responsibility for the apparatus is clearly vested in the anaesthetist and the prevention of catastrophe due to malfunction depends on his vigilance. Anaesthesia and hypoxia – which are quite distinct processes – each result in unconsciousness and it is the experience of the anaesthetist which guards the patient; warning signs may be missed by the inexperienced or even by the consultant if he is required to supervise more than one operating theatre. It is possible for an apparently satisfactory induction to be due not so much to the presence of anaesthetic as to the absence of adequate oxygen, and, unless this is corrected, the patient may suffer any of the long-term effects of hypoxia on being released to the normal atmosphere. Such confusion may result even from the use of the more simple agents such as nitrous oxide; there are particular hazards in dental practice in which, although anaesthesia is generally of short duration, cerebral hypoxia may be exaggerated by the sitting position. Severe shortage of oxygen during deep anaesthesia may be due to inadequate ventilation and can result in sudden death on the table due to heart failure. Again, conditions such as anaemia, haemorrhage or lung disease may have an important synergistic action.

Ill-effects from the actual anaesthetics depend upon their toxicity; this may be selective as to organ and some agents – e.g. the almost obsolete chloroform and cyclopropane – are particularly cardiotoxic. This, however, is not to say that such drugs should not be used by competent practitioners if they have other advantages; the delicate balance upon which good medical practice depends is well illustrated in this context.

Severe long-term effects may be seen in the lungs following general inhalation anaesthesia of any type – generally in the form of collapse of portions of the lung or of pneumonia. Fatal disease of the liver may also be attributed to the anaesthetic agent. Chloroform was especially implicated in the past but it is probable that its reputation was ill founded; any toxic effect of an anaesthetic on the liver is greatly potentiated by associated hypoxia and this was especially true of that old agent. Therapeutic dilemmas also arise using modern drugs. Halothane is judged by most practitioners to be the best 'general' anaesthetic agent available. But it seems possible that repeated administration of anaesthetics of this group may load the liver with problems of metabolism to which it may succumb – particularly if the anaesthetics were repeated at very short intervals and the liver was previously unhealthy, for example, due to the effects of alcoholism.[6] The doctor must balance the advantage to the patient of a good anaesthetic agent against the possibility of subsequent liver damage; the important point is that this is a legitimate decision which only becomes unacceptable if the judgement is unconsidered.

Some patients are unduly susceptible to anaesthetics and may react abnormally. Malignant hyperpyrexia – or rapid and severe rise in body temperature – is one such example which can be associated even with

---

[6] There is very great controversy over this question. *See* for example Inman W. H. W. and Mushin W. W. (1974) Jaundice after repeated exposure to halothane: an analysis of reports to the Committee on Safety of Medicines, *Br. Med. J.* **1,** 5. The views expressed in this paper were contested in the USA by McPeek B. and Gilbert J. P. (1974) Onset of postoperative jaundice related to anaesthetic history, *Br. Med. J.* **3,** 615.

such simple agents as nitrous oxide.[7] Susceptibility to malignant hyperpyrexia, and probably to other forms of hypersensitivity, is genetically controlled; the importance of taking a good preoperative history is emphasized.

The unconscious patient poses special problems because he is unable to take correcting reflex action if an adverse situation arises. The commonest danger lies in failure to protect the air passages against inhalation of foreign material. Stomach contents may flow back into the mouth and air passages of a supine patient or the patient may vomit – particularly if there had been no preoperative sedation. Blood, swabs or even teeth may be inhaled without reflex coughing – there is an obvious potential association with dental surgery. Even without aspiration, the patient's tongue may fall back and cause suffocation. An acute asphyxial death may follow aspiration but survival can also be accompanied by an inflammatory process in the lungs of great severity associated with the acidity of the inhaled stomach contents; the aspiration of a solid object will cause collapse of a part of or the whole of the lung which will then be particularly susceptible to infection.

Occasionally, patients who have been operated upon may appear well for several days, until quite unheralded sudden death occurs. The cause is nearly always pulmonary embolism – a clot of blood, usually forming in a leg vein, detaches and lodges in the pulmonary artery. The formation of such clots is naturally associated with immobility in bed and, while every prophylactic care may be taken, occasional instances are inevitable; death is effectively due to natural causes.

The spectacular nature of fires and explosions probably leads to exaggeration of their frequency; nevertheless, very considerable effort must be put into their elimination. Cyclopropane and ether are highly inflammable, especially when combined with oxygen; it would be desirable to use gases which will not burn and this is one reason for the preference for halothane. If explosive gases are used, the concurrent use of electric tools or operation by diathermy must be severely limited and all equipment for lighting the inside of the body must be battery-powered. The main danger, however, lies in the static spark which cannot be anticipated; preventive measures include the use of conducting rubber equipment, the use of conducting materials for the floor and the maintenance of a relatively humid atmosphere.

Special Factors relating to Intravenous Anaesthesia
Anaesthesia is often induced by the injection of ultra-short-acting barbiturates of which methohexitone is the most commonly used. Occasionally, the whole surgical procedure may be covered by this method.

---

[7] *See* Ellis F. R. et al. (1974) *Br. Med. J.* **4,** 270.

Barbiturates have a profound effect on the blood pressure and on the action of the heart; as a result, they must be used with particular care in the elderly and unfit. There is no physiological control over the absorption of a substance injected into a vein, the whole dose is instantly available for transmission to the tissues and it cannot be removed; everything depends, therefore, on the skill of the injector.

Intravenous barbiturates also act on the respiratory centre which is affected by overdose so that the breathing becomes ineffective. Moreover, a tendency to uncontrolled reflex spasm is especially marked under barbiturate anaesthesia and any irritation of the throat may result in spasm of the glottis and suffocation of the patient. A lengthy intravenous anaesthetic can, therefore, be dangerous, as the anaesthetist's attention may be unduly taken up with the locus of injection at the expense of the airway.

The hazards of intravenous anaesthesia are most dramatically illustrated in the field of dental surgery where, despite recommendations to the contrary,[8] the single-handed anaesthetist/surgeon is not uncommon. Although the practice has been defended by experts, several deaths have been reported which make very clear the difficulty of performing two expert functions at the same time; coincidental complications with resuscitative apparatus have also been described.[9] Coroners' inquests have revealed some dramatic examples of hazards related to the maintenance of apparatus or the training of assistants, including unnoticed breakage of the tap on the oxygen cylinder or lack of oxygen dictating the summoning of help from the fire brigade; one assistant is reported as stating that she 'had not been on any course but had trained by watching others'.[10] From the medico-legal aspect, such circumstances are of far greater significance than are the physiological problems of anaesthesia.

Hazards associated with Relaxant Drugs

The use of relaxant drugs, which has opened up major surgery to a wide group of patients who might well have died under a comparably effective unassisted general anaesthetic, is not without hazard – mainly because of concurrent paralysis of the respiratory muscles. This is immaterial during the operation as the anaesthetist will be using, or have available, artificial respiration; nevertheless, persistent failure to breathe after the operation is not uncommon. Although this can be treated, the danger lies in relapse after the patient has left the expert

---

[8] Ministry of Health (1967) *Dental Anaesthesia, Report of Joint Sub-Committee of the Standing Medical and Dental Advisory Committee on Dental Anaesthesia.* London, HMSO.

[9] *Br. Med. J.* (1975) Death in the dental chair. **1**, 293.

[10] *Br. Med. J.* (1974) **4**, 352.

hands of the anaesthetist. Paralysis of the throat muscles may also occur and the danger of inhalation of regurgitated stomach contents is increased by the use of muscle relaxants.

THE EXPERT WITNESS

The pathologist's evidence in a case of death during an operation may well be limited. There will be little difficulty if death has resulted from a frank surgical mishap – the result, say, of failing to secure adequately an artery of moderate size is very obvious. Beyond this, the findings and interpretations become progressively less dogmatic. Thus, the presence of a tooth or a swab in the main air passages may be simple to demonstrate, but to state with certainty that death resulted from vagal stimulation as a result of their presence is very much harder. Vomit may be found in the trachea but it may be extremely difficult to decide whether this was the cause of, or the result of, a hypoxic death.

The pathologist will seek and demonstrate any pre-existing disease. But having done so, the standard dilemma in the interrelationship of disease with any accident remains to be solved – was it causative, contributory to or purely incidental to the death? It is seldom easy to make the choice with certainty and a cautious approach by the witness may be a sign of experience rather than of indecisiveness. If disease discovered is considered significant, further consideration must be given as to whether it was noted or, if not, should have been noted before the operation.

The real problem lies in the fact that the majority of operation deaths, and certainly most of those correctly regarded as 'anaesthetic deaths', will be of a physiological nature. There will be no anatomical evidence available to the pathologist and much of his opinion must be based on exclusion and reasoning. One cannot do better than quote Simpson:[11] 'The pathologist is bound to rely in part on what he is told of the events leading to death, for functional lapses like fall in blood pressure, cardiac arrhythmia, spasm of the glottis, or vagal inhibition leave no trace at autopsy.'

The post-mortem in such cases is incomplete without toxicological analyses designed to disclose a positive overdose of anaesthetic or other therapeutic agent, and it is important that both the pathologist and the analyst be properly informed as to the drugs which have been administered. Specimens should also be taken to assess any biochemical or enzymatic abnormalities which may have caused the catastrophe or which may indicate its mechanism; due regard, must, however, be paid to post-mortem changes which may affect the analytical result. But even

---

[11] In *Forensic Medicine*, 7th ed. p. 143.

with maximum investigation, the pathologist is often able to do little more than decide 'death was due to anaesthesia but there is no [or, and there is] evidence that the anaesthetic was given incorrectly'.

It is inescapable that the true answer will probably not be reached in the absence of full and frank discussion between surgeon, anaesthetist and pathologist. This is most likely to be attained in an atmosphere in which all parties are working together for the good of future patients; such a state is more easily achieved under the Scottish system of investigation and was clearly the objective of the Brodrick Committee.

In eliciting expert evidence, the advocate should remember that the pathologist is seldom an expert clinician. He is often pressed to state whether an operation or anaesthetic procedure was good or proper; his correct attitude is to refuse to be drawn unless he has a special knowledge or unless the matter is of great simplicity.

RESPONSIBILITY FOR THE PATIENT AT OPERATION

It is almost impossible to lay down dividing lines of responsibility between the surgeon and the anaesthetist which can be applied as a generalization. Decisions taken can only be assessed in the light of the particular circumstances. The operating theatre in some ways resembles the flight deck of an aircraft – the captain is undoubtedly in command and takes ultimate decisions but it would be an unusual man who disregarded the advice of his navigator without careful consideration.

On this analogy, the surgeon is the captain and is ultimately responsible for the decision to operate, the extent of the operation and for any decisions as to whether to complete or abort his intended routine. But in making these, he will be advised by the anaesthetist as to the patient's preoperative physical state and his condition during the operation. The anaesthetist is responsible for the functioning of the anaesthetic apparatus, for maintaining adequate anaesthesia and adequate respiratory function during the operation and for ensuring that the patient is fit to be returned to the ward.

The most 'twilight' area of authority lies in the maintenance or resuscitation of the patient by means of intravenous fluid replacement therapy. Generally, this would be regarded as a function of a member of the surgical team, but during the operation it may be so much a part of maintaining the patient's physical state that the anaesthetist assumes responsibility.

FLUID REPLACEMENT THERAPY

The body subjected to operation may be deficient in fluid for any of three reasons:

   a. The condition requiring treatment may have precipitated fluid loss – e.g. haemorrhage from a ruptured vessel in a stomach ulcer.

   b. The operation itself may lead to significant loss of fluid. All operations incur some blood loss and it is the mark of the good surgical team to reduce this to a minimum. But fluid loss is to be anticipated even in the best of hands in many procedures.

   c. The condition of hypovolaemic shock may be present before, or arise during or after, the operation.

Hypovolaemic shock may result from active blood loss, from severe pain, from burning, from crushing, from circulating toxins or, indeed, from any condition in which the body's physiological defences are overstretched. Whatever the precipitating cause, fluid is removed from the circulation and is either lost to the exterior or left stagnant in the tissues; the effective volume of the blood is reduced. If whole blood is lost, there is reduction in the number of oxygen-carrying cells; if only plasma is lost, the blood thickens and the red cells circulate inadequately. In either case, oxygenation of the tissues is impaired and fluid loss from the consequently damaged capillaries is accentuated. This vicious cycle is compounded by increasing failure of the heart to cope with the excessive demands imposed upon it and death follows. Recovery from prolonged shock is often accompanied by acute renal failure.

Treatment or prevention of the 'cycle' lies mainly in replacing the volume of circulating blood by the intravenous infusion of artificially prepared solutions of electrolytes, of simulated or natural plasma or of blood.

Infusion of Fluids other than Blood

The choice of fluid for infusion depends on careful biochemical monitoring. The laboratory will advise as to the degree of fluid loss, as to the particular electrolytes required and as to the efficacy of treatment. There is no purpose in detailing the methods involved save to say that they are complicated and ideal surveillance may well be beyond the capabilities of a small hospital; in such circumstances, the control of fluid balance has to depend on clinical judgement aided by a fluid balance chart which must be kept to give some quantitative, albeit rough, guide.

Subsequent problems arise from the possibilities that the infusion given contained the wrong electrolytes or that either electrolytes or fluid were given in inadequate quantity to achieve cure. An equally important error is to use too much fluid so that the heart is embarrassed by hypervolaemia – too *great* a circulating blood volume. More fluid then escapes into the tissues and, in particular, into the lungs – the patient is effectively drowning in his own fluid. This condition of overhydration has been regarded as a *novus actus interveniens*.[12]

The transmission of a type of jaundice involving the virus-like particle known as Hepatitis B Antigen (HB_sAg) is a particular hazard of transfusing human plasma. Before the agent was discovered, this dangerous form of liver disease was sufficiently common as to almost eliminate human plasma in fluid replacement. It should now rarely occur because artificial plasma expanders, of which dextran is a typical example, are equally, if not more, effective and all blood donors are screened for being potential carriers of HB_sAg.

Hazards of Blood Transfusion

Chapter 18 described the well-demarcated blood group systems related to the red cell. Each system contains a minimum of two alleles and in most there are considerably more. The chances of transfused blood containing a 'foreign' antigen are, therefore, very high. The concept of rejection of non-self by the formation of antibodies has been discussed in Chapter 1. In general, the strength of the rejection reaction depends on the 'strength' of the antigen; from the point of view of blood transfusion reactions, the antigens of the ABO and Rhesus (CDE) systems are by far the most important. Nevertheless, repetitive exposure to the same foreign antigen of any 'strength' leads, in the end, to antibody production so that the effect of the lesser antigens increases as more transfusions are given; clinically, it becomes increasingly difficult to find donor blood which is compatible with the recipient.

The nature of antibodies must be considered if the hazards of blood transfusion are to be properly appreciated. The antibodies in the ABO system are, as described in Chapter 18, of 'naturally occurring' type and are found antithetically to the antigens. The four basic blood profiles can be summarized:

Blood Group	Antigen present on cell	Antibodies present in plasma
A	A[13]	Anti-B
B	B	Anti-A[13]
AB	AB	None[13]
O	O	Anti-A and Anti-B

Not only are the antigens and antibodies particularly reactive but, since the antibodies are already present, an incompatible ABO transfusion – for example transfusing group A blood to a group B recipient – will result in an immediate reaction.

---

[12] R. v. Jordan (1956) 40 C.App.R. 152. C.C.A.

[13] The complications introduced by subgroups of Group A have been described at p. 219. Patients of blood group A_2 and particularly of A_2B may contain Anti-A_1 in their plasma.

All other blood group antibodies are of simple 'immune' type which come into being only as a result of active stimulation by the specific antigen. The effect, say, of transfusing D+ blood into a D–(dd)[14] person will be to alert the body's defensive mechanism and to lay down the template of antibody production in preparation for a second attack. In all probability, there will be no clinical effect from the first 'incompatible' transfusion. Nevertheless, the body has been sensitized, antibody is now circulating and the next similar transfusion may result in an immediate reaction. The word 'may' is used advisedly, as antibody production is dependent on the capability of the recipient and on the 'strength' of the foreign donor antigen; a number of incompatible transfusions may be required to stimulate sufficient antibody to provoke a reaction to the lesser antigens. Immune antibodies are described by serologists as being either 'complete' or 'incomplete'. There is no clinical difference, but the latter require special methods for laboratory demonstration. In modern circumstances, it would be inexcusable to neglect to search for such antibodies prior to transfusion. In some blood group systems the bearing of a fetus of a different group from the mother is equivalent to a transfusion of similarly different blood.[15] The effects may be additive and it follows that a mismatched transfusion may have a profound effect on a woman's future child-bearing capacity. Accurate matching of blood is, therefore, particularly important in the case of female patients.

An incompatible transfusion may, as described, give no clinical signs but simply set the scene for the future. A mild antigen/antibody reaction will produce a rise in temperature, a 'rigor' and varying constitutional upset. A severe reaction, and certainly one associated with ABO incompatability, will result from massive destruction of blood within the vessels, the condition of shock will develop rapidly and the patient may die. Recovery from this, as from shock of any origin, may well be followed by acute renal failure.

The prevention of transfusion reactions depends on compatability testing in the laboratory. The techniques are immaterial here; all are well known to laboratory workers and are within the compass of relatively small departments. The lawyer must, however, understand the general principles.

The cells of the recipient are irrelevant in the context of transfusion reactions – their importance lies in indicating the group of the donor to be chosen. The plasma of the donor is similarly irrelevant because any contained antibodies are rapidly diluted in the recipient's body. Thus it is possible, and reasonable in an emergency, to transfuse Group O blood (the so-called universal donor blood) to a male recipient irrespective of his blood group. If the O blood is also D–, it could be used for a

---

[14] d is the allele to D and is apparently non-antigenic.

[15] The basis of haemolytic disease of the newborn (see Chapter 18).

female recipient, the calculated risk being the provocation of a transfusion reaction due to the presence in the recipient of an immune antibody other than anti-D. Such emergency practice is rarely undertaken; the delay due to testing offers less risk than does an unmatched transfusion and full compatibility is almost always assured.

This is done in two stages. Firstly, the donor cells are selected as being similar in ABO and CDE groups to those of the recipient. Compatibility of the recipient's plasma is then ensured by 'cross-matching' – the effect of mixing the actual donor cells with the actual recipient plasma (in practice, serum) is studied in the laboratory. The possibility of an immediate transfusion reaction can be excluded provided antibodies of both complete and incomplete type are sought by the most sensitive methods. Each donor unit (i.e. bottle or bag of blood) must be tested separately. This method does not exclude the possibility of sensitizing the recipient to one of the less important blood group antigens but testing for complete similarity of all blood group factors would be technologically impossible; provided cross-matching is undertaken regularly, the theoretical danger to the patient approximates to zero.

In practice, transfusions which are given and found to be incompatible by reason of inaccuracy of cross-matching are extremely rare; faults are far more commonly organizational in nature. The commonest mistakes include errors in transcription – due simply to clerical error or to the introduction of confusing terms such as 'group A serum' rather than 'anti-B serum'. Failure of the nursing staff to check the reference on the bag or bottle against the actual laboratory report on compatibility is another potent source of error which may be of catastrophic proportions. The presence of similarly-named patients in the ward may be disastrous if the donor blood is not checked against the patient's notes.

Such errors are compounded by the use of the telephone combined with trusting delivery of messages to intermediates – conditions which commonly obtain in an emergency. A famous instance, probably apocryphal, is quoted concerning a telephone message to the effect, 'We are sending up the blood for the melaena patient' – meaning 'for the patient with bowel haemorrhage'; the blood was transfused into a child with the first name 'Melina'.[16]

Not all reactions are due to antigen/antibody incompatibility. Some are due to infection of the unit of blood. It is most important that the storage cabinet be maintained at constant optimal temperature – cabinets should be fitted with alarm systems which operate if the temperature range is exceeded. Similarly, expiry dates must be scrupulously observed as blood which has degenerated may cause considerable

---

[16] Quoted by Taylor J. L. (1970) *The Doctor and the Law*, London, Pitman Medical, p. 110.

disability in its own right.

Finally, the blood may have contained pathogenic organisms other than HB$_s$Ag in life and these must be excluded before it is used – the best-known diseases transmissible through blood transfusion are malaria and syphilis.

The Expert Witness

Much as in the case of 'anaesthetic' deaths, the investigation of transfusion reactions requires the cooperation of all concerned and, again, the primary object must be to prevent similar mistakes in the future.

Inquiries must be made as to the method of cross-matching, the documentation, and the chain of orders by which the transfusion was given and as to the precise clinical presentation. A full investigation of the remaining blood in the container, including a bacteriological analysis, must be made and correlated with the serum obtained from the patient either while living or, if death occurs, at autopsy.

The anatomic pathological evidence will be directed to demonstrating signs of blood destruction, and these are particularly evident in the kidneys. At the same time, the contribution of the condition requiring transfusion to the death has to be assessed and, of course, the presence of unsuspected disease must be sought. In general, the precise cause of death is likely to be elucidated and suitable remedial measures can be introduced.

Appendix A
A Guide to Medical Terminology

PREPOSITIONAL PREFIXES

Prefix	Meaning	Example
A- or An-	Without	Anoxia = without oxygen
Ante-	Before	Antemortem = before death
Anti-	Against	Antiseptic = prevents sepsis
Circum-	Around	Circumoral = around the mouth
Contra-	Against, opposite	Contralateral = on the other side
De-	Away from	Dehydrate = remove water
Dia-	Through	Dialyse = to pass through a membrane
Dys-	Abnormal	Dysfunction = abnormal function
En- or Endo-	Within	Endotracheal = within the trachea
Epi	Outside	Epidermis = outermost part of the skin
Extra- or Exo-	Outside	Extradural = outside the coverings of the brain
		Exogenous = produced from outside
Hetero-	Different	Heterotopic = in the wrong place
Homo-	Similar	Homozygous = similar genes combined
Hyper-	Excessive	Hypertrophy = overgrowth
Hypo-	Too little	Hypotension = low blood pressure
Infra-	Below	Infraorbital = below the eye
Inter-	Between	Intercostal = between the ribs
Intra-	Within	Intrahepatic = within the liver
Juxta-	Beside	Juxtaposition = closeness together
Para-	Close to, around	Paravertebral = near the spine
Per-	Through	Percutaneous = through the skin
Poly-	Many	Polymorphic = many-shaped
Post-	After	Post-traumatic = after injury
Pre-	In front of	Prepatellar = in front of the knee cap
Proto-	First	Prototype = the original of the form
Retro-	Behind	Retrosternal = behind the sternum
Sub-	Beneath	Subcutaneous = beneath the skin
Supra-	Above	Supralabial = above the lip
Syn-	Together	Syndactyly = web fingers
Trans-	Through, across	Transplacental = across the placenta

SOME SUFFIXES

Suffix	Meaning	Example
-aemia	In or of the blood	Anaemia = no (or less than normal) blood
-algia	Pain	Neuralgia = pain in a nerve
-ectomy	Removal	Prostatectomy = removal of the prostate
-genic	Producing	Pathogenic = causing disease
-itis	Inflammation of	Laryngitis = inflammation of the larynx

Suffix	Meaning	Example
-logy	Study of	Pathology = study of disease
-megaly	Enlargement of	Splenomegaly = enlargement of the spleen
-oma	Tumour	Adenoma = a tumour of glands
-osis	Abnormal process other than inflammation	Fibrosis = proliferation of fibrous tissue (scarring)
-pathy	Abnormal structure or function of	Myopathy = abnormal muscle
-plasia	Growth	Hyperplasia = excessive growth
-stomy	Making a hole	Tracheostomy = artificial opening in trachea

ANATOMIC PREFIXES

Prefix	Relating to	Example
Aden(o)-	Glands	Adenitis = inflammation of glands
Angio-	Blood vessels	Angiospasm = spasm of the arteries
Arthr(o)-	Joints	Arthralgia = pain in the joints
Cardio-	Heart	Cardiomyopathy = abnormality of the heart muscle
Cerebro-	Brain	Cerebrospinal fluid = fluid surrounding the brain and spinal cord
Chol(o)-	Bile	Cholecystitis = inflammation of the gall bladder
Chondro-	Cartilage	Chondroma = a tumour of cartilage
Colo-	Large Bowel	Colostomy = making an opening in the colon
Costo-	Ribs	Costochondral = of the rib cartilages
Encephal(o)-	Brain	Encephalitis = inflammation of the brain
Enter(o)-	Intestines	Enteritis = inflammation of the intestine
Gastr(o)-	Stomach	Gastro-enterostomy = making a connecting hole between stomach and intestine
Haem(o)-	Blood	Haemothorax = blood in the thoracic cavity
Hepat(o)-	Liver	Hepatomegaly = enlargement of the liver
My(o)-	Muscle	Myasthenia = wasting of the muscle
Nephr(o)-	Kidney	Nephrosis = an abnormal process in the kidney
Pneumo-	Lung (or simply Air)	Pneumoconiosis = an abnormality of the lung associated with dust. Pneumothorax = free air in the thoracic cavity
Oste(o)-	Bone	Osteology = the study of bones

Note: American medical writing does not usually use diphthongs. Thus: Anaemia becomes Anemia; Tumour becomes Tumor; Oesophagus becomes Esophagus.

Appendix B
Reporting Deaths to Coroners

In deaths in the following circumstances the doctor is advised to inform the Coroner as soon as possible:

Sudden Deaths
When the cause is not clear or when the doctor cannot give a certificate because of nonattendance in the last illness.
  Not due to natural causes.

Accidents
In any way contributing to the cause of death.

Alcoholism
Chronic or acute.

Anaesthetics
Operations
Where it appears that either has caused or contributed to death, or where performed for any injury.

Drugs
Therapeutic or of addiction.

Foster Children
Industrial Diseases
Any pathological condition arising out of the nature of the deceased's employment, e.g. pneumoconiosis, Weil's disease and all diseases and poisons covered by the Factories Act.

Pensions
Where deceased has been in receipt of a disability pension.

Poisoning
From any cause, occupational, accidental, suicidal, homicidal and also food poisoning.

Stillbirths
Where there is any possibility of the child having been born alive.

To the above (from Camps F. E. and Purchase W. B. (1956) *Practical Forensic Medicine*, London, Hutchinson's Medical Publications) might be specifically added:
Deaths Due to Want, Exposure or Neglect
Obscure Infant Deaths

Appendix C
Conclusions of the Jury/Coroner as to the Death

Murder
Manslaughter
Infanticide
Killed himself
Attempted/Self-induced abortion
Accident/Misadventure
Execution of sentence of death
Justifiable or excusable homicide
Natural causes
Industrial disease
Want of attention at birth
Chronic alcoholism/Addiction to drugs
Aggravated by lack of care/self-neglect
Open verdict

Note: The concept of a Coroner's 'verdict' has been strongly criticized by the Brodrick Committee, *Report of the Committee on Death Certification and Coroners* (1971). Cmnd. 4810. London, HMSO, para. 16.37 *et seq.*

Appendix D
Deaths Reportable to the Procurator Fiscal

1. Any uncertified death.
2. Any death which was caused by an accident arising out of the use of a vehicle, or which was caused by an aircraft or rail accident.
3. Any death arising out of industrial employment, by accident, industrial disease or industrial poisoning.
4. Any death due to poisoning (coal gas, barbiturate, etc.).
5. Any death where the circumstances would seem to indicate suicide.
6. Any death where there are indications that it occurred under an anaesthetic.
7. Any death resulting from an accident in the home, hospital, institution or any public place.
8. Any death following an abortion.
9. Any death apparently caused by neglect (e.g. malnutrition).
10. Any death occurring in prison or a police cell where deceased was in custody at the time of death.
11. Any death of a newborn child whose body is found.
12. Any death (occurring not in a house) where deceased's residence is unknown.
13. Death by drowning.
14. Death of a child from suffocation (including overlaying).
15. Where the death occurred as the result of smallpox or typhoid.
16. Any death as a result of a fire or explosion.
17. Any sudden death.
18. Any other death due to violent, suspicious or unexplained cause.
19. Deaths of foster children.

Appendix E
Deaths Reportable after Investigation by the Procurator Fiscal to the Crown Office

i.   Where there are any suspicious circumstances;
ii.   where death was caused by an accident arising out of the use of a vehicle;
iii. where the circumstances point to suicide;
iv.   where the death was caused by an accident, poison or disease, notice of which is required to be given to any Government Department or to any Inspector or other officer of a Government Department under or in pursuance of any Act;
v.   where the death occurred in circumstances continuance of which or possible recurrence of which is prejudicial to the health and safety of the public;
vi.   where the death occurred in industrial employment;
vii. where the death occurred in any prison or police cell or where the deceased was in custody at the time of death;
viii. where death occurred under an anaesthetic in unusual circumstances or if there are features which suggest negligence;
ix.   where death was due to gas poisoning;
x.   where death was directly or indirectly connected with the actions of a third party whether or not criminal responsibility rests on any person; and
xi.   where any desire has been expressed that a public inquiry should be held into the circumstances of the death or where the Procurator Fiscal is of the opinion that a public inquiry should be held under the Fatal Accidents and Sudden Deaths Inquiry (Scotland) Act 1976.

Appendix F
Approximate Times of Appearance of some Centres of Ossification

Intra-uterine
1½ months—clavicle.
2 months—shafts of long bones.
3 months—ischium.
5 months—calcaneus.
6 months—manubrium sterni.
7 months—talus.
8 months—all segments of sternum.
9 months—lower end of femur, cuboid, head of humerus.
After Birth
1 month—head of tibia.
3 months—head of femur, lower end of tibia.
6 months—lower end of fibula.
7 months—lower end of radius, greater tuberosity of humerus.
10 months to 3 years—many of the small bones of hands and feet.
3 years—head of fibula, patella, greater trochanter of femur.
4 years—head of radius.
5 years—lower end of ulna.
Later Life
  8 years—olecranon.
  9 years—lesser trochanter of femur.
10 years—tibial tuberosity.
13 years—anterior spine of ilium, iliac crest.
15 years—ischial tuberosity, medial end of clavicle.

Note: While all these appearances are very variable, females are advanced compared to males throughout.

(Adapted from Krogman W. M. (1962) *The Human Skeleton in Forensic Medicine,* Springfield, Thomas.)

Appendix G
Union of Epiphyses

	Earliest age (years)	Latest age (years)
Humerus/lower end	15	18
Ulna/upper end	15	21
Ischial tuberosity	15	25
Radius/upper end	16	20
Scapula/acromion	16	25
Tibia/lower end	17	25
Fibula/lower end	17	25
Iliac crest	17	25
Radius/lower end	18	25
Ulna/lower end	18	25
Femur/head of femur	18	25
Tibia/upper end	18	25
Clavicle	18	25
Femur/lower end	19	24
Fibula/upper end	19	25
Humerus/head	20	25

(Adapted from Krogman W. M. (1962) *The Human Skeleton in Forensic Medicine*, Springfield, Thomas.)

Appendix H
Notification of Infectious Disease

The following diseases are notifiable to the Chief Administrative Medical Officer:

Anthrax
Cholera
Continued fever
Diphtheria
Dysentery
Erysipelas
Food poisoning
Leprosy
Leptospiral jaundice
Malaria
Measles
Meningococcal infection
Ophthalmia neonatorum
Paratyphoid A
Paratyphoid B
Plague
Poliomyelitis, acute paralytic
Poliomyelitis, acute nonparalytic
Puerperal fever
Relapsing fever
Scarlet fever
Smallpox
Tuberculosis, respiratory
Tuberculosis, nonrespiratory
Typhoid fever
Typhus fever
Viral hepatitis
Whooping cough
Yellow fever
Lassa fever⎫
Rabies   ⎬ added by regulation in 1976.

Local authorities may add to this list by virtue of Section 7 of the Infectious Disease (Notification) Act 1889. Rubella (German measles) is a fairly common addition.

Appendix I
Prescribed Diseases

Description of disease or injury	Nature of occupation
Poisoning by:	Any occupation involving:
1. Lead or a compound of lead	The use or handling of, or exposure to the fumes, dust or vapour of, lead or a compound of lead, or a substance containing lead.
2. Manganese or a compound of manganese	The use or handling of, or exposure to the fumes, dust or vapour of, manganese or a compound of manganese, or a substance containing manganese.
3. Phosphorus or phosphine or poisoning due to the anticholinesterase action of organic phosphorus compounds	The use or handling of, or exposure to the fumes, dust or vapour of, phosphorus or a compound of phosphorus, or a substance containing phosphorus.
4. Arsenic or a compound of arsenic	The use or handling of, or exposure to the fumes, dust or vapour of, arsenic or a compound of arsenic, or a substance containing arsenic.
5. Mercury or a compound of mercury	The use or handling of, or exposure to the fumes, dust or vapour of, mercury or a compound of mercury, or a substance containing mercury.
6. Carbon bisulphide	The use or handling of, or exposure to the fumes or vapour of, carbon bisulphide or a compound of carbon bisulphide, or a substance containing carbon bisulphide.
7. Benzene or a homologue	The use or handling of, or exposure to the fumes of, or vapour containing, benzene or any of its homologues.
8. A nitro- or amino- or chloro-derivative of benzene or of a homologue of benzene, or poisoning by nitro-chlorbenzene	The use or handling of, or exposure to the fumes of, or vapour containing, a nitro- or amino- or chloro-derivative of benzene or a homologue of benzene or nitro-chlorbenzene
9. Dinitrophenol or a homologue or by substituted dinitrophenols or by the salts of such substances	The use or handling of, or exposure to the fumes of, or vapour containing, dinitrophenol or a homologue or substituted dinitrophenols or the salts of such substances.
10. Tetrachlorethane	The use or handling of, or exposure to the fumes of, or vapour containing, tetrachlorethane.
11. Tri-cresyl phosphate	The use or handling of, or exposure to the fumes of, or vapour containing, tri-cresyl phosphate.

419

Description of disease or injury	Nature of occupation
Poisoning by:	Any occupation involving:
12. Tri-phenyl phosphate	The use or handling of, or exposure to the fumes of, or vapour containing, tri-phenyl phosphate.
13. Diethylene dioxide (dioxan)	The use or handling of, or exposure to the fumes of, or vapour containing, diethylene dioxide (dioxan).
14. Methyl bromide	The use or handling of, or exposure to the fumes of, or vapour containing, methyl bromide.
15. Chlorinated naphthalene	The use or handling of, or exposure to the fumes of, or dust or vapour containing, chlorinated naphthalene.
16. Nickel carbonyl	Exposure to nickel carbonyl gas.
17. Nitrous fumes	The use or handling of nitric acid or exposure to nitrous fumes.
18. Gonioma kamassi (African boxwood)	The manipulation of gonioma kamassi or any process in or incidental to the manufacture of articles therefrom.
19. Anthrax	The handling of wool, hair, bristles, hides or skins or other animal products or residues, or contact with animals infected with anthrax.
20. Glanders	Contact with equine animals or their carcasses.
21. (a) Infection by Leptospira icterohaemorrhagiae	Work in places which are, or are liable to be, infested by rats.
(b) Infection by Leptospira canicola	Work at dog kennels or the care or handling of dogs.
22. Ankylostomiasis	Work in or about a mine.
23. (a) Dystrophy of the cornea (including ulceration of the corneal surface) of the eye, (b) Localized new growth of the skin, papillomatous or keratotic, (c) Squamous-celled carcinoma of the skin, due in any case to arsenic, tar, pitch, bitumen, mineral oil (including paraffin), soot or any compound, product (including quinone or hydroquinone) or residue or any of these substances.	The use or handling of, or exposure to, arsenic, tar, pitch, bitumen, mineral oil (including paraffin), soot or any compound, product (including quinone or hydroquinone), or residue of any of these substances.
24. (Now covered by diseases 41 and 42)	

Description of disease or injury	Nature of occupation

Any occupation involving:

25. Inflammation, ulceration or malignant disease of the skin or subcutaneous tissues or of the bones, or blood dyscrasia, or cataract, due to electromagnetic radiations (other than radiant heat), or to ionizing particles — Exposure to electromagnetic radiations other than radiant heat, or to ionizing particles.

26. Heat cataract — Frequent or prolonged exposure to rays from molten or red-hot material.

27. Decompression sickness — Subjection to compressed or rarefied air.

28. Cramp of the hand or forearm due to repetitive movements — Prolonged periods of handwriting, typing or other repetitive movements of the fingers, hand or arm.

29.
30. (Now covered by disease 28)

31. Subcutaneous cellulitis of the hand (Beat hand) — Manual labour causing severe or prolonged friction or pressure on the hand.

32. Bursitis or subcutaneous cellulitis arising at or about the knee due to severe or prolonged external friction or pressure at or about the knee (Beat knee) — Manual labour causing severe or prolonged external friction or pressure at or about the knee.

33. Bursitis or subcutaneous cellulitis arising at or about the elbow due to severe or prolonged external friction or pressure at or about the elbow (Beat elbow) — Manual labour causing severe or prolonged external friction or pressure at or about the elbow.

34. Traumatic inflammation of the tendons of the hand or forearm, or of the associated tendon sheaths — Manual labour, or frequent or repeated movements of the hand or wrist.

35. Miner's nystagmus — Work in or about a mine.

36. Poisoning by beryllium or a compound of beryllium — The use or handling of, or exposure to the fumes, dust or vapour of, beryllium or a compound of beryllium, or a substance containing beryllium.

37. (a) Carcinoma of the mucous membrane of the nose or associated air sinuses. (b) Primary carcinoma of a bronchus or of a lung — Work in a factory where nickel is produced by decomposition of a gaseous nickel compound which necessitates working in or about a building or buildings where that process or any other industrial process ancillary or incidental thereto is carried on.

38. Tuberculosis — Close and frequent contact with a source or sources of tuberculous infection by reason of employment:

Description of disease or injury	*Nature of occupation*
	Any occupation involving:
	(*a*) in the medical treatment or nursing of a person or persons suffering from tuberculosis, or in a service ancillary to such treatment or nursing;
	(*b*) in attendance upon a person or persons suffering from tuberculosis, where the need for such attendance arises by reason of physical or mental infirmity;
	(*c*) as a research worker engaged in research in connection with tuberculosis;
	(*d*) as a laboratory worker, pathologist or person taking part in or assisting at post-mortem examinations of human remains where the occupation involves working with material which is a source of tuberculous infection.
39. Primary neoplasm of the epithelial lining of the urinary bladder (Papilloma of the bladder), or of the epithelial lining of the renal pelvis or of the epithelial lining of the ureter	(*a*) Work in a building in which any of the following substances is produced for commercial purposes:
	(*i*) Alpha-naphthylamine or beta-naphthylamine,
	(*ii*) Diphenyl substituted by at least one nitro or primary amino group or by at least one nitro and primary amino group.
	(*iii*) Any of the substances mentioned in subparagraph (*ii*), above if further ring substituted by halogeno, methyl or methoxy groups, but not by other groups.
	(*iv*) The salts of any of the substances mentioned in subparagraphs (*i*), to (*iii*), above.
	(*v*) auramine or magenta;
	(*b*) the use or handling of any of the substances mentioned in subparagraphs (*i*) to (*iv*), of paragraph (*a*), or work in a process in which any such substance is used or handled or is liberated;

Description of disease or injury	*Nature of occupation*
	Any occupation involving:
	(*c*) the maintenance or cleaning of any plant or machinery used in any such process as is mentioned in paragraph (*b*), or the cleaning of clothing used in any such building as is mentioned in paragraph (*a*), if such clothing is cleaned within the works of which the building forms a part or in a laundry maintained and used solely in connection with such works.
40. Poisoning by cadmium	Exposure to cadmium fumes.
41. Inflammation or ulceration of the mucous membrane of the upper respiratory passages or mouth produced by dust, liquid or vapour	Exposure to dust, liquid or vapour.
42. Noninfective dermatitis of external origin (including chrome ulceration of the skin but excluding dermatitis due to ionizing particles or electromagnetic radiations other than radiant heat)	Exposure to dust, liquid, or vapour or any other external agent capable of irritating the skin (including friction or heat but excluding ionizing particles or electromagnetic radiations other than radiant heat).
43. Pulmonary disease due to the inhalation of the dust of mouldy hay or of other mouldy vegetable produce, and characterized by symptoms and signs attributable to a reaction in the peripheral part of the bronchopulmonary system, and giving rise to a defect in gas exchange (Farmer's lung)	Exposure to the dust of mouldy hay or other mouldy vegetable produce by reason of employment: (*a*) in agriculture, horticulture or forestry; or (*b*) loading or unloading or handling in storage such hay or other vegetable produce; or (*c*) handling bagasse.
44. Primary malignant neoplasm of the mesothelium (diffuse mesothelioma) of the pleura or of the peritoneum	(*a*) The working or handling of asbestos or any admixture of asbestos; (*b*) the manufacture or repair of asbestos textiles or other articles containing or composed of asbestos; (*c*) the cleaning of any machinery or plant used in any of the foregoing operations and of any chambers, fixtures and appliances for the collection of asbestos dust; (*d*) substantial exposure to the dust arising from any of the foregoing operations.

Description of disease or injury	Nature of occupation
	Any occupation involving:
45. Adenocarcinoma of the nasal cavity or associated air sinuses	Attendance for work in or about a building where wooden furniture is manufactured.
46. Brucellosis	Contact with bovine animals infected by brucella abortus, their carcasses or parts thereof or their untreated products, or with laboratory specimens or vaccines of or containing brucella abortus, by reason of employment: (a) as a farm worker; (b) as a veterinary worker; (c) as a slaughterhouse worker; (d) as a laboratory worker; or (e) in any other work relating to the care, treatment, examination or handling of such animals, carcasses or parts thereof or products.
47. Poisoning by acrylamide monomer	Any occupation involving the use or handling of, or exposure to, acrylamide monomer.

(From *Notes on the Diagnosis of Occupational Diseases*. (1972) London, HMSO.)

Addendum
As from February 1976, viral hepatitis has been added to the list of prescribed diseases under the Social Security Act 1975. Angiosarcoma of the liver and osteolysis of the terminal phalanges of the fingers arising from exposure to vinyl chloride monomer were added in 1977.

Appendix J
Prescribed Occupations

PNEUMOCONIOSIS
1. Any occupation involving:
   a. the mining, quarrying or working of silica rock or the working of dried quartzose sand or any dry deposit or dry residue of silica or any dry admixture containing such materials (including any occupation in which any of the aforesaid operations are carried out incidentally to the mining or quarrying of other minerals or to the manufacture of articles containing crushed or ground silica rock);
   b. the handling of any of the materials specified in the foregoing subparagraph in or incidental to any of the operations mentioned therein, or substantial exposure to the dust arising from such operations.
2. Any occupation involving the breaking, crushing or grinding of flint or the working or handling of broken, crushed or ground flint or materials containing such flint, or substantial exposure to the dust arising from such operations.
3. Any occupation involving sand blasting by means of compressed air with the use of quartzose sand or crushed silica rock or flint, or substantial exposure to the dust arising from such sand blasting.
4. Any occupation involving work in a foundry or the performance of, or substantial exposure to the dust arising from, any of the following operations:
   a. the freeing of steel castings from adherent siliceous substance;
   b. the freeing of metal castings from adherent siliceous substance:
      i. by blasting with an abrasive propelled by compressed air, by steam or by a wheel; or
      ii. by the use of power-driven tools.
5. Any occupation in or incidental to the manufacture of china or earthenware (including sanitary earthenware, electrical earthenware and earthenware tiles) and any occupation involving substantial exposure to the dust arising therefrom.
6. Any occupation involving the grinding of mineral graphite, or substantial exposure to the dust arising from such grinding.
7. Any occupation involving the dressing of granite or any igneous rock by masons or the crushing of such materials, or substantial exposure to the dust arising from such operations.
8. Any occupation involving the use, or preparation for use, of a grindstone, or substantial exposure to the dust arising therefrom.
9. Any occupation involving:
   a. the working or handling of asbestos or any admixture of asbestos;
   b. the manufacture or repair of asbestos textiles or other articles containing or composed of asbestos;
   c. the cleaning of any machinery or plant used in any of the foregoing operations and of any chambers, fixtures and appliances for the collection of asbestos dust;
   d. substantial exposure to the dust arising from any of the foregoing operations.
10. Any occupation involving:
   a. work underground in any mine in which one of the objects of the mining operations is the getting of any mineral;
   b. the working or handling above ground at any coal or tin mine of any minerals extracted therefrom, or any operation incidental thereto;
   c. the trimming of coal in any ship, barge, or lighter, or in any dock or harbour or at any wharf or quay;
   d. the sawing, splitting or dressing of slate, or any operation incidental thereto.

11. Any occupation in or incidental to the manufacture of carbon electrodes by an industrial undertaking for use in the electrolytic extraction of aluminium from aluminium oxide, and any occupation involving substantial exposure to the dust arising therefrom.

12. Any occupation involving boiler scaling or substantial exposure to the dust arising therefrom.

Definitions

'Silica Rock' means quartz, quartzite, ganister, sandstone, gritstone and chert, but not natural sand or rotten rock.

'Foundry' means those parts of industrial premises where the production of metal articles (other than pig iron or steel ingots) is carried on by casting (not being diecasting or other casting in metal moulds), together with any part of the same premises where any of the following processes are carried on incidentally to such production, namely, the drying and subsequent preparation of sand for moulding (including the reclamation of used moulding sand), the preparation of moulds and cores, knock-out operations and dressing or fettling operations.

'Grindstone' means a grindstone composed of natural or manufactured sandstone and includes a metal wheel or cylinder into which blocks of natural or manufactured sandstone are fitted.

'Asbestos textiles' means yarn or cloth composed of asbestos or of asbestos mixed with any other material.

'Mine' includes every shaft in the course of being sunk, and every level and inclined plane in the course of being driven, and all the shafts, levels, planes, works, tramways and sidings, both below ground and above ground, in and adjacent to and belonging to the mine, but does not include any part of such premises on which any manufacturing process is carried on other than a process ancillary to the getting or dressing of minerals or the preparation of minerals for sale.

'Coal mine' means any mine where one of the objects of the mining operations is the getting of coal (including bituminous coal, cannel coal, anthracite, lignite and brown coal.)

ASBESTOS AND DIFFUSE MESOTHELIOMA
Any occupation involving:
  a. the working or handling of asbestos or any admixture of asbestos;
  b. the manufacture or repair of asbestos textiles or other articles containing or composed of asbestos;
  c. the cleaning of any machinery or plant used in any of the foregoing operations and of any chambers, fixtures and appliances for the collection of asbestos dust;
  d. substantial exposure to the dust arising from any of the foregoing operations.

BYSSINOSIS
Byssinosis is prescribed in relation to all insured persons who have been employed:
  a. in insurable employment at any time on or after the appointed day; and
  b. for a period or periods (whether before or after the appointed day) amounting in the aggregate to not less than ten years:
in any occupation in any room where any process up to and including the carding process is performed in factories in which the spinning or manipulation of raw or waste cotton or of flax is carried on.

FARMER'S LUNG
Any occupation involving exposure to the dust of mouldy hay or other mouldy vegetable produce by reason of employment:

a. in agriculture, horticulture or forestry; or
b. loading or unloading or handling in storage such hay or other vegetables produce; or
c. handling bagasse.

(From *Pneumoconiosis and Allied Occupational Chest Diseases*. (1967) London, HMSO.)

Appendix K
Diseases Notifiable to HM Inspector of Factories

The following industrial diseases, when contracted in a factory, are notifiable to HM Inspector of Factories:

Beryllium poisoning
Cadmium poisoning
Lead poisoning
Phosphorus poisoning
Arsenical poisoning
Mercurial poisoning
Compressed Air Illness
Anthrax
Chrome ulceration
Toxic jaundice
Aniline poisoning
Chronic benzene poisoning
Epitheliomatous ulceration
Manganese poisoning
Toxic anaemia

Appendix L
Form of Consent for Amniocentesis

We, the undersigned have requested that amniocentesis should be carried out. The risks and limitations of this procedure have been explained to us by...........
and we appreciate that the procedure may have to be repeated. We understand that the birth of a normal child cannot be guaranteed from the results of studies on amniotic fluid and its contained cells.

Signed ....

....

Date ....

Hospital ....

Case No. ....

Appendix M
Some Useful Equivalents of Weight, Capacity, Length and Temperature

Standard measurements in the form of SI Units are described in Appendix P. Many reports will, however, refer to more colloquial terms and the following may be found useful as an aid to conversion of these.

Weight
1 gram (g)	= 15·4 grains
1 kilogram (kg)	= 35·3 ounces (avoirdupois)
1 grain	= 64·8 milligrams (mg)
1 ounce (avoirdupois)	= 28·3 grams (g)
1 pound (avoirdupois)	= 438·6 grams (g)

Capacity
1 fluid ounce	= 28·4 millilitres (ml)*
1 gill	= 5 fluid ounces
1 pint	= 568 millilitres (ml)
1 gallon (Imp.)	= 4·55 litres (l)
1 litre (l)	= 1·76 pints
1 litre (l)	= 35·2 fluid ounces

Length
1 micron (μm)	= 10^{-6} metre (m)†
1 inch	= 2·54 centimetres (cm)
1 foot	= 30·5 centimetres (cm)
1 Ångstrom unit	= 10^{-10} metre (m)

Temperature
An interval of 1 degree Centigrade (° C) corresponds to 1·8 degrees Fahrenheit (° F)

To convert ° F to ° C: $\dfrac{F - 32}{9} = \dfrac{C}{5}$

Some parts of the Electromagnetic Spectrum
Ultraviolet	= 100–400 nanometres (nm)
Visible	= 400–800 nm
Infra-red	= 800–100 000 nm

---

* For all practical purposes 1 millilitre is equivalent to 1 cubic centimetre (cc or cm³).
† The symbol μ is also still used to express the micron.

Appendix N
Some Medical Qualifications in the United Kingdom

Primary Qualifications

LMSSA	Licentiate in Medicine and Surgery of the Society of Apothecaries.
MRCS, LRCP	Member of the Royal College of Surgeons of England, Licentiate of the Royal College of Physicians of London.
LRCP, LRCS (Edin. or Irel.)	Licentiate of the Royal Colleges of Physicians and Surgeons of Edinburgh or in Ireland.
LRCPS	Licentiate of the Royal College of Physicians and Surgeons of Glasgow.
MB (or BM), BCh (or BS or ChB)	Bachelor of Medicine and Surgery. Graduating degree awarded by Universities with Medical Schools.

Note. All qualifying degrees refer to both medicine and surgery but not every doctor practises major surgery. Many doctors are also qualified BA (or subsequently MA) or BSc; these are intermediate University degrees taken before clinical training.

Some Postgraduate Degrees

MD	Doctor of Medicine. Almost always obtained by thesis.
MS (or MCh or ChM)	Master of Surgery. Sometimes taken by thesis, sometimes by general examination.
PhD	Doctor of Philosophy. Obtained by thesis after a period of approved scientific research.
MSc	Master of Science. Obtainable in many scientific subjects related to medicine.

Such degrees indicate research in depth of a particular subject. They imply that there is some specific field in which the holder is an outstanding authority. Other special masterships are offered – e.g. in radiology.

Membership of the Royal Colleges and Faculties

Possession of these higher qualifications is certain evidence of specialization. They are obtained by means of a searching examination; only very rarely is 'membership' conferred by virtue of published work or reputation. The Colleges of Physicians in London, Edinburgh and Glasgow (Physicians and Surgeons) at one time conferred individual memberships; examinations are now on a United Kingdom basis. In general, members are elected to be fellows of individual colleges after a delineated period; the main exceptions are the Royal Colleges of Surgeons which confer fellowship by examination.

FRCS	Fellow of the Royal College of Surgeons
MRCP	Member of the Royal College of Physicians
MRCOG	Member of the Royal College of Obstetricians and Gynaecologists
MRCPath	Member of the Royal College of Pathologists
MRCPsych	Member of the Royal College of Psychiatrists
MRCGP	Member of the Royal College of General Practitioners
FFA RCS	Fellow of the Faculty of Anaesthetists
FFR	Fellow of the Faculty of Radiologists
FFCM	Fellow of the Faculty of Community Medicine

Postgraduate Diplomas
Both the Universities and the Royal Colleges issue diplomas on the basis of examination. The role of the diploma in indicating the narrower field of interest and expertise of the holder has been somewhat reduced by the growth of increasingly specialized Royal Colleges; in many cases, however, they are the sole indication of a particular proficiency while others may be looked upon as 'stepping-stones' to membership.
The following list is certainly not exhaustive.

DA	Diploma in Anaesthetics
D Av Med	Diploma in Aviation Medicine
Dip Bact	Diploma in Bacteriology
DCH	Diploma in Child Health
DIH	Diploma in Industrial Health
DLO	Diploma in Laryngology and Otology
DMJ	Diploma in Medical Jurisprudence
DO	Diploma in Ophthalmology
D Obst RCOG	Diploma in Obstetrics of the Royal College of Obstetricians and Gynaecologists
BAO	Bachelor of the Art of Obstetrics (given in Ireland)
D Path	Diploma in Pathology
DRCPath	Diploma of the Royal College of Pathologists
D Phys Med	Diploma in Physical Medicine
DPM	Diploma in Psychiatric Medicine
DPH	Diploma in Public Health
DMRD or T	Diploma in Radiological Diagnosis or Therapy
Dip Soc Med	Diploma in Social Medicine
DTM & H	Diploma in Tropical Medicine and Hygiene
DTPH	Diploma in Tropical Public Health
DTCD	Diploma in Tuberculosis and Chest Diseases

Appendix O
Report to Procurator Fiscal of Death associated with Anaesthesia and/or Operation

Sir,

We hereby report the death of . . . .

at . . . .(Hospital, Nursing Home, etc.) on . . . . . .date which was associated with anaesthesia and/or operation. (See Note 1.)

1. Full Name . . . . Age . . . . . Ward . . . .
    Home Address . . . .
2. Date admitted to Hospital, and time . . . .
3. Nature of Disease, Injury or Ailment for which operation was advised.

4. Was formal consent for operation and administration of anaesthetic obtained?
5. Was the operation of an Elective or Emergency nature? . . . .
6. Note on clinical findings of examination of Heart, Lungs and Urine.

7. Note on any concurrent pathological condition or ailment present, or other relevant pre-operative details.

8. What precautions and medicaments were used in preparing the patient for anaesthesia and the surgical or other procedure? Where applicable give quantities and times.

9. Anaesthetic:
    Date and Time: Administration started . . . . Stopped . . . .
    Details of agents and techniques used, including sequences and quantities.

    Remarks

    Anaesthetist
10. Operations:
    Date and Time: Started . . . . Finished . . . .
    Nature of operation proposed, performed, or in progress:

Remarks.

Operator.
11. Date, Time and Place of Death (*i.e.*, Theatre, Ward, etc.).
12. Details in chronological order of events immediately preceding death and of resuscitative measures undertaken.

13. Opinion as to Cause of Death, and any other general observations on the case:

Date. . . . .   Signature. . . . .
                                                                (Operator)
                                           Signature. . . . .
                                                                (Anaesthetist)
The Procurator Fiscal,
       . . . .

Notes:
1. Only deaths, the circumstances of which fulfil any one or more of the following conditions, should be reported on this form, *viz:*
    (*a*) Deaths which occur during the actual administration of a general or local anaesthetic, or during operation performed under a general or local anaesthetic, or
    (*b*) Deaths which are considered to be clinically due to the anaesthetic, or
    (*c*) Deaths which occur in the immediate postoperative period ordinarily not exceeding 12 hours following a general anaesthetic from which consciousness has not been regained.
2. Wherever practicable this form should be completed in consultation with any other Medical Practitioner specially concerned or specifically mentioned and forwarded to the Procurator Fiscal as soon as possible.
3. The Death Certificate must not be issued until instructions have been received from the Procurator Fiscal or his representative.
4. The completion of Question 13 is a matter of discretion; while it is to assist the Procurator Fiscal and his Medical Adviser to arrive at a certifiable cause of death, it is not in itself the certified cause of death.

Appendix P
Notes on the International System of Units (SI Units)

There is a general move to report laboratory results, etc., in terms of SI units (*Système Internationale d'Unités*) many of which will be unfamiliar. The following notes are not exhaustive but may be found useful.

The independent base units of SI are (physical quantity, name of unit, and symbol):

length	metre	m
mass	kilogram	kg
time	second	s
electric current	ampere	A
thermodynamic temperature	kelvin	K
luminous intensity	candela	cd
amount of substance	mole	mol

Decimal multiples and fractions of the units are formed by prefixes, with appropriate symbols (*see also* Appendix M):

10^{12}	tera	T	10^{-1}	deci	d
10^{9}	giga	G	10^{-2}	centi	c
10^{6}	mega	M	10^{-3}	milli	m
10^{3}	kilo	k	10^{-6}	micro	μ
10^{2}	hecto	h	10^{-9}	nano	n
10	deca	da	10^{-12}	pico	p
			10^{-15}	femto	f
			10^{-18}	atto	a

Other units can be derived from these—e.g. the SI unit of area is the square metre (m^2) and of volume the cubic metre (m^3). When there is a combination, the divider ('per') is shown by the use of negative powers. Thus:

speed = metres per second = $m\,s^{-1}$

acceleration = metres per second per second = $m\,s^{-2}$.

Several derived SI units have been given new and special names. Few of these are of great medical interest save, perhaps:

unit of force = newton = N = $kg\,m\,s^{-2}$ (i.e. mass × acceleration)

unit of pressure = pascal = Pa = $N\,m^{-2}$ (i.e. force per square metre).

Despite this, the common unit of weight (gram = g) and of volume (litre = l) will continue in use.

Slowly, therefore, reports will include less well-known terms—e.g.:

Blood pressure = 150/75 mmHg = 20/10 kPa

Amount of phenobarbitone = 10 mg/100 ml = 430 μmol l^{-1}.

It is even conceivable that a blood alcohol of 80 mg/100 ml will be reported as 17·4 mmol l^{-1}.

Temperature on the clinical scale is now preferably referred to in terms of degrees Celsius (° C). The units are identical with degrees centigrade.

Appendix Q
Weights of the Organs

Organ weights at various ages (in grams)[1]

	Lungs Men	Lungs Women	Brain Men	Brain Women	Heart Men	Heart Women	Kidneys Men	Kidneys Women	Liver Men	Liver Women	Spleen Men	Spleen Women
Newborn	51·7	50·9	353	347	19	20	24	24	124	125	8	6
0–3 mth	68·8	63·6	435	411	—	—	—	—	—	—	—	—
3–6 mth	94·1	93·3	600	534	—	—	—	—	—	—	—	—
6–9 mth	128·5	114·7	877	726	41	36	60	52	300	240	26	25
9–12 mth	142·4	142·1			54	48	72	65	400	390	35	34
1–2 yr	170·3	175·3	971	894	63	62	85	75	460	450	42	41
2–3 yr	245·9	244·3	1076	1012	73	71	93	84	510	500	48	47
3–4 yr	304·7	265·5	1179	1076	83	80	100	93	555	550	53	52
4–5 yr	314·2	311·7	1290	1156	95	90	106	102	595	595	58	57
5–6 yr	360·6	319·9	1275	1206	103	100	112	112	630	635	62	62
6–7 yr	399·5	357·5	1313	1225	110	113	120	123	665	685	64	67
7–8 yr	365·4	404·4	1338	1265	122	126	128	135	715	745	68	71
8–9 yr	405·0	382·1	1294	1208	132	140	138	148	770	810	73	77
9–10 yr	376·4	358·4	1360	1226	144	154	150	163	850	880	82	85
10–11 yr	474·5	571·2	1378	1247	157	168	164	180	950	950	91	93
11–12 yr	465·6	535·0	1348	1259	180	188	178	195	1050	1080	101	103
12–13 yr	458·8	681·7	1383	1256	202	207	196	210	1150	1180	111	112
13–14 yr	504·5	602·3	1382	1243	238	226	212	222	1240	1270	121	120
14–15 yr	692·8	517·0	1356	1318	258	238	229	230	1315	1330	135	127
15–16 yr	691·7	708·8	1407	1271	282	243	244	236	1380	1360	145	134
16–17 yr	747·3	626·5	1419	1300	300	247	260	240	1450	1380	152	140
17–18 yr	776·9	649·5	1409	1254	310	250	270	244	1510	1395	157	146
18–19 yr	874·7	654·9	1426	1312	318	251	282	247	1580	1405	160	151
19–20 yr	1035·6	785·2	1430	1294	322	252	290	248	1630	1415	162	155
20–21 yr	953·0	792·8		—								

[1] Boyd E. (1962) In: Altman and Dittmer (ed.) *Growth, Including Reproduction and Morphological Development*, Biological Handbooks, Federation of American Societies for Experimental Biology, Washington. pp. 346–348. Reproduced by permission of the publishers.

Index

Abortifacient drugs, 230
Abortion, 26, 225
  conscientious objection, 237
  criminal, (*Fig.* 17), 228–34
    by direct violence, 231
    instrumentation, 231
    legal position of doctor, 233
  historical background, 225
  legalized, incidence, 235
  natural, distinction from criminal, 238
  pathological evidence of death, 238
  Report of the Committee on the Working of the Abortion Act, 1974, 236n
  Roman Catholic viewpoint, 236
  Scottish law, 227
Abortion Act 1967, 73, 226, 228
Abortion (Amendment) Bill, 73, 235n
Abortion Regulations 1968, 235
Abortion (Scotland) Regulations 1968, 235
Abrasions, (*Plates* 3b, 4b) 96, 114–15
  self-inflicted, (*Plate* 4b) 98n
Acceleration injuries, 114–29
  intracerebral haemorrhage, 135
Accepted medical practice, definition, 391
Accidents
  aircraft (*see* Aircraft accidents)
  alcoholic, (*Tables III, IV*) 310, 311–14, 315–16
  as cause of disease, 124
  death from, diagnostic radiology, 336
  firearm, 109
  inquest conditions, 36
  major, identification of the dead, 47, (*Fig.* 8) 54
    inquest conditions, 36
  pedestrian, 114, 251, 314
  reconstruction of events, role of odontology, 372
  road traffic, (*see* Vehicular accidents)
  vehicular (*see* Vehicular accidents)
Accuracy, in quantitative assay, definition, 329

Adam's apple, 12
Adenosine triphosphate, role in rigor mortis, 58
Adipocere, 61
Adolescence, crime in, characteristics of offenders, 345
  determination of age, in the dead, 50
Adopted children, incest law, 265
Adoption Act 1958: AID child, 205
Adrenal glands, 27
Adrenalin, 27
Adult(s)
  determination of age, in the dead, 51
  sudden natural death, 89
    non-vascular causes, 92
  young, sudden natural death, 87
Adultery of doctor with patient, 379–80
Advertising, as professional misconduct by medical practitioner, 380
Advisory Council on the Misuse of Drugs, 287, 288
Advisory Group, on disposal of fetuses, 73
Affinity as grounds for annulment of marriage, 201, 201n
Age and ageing
  estimation, by dentition, (*Fig.* 23) 366, 368
  in the dead, 50
  of wounds, 4
  personality changes, 349
Agriculture (Poisonous Substances) Act 1952, 273
Agriculture (Safety, Health and Welfare Provisions) Act 1956, 186n
Aircraft accidents (*see also* Vehicular accidents)
  diagnostic radiology, (*Plate* 20) 337
  alcoholism and, (*Table III*) 310, 315–16
  escape equipment, 120
  identification of dead, 54
  in-flight explosion, 112
    decompression, 162
  injurious forces involved, 114

Head injury—*continued*
  long-term effects, 137
  personality change from, 350
  prevention, 137
  related to accident, 131
Health and Safety at Work, etc. Act
  1974, 187
  on radiation, 341*n*
Health and Safety Commission, 187
Health Service Commissioner, functions,
  388
Health Services and Public Health Act
  1968, 79*n*
Heart
  anatomy and physiology, (*Fig.* 2) 7
  compression injury, (*Fig.* 12) 116
  disease, asymptomatic, 121*n*
  enlarged, sudden death from, 91
  failure, 156
  inhibition of action, cause of sudden
    death, 86
  muscle disease, 88
  pathological sequelae of traumatic
    injury, 125
  vagal inhibition, of criminal abortion,
    232
  weight, 436
Heartbeat, in definition of death, 144
Heat exhaustion, 170
Heat stroke, 170
Heilbron Committee, on rape, 255
Helmets, protective, 137
Helminths, definition, 75
Hepatitis, 18
  B antigen, in plasma transfusion, 406
Herbicide poisoning, 274
Herniation, brain, 136
Heroin addiction, 296
  medical effects, 304
Heterozygous state, (*Fig.* 14) 211
Hippocratic Oath, 381
Homicide
  by burning, 165
  of child (*see also* Abortion), 228, 240
  definition, 94
  by destruction of aircraft in flight,
    112
  diagnostic radiology, 337
  by drowning, 172
  gunshot, characteristics, (*Plates* 6, 7)
    108, 110
  head injury, 130
  suspects, suicide rate, 352
Homicide Act 1957
  on diminished responsibility, 358
  on rape, 259*n*
Homosexual offences, 265
  age factor, 257
Homozygous state, (*Fig.* 14) 211
Hormones, 26

abortifacient, 230
feed-back mechanism, 33
Hospital Authorities, liability for actions
  of staff, 386
Hospital Order, 359, 361
Human Tissue Act 1961, 71, 141
  suggested amendment, 145
Hunger strike, 176
Hydrocarbon poisoning, industrial, 271
  aliphatic hydrocarbons, 272
  halogenated hydrocarbons, 272
Hydrogen Cyanide (Fumigation) Act
  1937, 160
Hydrostatic test of lungs, 241
Hymen, anatomy, 25
Hyoid, 12
Hyperkalaemia, of drowning, 171
Hypertension, 20, 89
Hyperthermia, death from, 171
Hypoglycaemia, 27
Hypospadias, 199
Hypostasis, 61
  colour, guide to mode of death, 62
  differential diagnosis, 62
  pneumonia, 14
Hypothermia, 174, 315
Hypoxia
  in aircraft accident, 162
  of inhalation anaesthesia, 399

Iatrogenic poisoning, 276
Identification commission, for major
  disasters, (*Fig.* 8) 54
Identification of dead and remains,
  (*Plate* 1a; *Fig.* 8) 47–55
  dental, (*Figs.* 23, 24) 364–72
  laboratory analysis, method, 326
  major accidents, 47, (*Fig.* 8) 54
  purposes, 48
  radiological (*see* X-rays, identification
    of dead)
  single unknown body, 48
Illusion, definition, 352
Imipramine, distribution in body, 331
Immersion in water, effect on rate of
  putrefaction, 60
Immune reaction, 21
Immunity, 21
Immunization, 80–3
  antivenin, 282
  hazards, 80–2
Immunology, in identification of dead,
  49
Immunosuppression, in organ trans-
  plantation, 139
Impotence, 200
Inborn errors of metabolism, 32, 245
Incest, 264
Incest Act 1567, 264
Indecency with Children Act 1960, 255

Lungs
anatomy and physiology, 12
assessment of nodules, in pneumoconiosis, 182
diseases (*see also specific diseases*), 13
cause of asphyxia, 157
hydrostatic test, 241
injuries, to types, 14
long-term effects of inhalation anaesthesia, 400
in neonatal death, 241
size, 12*n*
weight, 436
Lutheran antigenic system, 220
Lymphatic system, 11
Lympho-reticular system, 5

McNaghten Rules, 357
Major accident
identification of the dead, 47, (*Fig.* 8) 54
inquest conditions, 36
Malaysia, medico-legal system, 43
Mandrax, 298
Manic–depressive psychosis, 352
Manslaughter, alcoholic, 316
March haemoglobinuria, 191*n*
Marihuana, 298
Marriage
medico-legal aspects, 199–210
Othello syndrome, 354
sexual offence within, 258
Marriage (Enabling) Act 1960, 201*n*
on incest, 265
Mass spectrophotometry, 326–8
Matrimonial Causes Act 1973, 198*n*, 204, 208*n*, 363
Measurements, standard equivalents, 430
Medical Appeal Tribunals, 180
Medical Code, 381
Medical ethics, 380–93
Medical Examiner (USA), 38
Medical history, in identification of the dead, 52
Medical practice, legal aspects, 377–93
Medical qualifications, UK, 431
Medical records, confidentiality, 385
Medical Referee, role in cremation, 70
Medicines Act 1968, 230, 275, 284, 286–7
Medicines Commission, 275, 287
Medico-Legal Institutes, Europe, 37
Medico-legal systems, comparative, 34–46
analysis, 44
Menstrual cycle, lengths, 202
Mental deficiency
in case of rape, 256
as grounds for annulment of marriage 201

Mental disorder
civil actions, 363
legal framework, 360–3
Mental handicap, 347
Mental Health Act 1959, 360–3
Mental Health (Scotland) Act 1960, 360–3
Mental hospitals, freedom of patients, 362
Mental illness, 348–54
Mescaline, 298
Mesothelioma, from exposure to crocidolite, 185, 185*n*, 426
Metabolism, definition, 31
inborn errors of, 32, 245
Metabolites, drug, in laboratory analysis, 331
Metal poisoning, 271, 330
Methadone, substitution of heroin, 297
Methanol (*see* Methyl alcohol)
Methyl alcohol, 318
Methyl bromide poisoning, industrial, 272
Methyl chloride poisoning, industrial, 272
Methylated spirits, 318
Mineral Workings (Offshore Installations) Act 1971, 186
Mines and Quarries Act 1954, 186, 187
Minors, consent to examination and treatment, 382
rape of, 256
Misuse of Drugs Act 1971, 122, 284, 287–92
Misuse of Drugs (Notification of and Supply to Addicts) Regulations 1973, 291, 384
definition of addict, 294
MNS antigen system, (*Fig.* 16) 216
Mobility of organs in relation to injury, 3
Mononuclears, 11
Morphine addiction, 296
Mosaicism, 198
Motor car exhaust, carbon monoxide poisoning, 158, 269
Motor cycle accidents, protective helmets, 138
Mule spinner's cancer, 272
Mummification, 61
Murder (*see* Homicide)
Muscle, types, 27, 29
Musculoskeletal system, 4, 27–31
Mutation, genetic, 214, 214*n*
radiation-induced, 342
Myocarditis, 88

Naphthylamine poisoning, 272
National Health Service and doctor, legal aspects, 386

448   INDEX

National Health Service (Scotland) Act 1972, 79n
National Insurance Commissioner, 179, 180
National Radiological Protection Board, 341n
Neck wounds, stab, 102
  subarachnoid haemorrhage following, 134
Neglect, death from, 175
Negligence, professional
  in boxing, 190, 190n
  in immunization, 81, 82
  legal aspects, 390–3
  routine X-ray examination, 339
Nembutal, 297
Nephrosis, 22
Nervous system, 4
  anatomy and physiology, 14–17
New Hampshire formula of 1865, on criminal responsibility, 357
New Zealand, medico-legal system, 42
Nicotine, agricultural, poisoning, 274
Nitrates, in gunshot investigations, 110
Nitrobenzene poisoning, industrial, 271
Nitrogen narcosis, 195
Nitroglycerin poisoning, industrial, 271
Non-contact sport, sudden death in, 190
Non-ionizing radiations (see also X-rays) 340
North Sea exploration, fatal accidents, legislation on, 40
Notifiable disease, industrial poisoning (see also Communicable disease), 270, 428
Notification of Addicts Order 1968, 384
Notification of Pesticides Scheme 1955, 273
Novus actus interveniens, 128, 143
'Noxious thing,' definition, 230
Nuclear power, radiation hazards, 343
Nullity of marriage, 199–201
Nutritional state, in death from neglect, 175

Occupation(s)
  of carriers of infectious disease, 79
  effect on teeth, 369
  prescribed, 425–7
  safety regulations, 186
Occupational disease, 179
  cancer, 272
  radiation, 341
Odontology (Figs. 23, 24) 364–76
Oedema
  of asphyxia, 148
  cerebral, 136
  pulmonary, 155
Offences Against the Person Act 1861, 93, 105n

on abortion, 225
on homicidal poisoning, 279
on sexual offences, 255
Offices, Shops and Railway Premises Act 1963, 186n
Official Register (of medical practitioners), 377
Opium addiction, 296
Organochlorines, 274, 274n
Organophosphorus poisoning, 274
Organs, weights, 436
Ossification, 30, 50, 416
  centres, (Plate 15) 240, 334
  approximate times of appearance, 50, 416
Othello syndrome, 354
Overcrowding, cause of asphyxia, 161
Overhydration, hazard of surgery, 405
Overlaying of children, 250, 315
Oxygen
  poisoning, of divers, 195
  requirement, in states of low metabolism, 174
  role in the respiratory system, 12

P antigenic system, 220
Pancreas, 18
  damage to, causes, 19
  insulin secretion, 27
Paraffin test, in gunshot investigations, 110
Paraquat poisoning, 274
Parathion poisoning, 274
Parathyroid gland, 27
Parentage, tests, (Fig. 16, Table II) 214–24
Paternity
  circumstantial evidence, 201
  exclusion, governing principles, (Fig. 16, Table II) 215
  testing, principles, 215
Patient transfer, between NHS doctors, 386
Patients' rights, 388n
Pedestrian traffic accidents, 114
  alcoholism, 314
  young children, 251
Pelvis, bones, (Fig. 7) 49–50
  fracture, 118
Pentobarbitone, 297
Peripheral nervous system, anatomy and physiology, 14
Peritoneum, 18
Perpetuities and Accumulations Act 1964, 201n
Personality
  ageing process, 349
  disorders, 346
  effects of brain damage, 349, 350
Pesticides, toxicity, 273

Petechial haemorrhage, 147
  following natural death, 148
pH, definition, 32*n*
Pharmacy and Medicines Act 1941, 230
Pharmacy and Poisons Act 1933, 284
Phenotype, definition, 213
Phenylketonuria, 245
Phosphatase, staining, 224
Physiology, 6–33
Pituitary gland, 26
Place of work, definition for insurance
  purposes, 178
Placenta, 8
Planes of body, (*Fig.* 1) 2
Plasma, 10
  transfusion, Hepatitis B antigen, 406
Plastic bag suffocation, 149
Pneumoconioses, 14, 181–5
  complicating conditions, 182
  definition, 180
  post-mortem dissection, 183
  prescribed occupation, 425–6
  X-rays in, (*Plate* 13b) 182
Pneumoconiosis Medical Panel, 182,
  183
Pneumonia, hypostatic, 14
Pneumonitis, post-immersion, 173
Poisonous berries, 278
Poisons and poisoning, 268–83
  accidental, 278
  agricultural, 272
  asphyxia, toxic (*Plate* 12) 157–61
  categories, 268
  drug, 275–8
  environmental, 268
  exhumation procedure, 69
  food, 78*n*, 281
  gastro-intestinal effects, 18
  homicidal, 279
  iatrogenic, 275–8
  industrial, 270
    notification, 186
  inhaled, 270
  insect bites and stings, 283
  laboratory investigation, 321–33
  legislation, 284–92
  marine animals, 196
  natural, 281
  naturally injected, 282
  nonmedical, sale to public, 284
  and putrefaction, 60
  rodenticides, 280*n*
  role of enzymes, 32
  snakebite, 282
  suicidal, 275–8
  threshold limit values, 270
  venomous, 282
Poisons Act 1972, 284
  Poisons Rules, 274, 284
  Schedules, 285

Poisons Board, 285*n*
Poisons List, 285
Poisons Rules (*see under* Poisons Act)
Pollution, atmospheric, 268
  by specific elements, 269
Polymorphonuclears, 11
Possession of body, definition, in trans-
  plantation of organs, 142
Postconcussional states, 350
Postcontusional states, 350
Post-mortem artefacts, (*Plate* 2a) 62–4
Post-mortem changes, 56–64
Post-mortem injury, (*Plate* 2a) 63
Precipitin test, in identification of the
  dead, 49
Precision, in quantitative assay, defini-
  tion, 329
Precognition of witnesses, by the
  Procurator Fiscal, 39
Pregnancy
  age limits in law, 201
  concealment, 239
  duration, 202
  ectopic, 88
  effects of immunization, 81
  medico-legal aspects, 201
  pathological evidence, 237
  premature end, statistics, 228
  X-ray hazards, 344
Prescribed diseases, 419–24
Prescribed occupations, 425–7
Prescription, of controlled drugs, (*Fig.*
  18) 289
Preservatives, of biological specimens,
  321
Pressure abrasions, 97
Pressurization, prevention of diving
  accident, 196
Preventive medicine, role of pathologist,
  119
Private practice, legal position of doctor,
  388
Probation order with condition of
  treatment, 360
Procurator Fiscal
  deaths reportable, to, 38, 414
  functions and duties, 38–40
Professional misconduct of medical
  practitioners, 379
Professional secrecy (*see* Confidentiality,
  professional)
Progressive massive fibrosis, 182
Prostaglandins, as abortifacients, 230
Prostatism, 24
Protection of Animals Acts 1911–1927,
  274*n*
Protection of Birds Acts 1954–1967,
  274*n*
Protozoa, definition, 75
Psychedelics, 298

Schizophrenia, 353
Scorpion sting, 283
Sealed and Unsealed Source Regulations, 341*n*
Seat belts
  crutch strapping, 120
  insurance and legal implications, 115
  syndromes, 119
Select Committee on Violence in Marriage, 209*n*
Self-neglect, 175
Semen (*see also* Artificial insemination)
  staining, examination, 224
  in rape, 262
Senses, alteration by drugs, 298
Sepsis, following criminal abortion, 233
Serum, 10
  blood groups, 220
Sex
  change, surgical, 199
  determination, 198
    evidence of skeleton, 31
    in the dead, 49
    in sport, (*Plate* 14) 192
  disputed, 198
Sex hormones, 27
Sex linkage, (*Fig.* 15) 212
Sexual intercourse, unlawful, as distinct from rape, 256
  definition, 258
Sexual offences, 255-67
  age and consent, 255
  by mentally handicapped, 348
  psychological abnormality, 356
Sexual Offences Acts 1956–1976, 255, 256
  on incest, 264
Sexual Offences (Scotland) Act 1976, 255, 256
  homosexual offences, 265
  resistance to rape, 260
Shark hazards, 196
Ships, deratting regulations, 78
Shock
  effects, 22
  electric, determinants, 167
  surgical, 6, 164
Shoplifting
  in aged, 350
  by manic–depressive, 352
Shotgun
  calibre, terminology, 105
  injuries, 105
    estimation of distance, 106
SI Units, 435
Sickle cell anaemia, 11
  fitness for sport, 191
  gene, ethnic variations, 223*n*
Silicosis, 184
Simultaneous death, 125–8

Singapore, medico-legal system, 43
Site of election, of suicidal gunshot wound, 109
Skeleton
  abnormalities, in comparative radiological identification, 335
  as evidence of sex, 31
  major relationships, (*Fig.* 5) 27
Skeletonization, stage of decomposition, 61
Skin diving, limits, 196*n*
Skull
  anatomy and physiology, 29
  base
    fractures, (*Plate* 9) 131
    inner surface, (*Fig.* 6) 29
  fracture, 130
  sinuses, in comparative radiology (*Plate* 19) 335
Sleep, coronary death during, 92
Smog, 268
Smoking (*see* Cigarette smoking)
Snakebite, 282
'Snow', 295
Social Security Act 1975, 178
Sodium amylobarbitone, 297
Sodium amytal, 297
Sodomy, 265
Solar plexus pressure, effect, 16
Spasm, cadaveric, (*Plate* 1b) 59, 108, 173
Spectrometry, of metals, 330
Spectrophotometry, analysis of drugs, (*Figs.* 21, 22) 326–8
'Speed', 295
Spermatozoa
  characteristics, 24
  duration of viability in vagina, 258, 258*n*
  evidence following sterilization, 207
Spider bite, 283
Spina bifida, 245
Spinal anaesthesia, 397
Spinal cord
  anatomy, 15
  covering matter, 16
  damage, effects, 14, 118
Spine
  anatomy, 29
  in deceleration and acceleration injuries, 117
Spleen, 11
  damage, 117
  weight, 436
Sport, medico-legal aspects (*Plate* 14) 188–97
Sri Lanka, medico-legal system, 44
Stab wounds, (*Plate* 5; *Fig.* 11) 99
Staines, Trident aircraft accident, 122
Staphylococcal food poisoning, 281